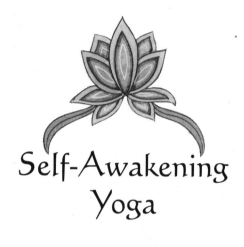

Self-Awakening Yoga

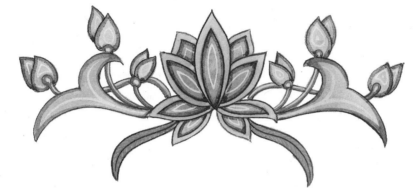

Self-Awakening Yoga

The Expansion of Consciousness
through the Body's Own Wisdom

Don Stapleton, Ph.D.

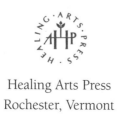

Healing Arts Press
Rochester, Vermont

Healing Arts Press
One Park Street
Rochester, Vermont 05767
www.InnerTraditions.com

Healing Arts Press is a division of Inner Traditions International

*Note to the reader: The movement inquiries in this book and CD are intended as informational guides.
The approaches described herein are meant to supplement, and not to be a substitute for, professional
medical care or treatment. They should not be used to treat a serious ailment without
prior consultation with a qualified health care professional.*

LIBRARY OF CONGRESS CATALOGING-IN-PUBLICATION DATA

Stapleton, Don.
Self awakening yoga : the expansion of consciousness through the body's
own wisdom / Don Stapleton.
p. cm.
ISBN 0-89281-183-8 (pbk.)
1. Hatha yoga. I. Title.
RA781.7.S725 2004
613.7'046—dc22
2004010144

Printed and bound in the United States at Capital City Press

10 9 8 7 6 5 4 3 2 1

Photographs by Rodrigo Oviedo Villalobos, Tierra Fértil
Models: Amba Stapleton and Don Stapleton

Compact disk design and photographs by Rodrigo Oviedo Villalobos
Technical production and animation by Johann Pereira

Text design and layout by Virginia Scott Bowman
This book was typeset in Berkeley and Avenir with Kabel, Caliban,
and Calligraph 421 as the display typefaces

To Amba, my cherished life companion

Contents

Acknowledgments

My heartfelt gratitude:

To my family members, whose personal gifts in the lessons of love inspire me to follow my aspirations: my son, Jonathan; my parents, Joe and Mary Stapleton; my sisters, Kay Flynt and Sharon Hicks; my second family, Marilyn and Earl Henderson, Sr., Ginger, Danny and Earl, Jr.

To all my teachers, mentors and guides, especially Yogi Amrit Desai, my guru in the paradox of love; Swami Kripalu, who is the embodiment of living yoga; and Guillermo Cuellar, my first yoga teacher.

To Ann Hunt, Richard Jordan, and all of the Nosara yoga teachers, who, through your love for learning and enthusiasm for teaching, bring magic to all who take part in Nosara Yoga Institute.

To my compatriots in the Kripalu and Omega communities, for your friendship and encouragement along my journey.

To Susan Davidson, who taught me to listen for my muse, and whose creative genius for refining, collaborating, and editing has nurtured this work into fruition; to Ehud Sperling and Jon Graham, who placed their faith in me; and to the entire team at Inner Traditions, whose collective effort encourage diversity in our evolutionary vision.

To Rodrigo Oviedo Villalobos and Johann Pereira of Tierra Fértil, for your tireless creative support in producing the photos in this book as well as the technical production, music and graphic design of the accompanying CD.

To Robin and Marsha Williams, whose kindhearted support has made it possible to launch Nosara Yoga Institute as a haven for nurturing the creative spirit through yoga education.

To all who have given the generosity of your time and participation throughout my thirty years of conducting yoga classes, workshops and teacher trainings—the gifts of your shared genius are now offered to those who hold these pages.

Prologue: Your Body as Earthen Vessel

mud \\'məd\ **n.**: wet, sticky, soft earth, as on the banks of a river

hut \\'hət\ **n.**: a small, cozy house, shelter, or cottage

adobe \ə-'dō-bē\ **n.**: a sun-dried brick of clay and straw used to build a structure

MANY WISDOM TRADITIONS THROUGHOUT HISTORY CONSIDER the body to be a temple for the spirit. In order to create a conscious and functional relationship with the body, I prefer to begin with an image that is less grandiose than a temple. A temple is an awesome destination. Going to a temple requires that I leave my home and my everyday life to seek contact with the divine. There are times and places for this journey, moments in life when a pilgrimage to a place beyond home is desirable and appropriate exactly for the separation from everyday life that it affords. But I choose not to approach the body in this manner.

Rather than a temple of magnificent marble columns and lofty spires, I am inviting you into an image of your body that is more personal, more like a cozy seat in front of a hearth shared with your most trusted friend. This trusted friend beside you is yourself—not the icon of a supreme being, not an authority on mystical transcendence, but your own inner advisor.

When my wife, Amba, and I were making plans to build a home in the jungle on the Pacific coast of Costa Rica, I attended a seminar on the contemporary uses of adobe in Central America. I grew up in the American Southwest where some of the adobe buildings—earthen structures made of clay and straw and built a thousand years ago—are still standing today. Since as far back in my childhood as I can remember, being inside these adobe homes has always given me a cozy, secure feeling, like being taken into an earthen womb.

As part of the seminar we took a field trip to an ancient village in Costa Rica to see homes that have been standing for more than eight hundred years, surviving earthquakes, volcanic eruptions, and torrential storms. Passing through the portal into one of the earthen cottages, I was overcome by a vivid awareness of the many human activities that this profoundly simple home had seen. Inside the intimacy of that magical hut, where the walls reverberated with the energy of living human community, I sat down on the floor in front of a sculpted fireplace and conceived the vision of yoga that I share with you in this book.

Different from the many views present in the world of yoga today, I want to provide a perspective that comes from an inquiry into who you already are, to present a mirror for you to behold the power, beauty, and wisdom that live inside you. In my thirty years of practice in spiritual and body-based disciplines, the experiences that have made the most profound difference in my life are the ones that awaken from a place deep inside my own being.

I begin this book with the metaphor of a humble adobe hut to underscore the experience of timelessness and simplicity that we, as human beings, can have while living in our earthen, fleshly bodies. The simple beauty of a mud home is a symbol for the journey presented herein: I desire that the time you invest in the inquiry of Self-Awakening Yoga will result in a deeper appreciation for the flesh-and-blood haven of your own body. I intend nothing less than a coming home to the comfortable security of your hut, your cozy shelter within.

Yoga is often presented in the West as a way to "get better." With promises of physical prowess, heavenly states of consciousness, and the attainment of powers of concentration and self-mastery, yoga is frequently undertaken with ardent hopes for a better body, stronger control of mind and emotions, and the dream of a life beyond mundane human experiences. However, embracing the technology of yoga—and the authority of the yoga teacher—can easily become another way of separating ourselves from our natural wisdom by encouraging us to look outside ourselves for the peace and harmony we seek. To return to our natural state of being at ease in our bodies entails a personal journey that does not require traveling beyond ourselves to find the means for expanding into our fullest evolutionary potential. To come home to ourselves calls for returning to the original creativity that permits us the freedom and benevolence of spirit to begin with ourselves as we already are.

For the many years that I taught art-education courses I made it a priority to organize a field trip early in the semester to the closest deposit of clay I could find. With forty university students caravanning to a vacant field or remote river, we would arrive amid a lot of noise—doors opening, trunks popping up, shovels and buckets clanging, and a chorus of the requisite "Why are we here?" questions. When I determined that I could be heard above the hubbub, a hush gave way to my pronouncement. "As elementary teachers, our culture entrusts our children into your care. You have a responsibility to help children develop a comfortable relationship to nature and the world in which they live."

"But Professor Stapleton, do we have to get muddy to learn how to teach this? And what about the gnats and grasshoppers out here?"

I encouraged everyone to notice the discomforts as obstacles to feeling at home in these unfamiliar surroundings. How can teachers provide an experience to their students that they have not integrated within themselves? And how else can we enter into an experience of the unknown unless we are willing to pass through the initial discomforts of each moment in a new situation?

Every "clay day" unfolded in an amazingly consistent manner: the fascination of discovery became absorbing to the point that nagging annoyances faded to the background. We became original humankind searching for the oldest material shapeable by human hands—clay. By digging for clay we were participating with the funded wisdom of our entire human ancestry.

Maybe it was the sensual allure of clay on bare feet that caused the first human to stoop down and pick up the sticky mass with his or her hands. Maybe it was in scraping the clay off the feet that a natural fascination for squeezing and squishing the malleable stuff emerged. How many lifetimes were spent in playful, idle fascination with the material itself before clay became useful? All conjecture aside, we know that at some moment in time an important discovery was made: when the pliable lump of earth was left by the fire, it hardened. Based on this realization, hunter-gatherers were able to create bowls and jars—vessels essential for transporting provisions from place to place.

For elementary teachers-in-training to smell the loam of earth, to feel the sensation of raw clay in their hands, to fathom the depths of human creativity involved in one single click on the evolutionary wheel I was willing to make sandwiches and journey with them to the edge of the South Florida marshlands. I withheld from my temptation to answer their inevitable "Why are we here?" question with the predictably professional answer: "We are here to discover that clay comes from some place other than a plastic bag in Wal-Mart." I wanted more for them than simply an enhanced understanding of a material that was going to be used in their classrooms. I hoped that clay day would set the mood for awakening an inquiry into our innate creativity and the learning process.

Once, in a lecture to a group of my graduate students, Buckminster Fuller characterized the room we were sitting in as a rectilinear box. He pointed out that, in our human desire to compartmentalize our knowledge, we went so far as to create our homes and workspaces as boxes in which we organize and "store" ourselves. In contrast, early homes were caves, lean-tos of branches and grass, organic forms sculpted from mud bricks—all manner of construction to shelter our bodies from the wide-open ceiling of sun and stars. The great inventor and architect's point was that the shape of the space in which we live actually shapes our consciousness. Fuller proclaimed the glories of living and working in shapes and structures that come from an organic interaction with nature; his favorite dwelling for human beings was the dome.

Years of yoga later I am ever grateful to Buckminster Fuller for his simple message that day. He provided insight into my experience of living in a bodily home, a home that is constantly shaping and reshaping my consciousness. Our bodies, like the clay we impress with the designs and shapes of our imagination, are infinitely malleable. We are the beings endowed with the ability to both shape and be shaped by the worlds in which we live.

The word *adobe* is not indigenous American or Spanish, as I had always thought. *Adobe* is an Arabic word that found its way into use throughout the world, from Africa to Israel, from India to Costa Rica, from Santa Fe to Peru. In all those places, *adobe* refers to huts and cottages that are constructed of mud bricks.

In my estimation, the word *yoga* has a similar universality. As I watch the word *yoga* enter mainstream culture, I appreciate its wide reference to a multitude of practices and modalities that share the foundational intention of bringing about integration of all aspects of one's being through a combination of physical and mental practices that both expand self-awareness and produce spiritual attunement. In addition to thirty years' experience teaching yoga in the United States, Europe, Canada, and Costa Rica, I also taught yoga in India, the land where yoga originally emerged. I was amazed to observe that hatha yoga is as foreign to most people living on the Indian continent as cowboys are to contemporary Texans. The bodily approach to yoga has frequently taken the lowest rung of respectability among the pious yoga practitioners in India; only recently have hatha yoga classes become available to the modern, health-conscious generations in India. I learned Zen Hara Yoga from Koji Yamamoto, a hara yoga master who had relocated from his home in Japan to teach in Manhattan. When I accepted an invitation to teach hara yoga in Japan, a culture known for its awesome focus on meditation, I was forewarned that the last thing my hosts wanted to learn was yet another way to sit and be still. They wanted to release seriousness and have fun and were deeply grateful for the lighthearted range of hara yoga and movement practices that evoked a deep belly laugh.

In such a multicultural climate of cross-pollination, we see exercise and fitness trends embrace the concept of yoga movement. We see popular fusions such as yogaerobics, power yoga workouts, Yoganetics, Acu-yoga, Yogalates, and many varieties of yoga therapy. Yoga fitness vacations blend the practices of multiple disciplines with adventure travel to offer fresh insights into the inquiry of yoga.

Freeing the term *yoga* and yoga experiences from their culture-bound and tradition-bound moorings is not a new phenomenon. According to folklore surrounding the shamanic origins of yogic practice, the secrets of yoga emerged in the covert experiments of individual practitioners who were searching for a deeper relationship to their own inner nature than was acknowledged in the dominating and often oppressive Vedic culture. The diverse practices forming the web of yogic knowledge grew out of the compelling urge for individuals to delve into the mysteries encoded within the layers of one's own experience of self, independent of pervading cultural beliefs and norms of the time. To protect their autonomy and to ensure their freedom to make this inner journey, the early yogis lived outside the culture, often in the surrounding forests and caves. The clandestine encounters between these earlier practitioners began to yield a common understanding that, although their inquiries into self-awareness were idiosyncratic, there were patterns of similarity emerging that resulted in an evolutionary progression toward expanding consciousness.

Our sense of who we are as individuals develops within the context of our culture's wisdom, history, and traditions. But hidden in the nature of being identified within any group—be that family, religion, or culture—is the seductive force that homogenizes all idiosyncratic differences into the unifying characteristics of the group. To come to intimately know ourselves as individuals requires turning inside to identify personal meaning and fulfillment.

In looking to the historic traditions of yoga as a map for making the inner journey, I have discovered that unless I look to the early spirit of inquiry and creativity modeled in the origins of yoga, I am likely to get caught up in the expectations inherent in the contemporary versions of yoga that are cycling through our culture at the moment. Many popular forms of yoga are offered with such fundamentalist zeal that personal inquiry is discouraged and experimentation with the traditional form is met with caution and fear.

"Medical-model yoga," or yoga that is taken on for the purpose of fixing or curing specific ailments, has become so common that many people look to the yoga teacher in the same way they would look to a doctor, physical therapist, or other health specialist for diagnosis, treatment, and prescription for their ills. What appears on the surface to be an alternative modality for health care can in fact be used to reinforce dependence on an external authority, displacing our power and responsibility outside ourselves rather than drawing us toward our inner resources to find strength and balance.

Routinized or formulaic approaches to yoga that do not vary with the individual or take into account the developmental needs that arise at different stages of life can become internalized as a substitute for genuine self-inquiry into what stimulates our evolutionary capacities toward growth and change. Traditionalists, who prefer to keep yoga pure to the customs of a particular school or historical form from India are at a loss to account for the often contradictory and widely differing interpretations of yoga's fundamentals. I view yoga as an evolving inquiry rather than as a six-thousand-year-old science or religion that must be historically reconstructed to be of use in our growth as human beings on the planet at this time. Drawing from my background as a visual artist, I have come to view yoga as an art—like the art of painting, for example. If you want to learn to paint, you begin with the style and materials of the teacher who introduces you to the experience. You learn the basics of the teacher's approach, and then you open into the wider field of experience by studying many artists, styles, and traditions. If you prematurely fixate on the style of one school or one teacher, your personal style will be out of reach. The benefit of practicing yoga with many different teachers is that each gives you a window to view your unique, subjective capacities and further the development of your own yoga practice.

Self-Awakening Yoga is a synthesis of principles and practices developed in my journey toward unlocking the power of learning through direct listening to the body. As a professor of art education, I searched for methods of teaching that nurtured the creativity in students who, for the most part, had been conditioned to see themselves as incapable of inventing images that were personally expressive. As the head program developer of yoga teaching at Kripalu, one of the worlds' largest yoga centers, I nurtured an environment that empowered teachers and students to draw from their personal yoga journeys for creating experiences that would inspire and sustain lifelong learning.

The explorations and inquiries herein are offered to you as a launching point for developing your own yoga. As you enter into this creative process, you are fueling your personal evolution while simultaneously participating with yoga's continual evolution. The self-knowledge you gain from undertaking the inquiries of Self-Awakening Yoga can provide a foundation for entering into any form of yoga practice without abandoning contact with your inner guidance or neglecting the wisdom flowing from your organism.

In returning to the comfort of yourself as you already are you may be astonished to discover that the expansion of consciousness can occur easily and comfortably each and every time you enter the "mud hut" of your inner home, rather than taking years to attain. As you develop your ability to listen to your body by following your sensations, you may notice yourself entering into direct communication with your inner self. The inquiries in this book can help you attune to the pulse of your inner being by increasing your overall sensorial awareness. By turning homeward for authority in your yoga practice, you may begin to regard your body as a place of refuge, renewal, and self-regeneration. As the opportunity arises to sense that your body is not just a house that you enter from time to time but that it is a home, you may begin to rely on your body as a place that is continuously being fashioned by you to fulfill your needs and to make deep contact with the unfolding layers of yourself.

One story goes that God planted his hands in a lump of clay to fashion an image in his own likeness then breathed the breath of life into his handiwork. If we are to participate with the creative force moving through all of creation, isn't it possible that we have the innate capacity to shape the world in which we live from the inside out?

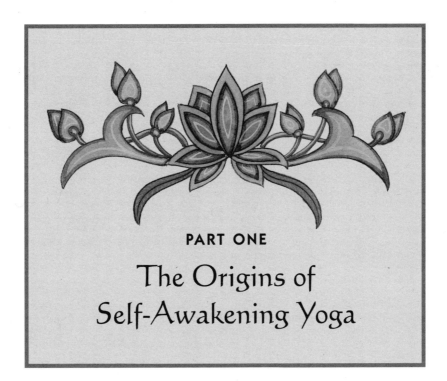

PART ONE

The Origins of
Self-Awakening Yoga

1 The Path to the Teacher Within

SOME FIRST-LOVE EXPERIENCES HAVE NOTHING TO DO with another human being. My first love emerged with a blank piece of paper when I discovered that I had the power to create a world by moving my drawing pencil across the page. My second love grew naturally out of the first—the love of enticing others to exercise their creative minds. To this end, I became an art teacher. I was introduced to my third love while teaching undergraduate and graduate-level courses in art education, the philosophy and psychology of creative development, and natural crafts at the University of South Florida.

This strange new love was yoga. But it was not an experience of love at first sight.

Being an artist, I accepted the conventional premise that extremes in lifestyle were part of the creative process. Excessive work, an imbalanced diet, and recreational dabbling with various mood-enhancing and mind-expanding drugs were behaviors begun in graduate school and continued as underground habits in my life as a professor. As befit the subject of our study—an exploration of the creative process—each group of students turned into a community; my friendship with many students outgrew our formal roles. As truly good friends will do, over time a few students pointed out to me that I could stand to get a lot healthier; I could clean up my diet and should quit smoking.

The truth of what they were telling me came as a wake-up call the night I ventured into my first yoga class. I expected to feel better after one class, but the class was torture—I was horrified at the simple things I could not do. Used to smoking a pack and a half of Marlboros every day, I could not even take a deep breath.

It was a year before I returned to a yoga class. That was a long year of going inside myself to realize that if I were to continue the same unwholesome patterns for much longer, I would quickly become an old man. Changing my detrimental habits and quitting smoking were not decisions that I consciously made and worked at; yet, over the course of that year following my introduction to yoga, my lifestyle began to change. My "confrontation" with my lifestyle habits had come in a package, complete with a few practices from that first yoga class that provided a structure for me to work with myself. A year later, when I went to my second yoga class, I was ready to open into a new life.

Over time my love for yoga grew. My enthusiasm drew me to study with many masters, including Ram Dass, who gave a weeklong retreat at the Ocala National Forest in Florida in 1975. By that time I was teaching yoga; I was searching for instruction that would further my personal practice and also give me insight into teaching others.

Ram Dass is a witty, brilliant, and totally engaging teacher. He was a student of yoga—not a guru. He was not recruiting disciples. He was dedicated to transmitting his passion for the journey of transformation that came through the path of yoga, which for him was centered in social service.

At that retreat we chanted, danced, and sat for hours listening to Ram Dass's stories. We sipped barley soup and ate brown bread in silence. We sat for meditation at 4:00 every morning, and after breakfast we were instructed in the familiar yoga postures that I was already teaching. I felt at home with the three hundred people who were sharing this experience of spiritual education, American style.

One evening, as Ram Dass was leaving the dining hall, I cornered him with a question about my conflict between teaching art and teaching yoga. His message was that I appeared to be seeking yogic awakening in a mental way and that I could not skip the first step of opening my heart. He encouraged me to follow the path with heart.

I admit that I felt embarrassed about not already knowing how to do what Ram Dass was suggesting. I could perform postures. I could sit still and meditate. I could accomplish whatever willful practice I decided to do that was good for me. But open my heart? I had no idea how to approach the task.

"A path with heart"—although I was embarrassed and perplexed, this disturbing advice was to become a guiding force in my life.

In January of 1976, a few months after being with Ram Dass, I met Yogi Amrit Desai at a retreat at Swan Lake, outside of Gainesville, Florida. Some friends from my yoga circle were going to the retreat, making it convenient and comfortable for me to "check out" another guru.

Upon arriving at the retreat grounds early in the afternoon, the guru's disciples and staff were instantly obvious; they all were dressed in white clothing. Retreat guests lined up at the registration and souvenir tables. Among the assortment of items for sale were prayer beads, audiotapes, and bundles of incense, the scent of which permeated all the buildings and grounds surrounding Swan Lake. The spicy fragrance was alluring—to this day I remember that scent and the feelings associated with experiencing it for the first time.

The grand hall filled fast. I positioned myself close to the central aisle. Everyone sat on the floor quietly waiting for the program to begin. A woman dressed in a white sari stood to take the microphone; she gave us instructions about how to stand when the yogi came into the room. She then led us in meditation until Yogi Desai arrived. I opened my eyes to scrutinize the woman more closely—she was continually readjusting the slippery yardage of her sari to cover her bare midriff. As she settled into her role it became clear that she was in charge of the retreat and would be telling us what was what for the weekend.

I was startled by the loud noise announcing the yogi's arrival. A man was blowing through a hole in a conch shell as though it were a trumpet. Everyone jolted up to standing for the yogi's arrival. I strained to see what was happening. The group quickly swarmed toward the center aisle. I feared that I would be pushed over the line of flower petals that delineated the boundary of the runway, and I knew by the demeanor of the woman who had given us our instructions that crossing that boundary would be a terrible transgression. I dug in my heels and held the line.

As he smoothly proceeded toward me, his pumpkin-colored robes swaying, I became utterly entranced. To the dissatisfaction of my analytical eye, I could not determine the origin of the yogi's movement. In years of drawing live models, my eye had been trained to observe lines of movement that transfer through the body from a point of origin or intention. Yet, as he approached, I could not determine what was moving this man. He appeared to be floating, his body hanging from his head like a string hanging from a helium-filled balloon. What was moving this man? How could a body move with such effortlessness?

I remember the exact moment in which I realized that Yogi Desai embodied a possibility for me—that I, too, could be inside myself in the same effortless way that the yogi inhabited his body. In that moment of realization I comprehended that my body was *meant* to move in the natural way that he was moving. I was infused with an instant understanding of the purpose of yoga. I knew that my life would be about yoga from that moment on.

Yogi Desai glided to the front of the hall and bowed to the giant photograph of his guru, Swami Kripalu, which stood on an easel surrounded by flowers and potted plants. All the people in the room went to their knees. Yogi Desai then stood up, put his hands together as if in a prayer, and looked out at us. Even though an ocean of people surrounded me, I felt the yogi looking directly at me.

The trancelike state began to modulate as the guru straightened his robe and sat down in a draped chair. Two stagehands quickly brought out a coffee table and a wood-box pump organ. The yogi explained that he was going to lead us in a chant with Sanskrit words. Since we did not understand what the words meant, he admonished us not to try too hard to interpret them. "You do not need understanding to enter the doorway to experience. Chanting is an experience of becoming enchanted— so relax and enjoy."

I was taking pleasure in the melody, clapping my hands and moving to the rhythm of the chant: "Om Namo Bhagavate Vasudevaya." At first only a handful of people were standing up to dance. As the room started stirring to the beat of the drums, many more joined in the magic of the dance. Behind my closed eyes, and being absorbed in my own movement, I didn't notice how others were being affected by the chanting until a woman sitting beside me began to cry. I opened my eyes to see her crying give way to shaking. I abruptly sat down. All around me people were entering into myriad intensifying expressions—uncontrollable laughing, weeping, howling, quivering, and jolting from one spontaneous yoga posture into another. Some people seemed to be entering torturous emotional states while others moved slowly into angelic stances, with expressions of rapture and bliss on their faces. Surrounded in the chaos of wild movement and the sounds of heavy breathing gone out of control, I had long since stopped chanting and stared with dismay at what I was witnessing.

I had heard about holy rollers, people at tent revivals who worked themselves into trance states and then handled snakes and spoke in tongues and danced wildly with an infusion of the Holy Spirit. The only way to make sense out of this commotion was to reference those stories from childhood, stories that I had taken to be at least an extension of the truth, if not pure myth. I squirmed to find an anchor in the midst of the tumult.

When Yogi Desai stopped chanting, the room immediately returned to stillness. The audience rapidly shifted into an attitude of normalcy, as though nothing unusual had just occurred. I was shocked. I clearly did not understand what was going on.

Yogi Desai stood up and shook out his robe, then sat back down. A big grin came over his face. I felt relief that he was grinning. I interpreted his smile to mean that he, too, thought the previous display was strange.

For the next half hour he talked about a mysterious life force called *prana* that could be awakened by chanting or doing yoga. I remember him saying something to the effect of: "When prana awakens, it has an intelligence all its own and will make your mind and body do some pretty strange things. In yogic terms, this process of awakening prana is called *purification*. Awakened prana has the effect of a detergent on your whole being and will leave you balanced, *if* you let it do its thing. If you try to stop it, you will be left with your fears and blocks as before. If you surrender to the flow of energy as you experience it naturally, it will always bring you into a harmonious relationship between body and mind."

He stated that those of us who didn't respond to the chanting were controlling our experience. It wasn't until he asked people to come to the front of the room and share their experiences that I began to feel more comfortable with the phenomenon I had witnessed. Like myself, here were ordinary people who had not expected anything to happen; unlike me, those who were now speaking had found themselves letting go into primal impulses that somehow became activated through the chanting. Remembering my trancelike experience when the yogi first entered the room, I began understanding that each person's prana could be awakened in a manner that suited his or her own personality and history at that moment.

By the end of the first morning's session I decided that I liked this yogi. I certainly did not understand everything that had happened, but I was willing to bypass my instinctual reflexes to judge and criticize what I did not understand.

After lunch the director arranged us in a big circle in the middle of the room. The roadies rolled out a large Oriental carpet and brought a microphone. We received our instructions to stand when the yogi entered the room, and to sit, kneel, or stand in concentric rings so that everyone could see what was happening in the middle of the circle.

We chanted for an hour. Finally the conch blew and in bounced Yogi Desai wearing white polyester pants and a nylon turtleneck. He was buoyant and full of fun. After bowing to his teacher's picture, he sat in the middle of the rug and explained that he was going to give us a demonstration of his yoga. He asked us to stay relaxed but alert while watching him.

Yogi Desai drew his legs into the lotus position and closed his eyes. Slowly his hands moved toward his face, a movement so prolonged that I didn't register the moment until his hands touched his skin. I was mesmerized. Soon I noticed his hands cupping his eyes. I fixated on the large sparkling reddish-purple stone he wore in a gold ring on his right hand. As I opened into the experience of this mesmerizing dance, the yogi's body began to move into various postures and positions that I did not recognize from my yoga training. What he was showing us felt more like a sacred temple dance than a Sun Salutation. Yogi Desai moved like a cat stretching, then like a serpent undulating. The rhythmic sound of his breath became louder as his ribs and chest began to open like a bird expanding its wings. The quality of his movement and his reverential attitude transmitted a great lesson about where yoga came from in the human psyche.

Becoming entrained with the guru's movement, I had the feeling that I was in the center of the circle, being moved by prana. I felt his relaxation and his peace. He achieved such a state of purity in being that I became concerned for his safety. Similar to watching a tiny baby move, he was so vulnerable that I wanted to protect him. I remember thinking that the world is not a safe place for such openness.

I don't know how the yoga flow ended; at some point I closed my eyes and was drawn very deeply into the cave of myself. I lost awareness of being in a room with other people and had the deepest rest I'd ever experienced while being awake.

When I opened my eyes Yogi Desai was seated in stillness. He opened his eyes and took the microphone. He said that it was difficult to speak after going so deep. He stood up and moved to his chair, which had been brought into the circle. Like little children with a kindly grandfather, everyone quickly scooted to sit as close to him as possible.

Then Yogi Desai explained that this yoga, which he called meditation in motion, couldn't be "learned"—that one's awakened prana was the only teacher. These words rang true for all that I had witnessed that day. Yogi Desai told the story of how his prana had first awakened during an experience with his guru, Swami Kripalu, when he was a boy of fifteen in India. The experience was strange to him at that time in his life, so he tucked the memory away and soon forgot about it. He did not experience the awakening of prana during his yoga-posture practice until years later when he had moved to the United States and was teaching traditional yoga classes in Philadelphia. One morning, performing his usual sequence of traditional postures, Yogi Desai became aware of the urge to move from a place deep inside his body. Surrendering to that urge, he was transported into a timeless state of consciousness. In this first experience of meditation in motion, his body moved in ways he had never imagined and there were no limits to his ability to stretch into whatever movement flowed from the previous one. Yogi Desai explained that since the time of this powerful awakening through the posture flow, his whole purpose in life was to teach about the awakening of prana as the basis for yoga practice. He created Kripalu Ashram in Sumneytown, Pennsylvania, as a place for people to live and study yoga with him. That afternoon there would be a meeting for those who were interested in finding out more about Kripalu.

Many people shared their experiences and asked the guru questions about their personal practice of yoga, which he answered with brilliant insight. I could not wait to go to the meeting.

That afternoon those of us assembled for the meeting crowded inside a small living room of the mobile home where Yogi Desai was staying. He wanted to know our names and where we were from. He wanted to answer any questions we had about living at Kripalu Ashram. One self-conscious person after another began a personal introduction with stuttering, unfinished sentences, and tongue-tied attempts to express the simplest facts. Everyone was at a loss to be herself or himself in the presence of someone who seemed so perfected.

Gradually the melting ice gave way to a warmer exchange. By the time it was my turn the hard-earned freedom of speech in the room had opened a doorway for me to speak from my heart. I asked the guru if he would come to my university to give a yoga lecture and demonstration before returning to his ashram. I told him that I was interested in visiting his ashram but that I could not leave a job that I loved so much. He seemed genuinely interested in me and in my invitation. He revealed that he, too, had been trained as an artist and that he would enjoy seeing my work.

In those few moments of exchange, the guru became a real person to me. He ceased being the godlike king on a throne in heaven, as the set-up of his stage in the large hall had been designed to make him appear. He did not feel to me to be the guru I was searching for. But I was interested in becoming closer to someone who loved both yoga and art.

On Tuesday afternoon a white Gremlin pulled up in front of my house. I observed that the rosy-cheeked lady in charge of the weekend was driving. She was wearing sunglasses and a big smile. She introduced herself as the guru's administrator, Krishna Priya. Yogi Desai got out of the car and straightened his white tunic. He was wearing white from head to toe, including white patent leather loafers with gold buckles. He was grinning widely.

I was so nervous that I hugged him with both arms. I felt awkward about being completely unfamiliar with the protocol. I did not want to offend him, but there I was hugging him like he was Bob Barker and I had just won *The Price Is Right*. I could not apologize enough for the outburst, although he laughingly assured me that it happened all the time.

He was surprised and delighted with the mood of my artist's hideaway—turn-of-the-century Florida funk. The cypress-frame cottage was situated at the end of the road at the edge of the Hillsborough River. The oaks and elms were draped with moss and bromeliads. Flowering hibiscus, camphor bushes, and banana palms surrounded my house. I toured the yogi around the grounds and showed him where the alligator came ashore last winter. I showed him the geodesic dome, which was built as an art project by some of the university students.

As we were walking, Yogi Desai put his arm around my shoulders and told me that he felt very connected to me. He told me that I would love his ashram and was wondering if I had considered moving to Kripalu. I loved teaching art and was not considering leaving my position at the university. "Are you happy?" he asked, "really happy?" I hesitated. I don't remember anyone in my life ever asking me that question, point blank. In my hesitation, he moved in with a clincher that was to precipitate the meltdown of my life as I had known it up until that moment.

"Lots of people are partially happy with the success of a job and fame from accomplishment in the world. But when you go to bed at night, can you say that you have lived that day from your heart? Have you ever made a decision in your life based on your heart?"

I was living a solitary life. The truth was that I went to bed many nights feeling very lonely. Although I was close to people in yoga class and with students and colleagues, I was living a life in which I was alone and separate much of the time. I had many unspoken questions about the direction of my life, questions that the yogi had touched upon in his lectures at Swan Lake. And in two minutes he had zeroed in on my insecurity.

"Have you ever made a decision in your life based on your heart?" he asked again. I had no answer to his question. My eyes welled up with tears, and I could not avoid the penetrating incision of his gaze. I stood revealed and speechless. Ram Dass had told me to seek a path with heart—that I could not get to yogic awareness without first making the journey through my heart. Now here was the identical message, coming through loud and clear. And I realized I had no idea how to open my heart. In an instant, all of my efforts and accomplishments in life dissolved into large, barely-held-back tears.

I might still be standing there if it had not been for Krishna's approach. I was embarrassed by the sudden intimacy I was sharing with the yogi. When I saw Krishna out the corner of my eye, I began chattering nervously. I talked about my neighborhood, an enclave filled with artists and bohemians. Neither of the two was familiar with Jack Kerouac, who had written *On the Road* in a cottage around the corner. Down the road were the sulfur hot springs. Tranquillo Coffee House, our local food co-op, and even the dog tracks were within a five-minute walk. I was advancing facts about my external world in an attempt to communicate that I was not a religious person destined to lead a cloistered life in an ashram. I wanted them both to know that I was a person of the world. But internally I was shoring up against the tidal wave of feelings that was roaring in my belly.

The yogi had nailed it. At the age of twenty-one I had gone straight from undergraduate school into a doctoral program. Because I desired to teach at the college level, an advanced degree was essential. My life plan was all very rational. I was awarded a fellowship at Penn State, which provided a financially comfortable situation for undertaking my studies. Along with the prestige of the fellowship came a highly competitive environment in which I had to work very hard to prove my worth—I had to continuously secure my status in the graduate school pecking order so that I would be assured a job when I finished. Although artistic expression had always been a means for me to explore my inner world, it had also become a way to exploit my inner world for gain. Where was the heart in all of this?

My tongue was thick and my head was spinning. After showing Yogi Desai the last few works of my art collection, we ambled toward the door. Krishna Priya brought the car around and I bid them farewell until the evening. Long after the final good-bye wave I remained standing there, wondering what was happening to me.

Guillermo, my yoga teacher, was relocating at the time of Yogi Desai's visit and was passing through Tampa for good-byes on his way to Amherst. I invited Guillermo to ride with me to escort the yogi to the auditorium where he would be speaking that night.

When we arrived at room 217 of the Red Carpet Inn, Yogi Desai was not quite ready. We waited on the landing outside his room. When he called us in, Krishna Priya was tidying up from their supper. The room smelled of Indian curry. I introduced everyone and bragged on the yoga-flow demonstration I had seen at Swan Lake. I explained to Amrit that Guillermo was my yoga teacher. The yogi insisted on moving the furniture aside and giving Guillermo a short demonstration of his prana-awakening yoga. This was great! A personal posture flow for my yoga teacher and me!

I think it was the moldy smell permeating the carpet of room 217 that distracted me; this time I did not go into a deep ecstatic state while watching the yogi. Guillermo was moderately impressed. I could tell that we were both beginning to worry about the time. We moved the bed back into place and hurried the yogi and Krishna Priya out the door to our car.

When we walked through the doors of the room at the university where the presentation was to be held, I felt relieved. My gang had done its job. There was a nice crowd, an interesting chair for the yogi, and a few potted plants. We made our way to the front; I briefly welcomed the group and introduced Yogi Desai. Before sitting down, the yogi surmised that his chair would be too low to see everyone and complained that it looked uncomfortable. He spied a table in the corner and we brought it over. We pulled the Indian bedspread off the chair and spread it over the table. He slipped out of his sandals and crossed his legs as he lifted himself to sit on the table. There was no microphone so he had to speak loudly.

Yogi Desai led a guided meditation and asked us to massage our faces and make some sounds. He taught us to make the ocean-sounding breath, *ujjayi*. He performed a condensed version of his posture flow, his hands moving very slowly toward his face and then circling the space around his torso. He looked tired under the glare of the fluorescent lights.

At the end of the two-hour session we strolled silently under billions of stars. The scent of orange blossoms filled the air. Guillermo and I escorted the yogi and his administrator to their Gremlin and reminded them of the route home. Amrit seemed pleased with himself and with the evening's turnout, although his voice was strained from having to project without a microphone. I hugged him good-bye and thanked him for coming.

In all honesty, I was relieved when it was finally over. To say that those five days had been intense would be an understatement. I was glad to get back to my routine. I longed to return to my safe world of the known.

Months before his leaving, Guillermo had asked me to take over his yoga classes. I agreed with some reluctance, but soon found myself fascinated with the new arena for teaching. Now, on the evenings when there was no yoga class I drew a warm bath and listened to a tape that I had purchased at the souvenir table at Swan Lake. It was the yogi leading a familiar series of postures that he recommended we do every day for the rest of our lives. That seemed to me to be an unreasonable request. But I did listen to the tape over and over again while soaking in the bathtub, looking at the shadows and the evening light filtering through the window.

I was different, and I knew that. But what had changed? A few days of listening to the tape made me realize that I missed the yogi—patent leather shoes and all. There was the childlike way he engaged in life, in the simplicity of the moment. There was his uninhibited grin, his way of being so comfortable talking to large groups of people. I started to shift from thinking of him as a big brother to thinking of him as a really wise man—perhaps even my guru? I was being very careful not to scare myself.

My house began to seem bigger and emptier.

Eventually I stopped drawing a bath and gave in to doing the postures as I listened to the tape of guided instructions. I enjoyed hearing Yogi Desai's voice and the way he led the explorations. More important to me than following the sequence of postures as he guided them was feeling prana beginning to awaken in me. My ability to concentrate on internal sensations was deepening.

As I began to let go of the struggle for achieving goals in my posture flow, I noticed that a friendly relationship was developing between my body and me. The best part was when the tape clicked off and I gave myself the time to see what my body would do if I didn't try to control it. Some days I just lay there rocking from side to side, or would go into Child pose and sing to myself. Other days I astonished myself with the way prana moved me into unexplored positions, sensations, emotions, and insights. The willful yoga I had been practicing to this time began to seem more like exercise, whereas letting myself enter this meditation in motion by following the movements of prana was awakening me to curious experiences of myself. I became fascinated at the possibility of entering experiences in which I did not know what would happen next. This form of self-inquiry was beginning to feel like daily nutrition.

My inevitable visit to Kripalu Ashram did not come immediately. I had unfinished business at Penn State. I returned to the campus in May of 1976 to conclude my doctoral dissertation. Seeing my efforts at completing my dissertation heading for the bone pile, along with many of my classmates', was a nagging threat. I had one year left on the six-year finishing clock. I could extend the deadline, but I felt my life would keep dragging on without completing this degree.

My dissertation was a study of creativity, specifically examining the dialectic between artistic capacity as learned behavior and artistic capacity as an inborn dimension of human intelligence. From my research I had come to the point of view that visual expressiveness is as innate a capacity in human beings as the capacity for speech and movement.

We all know people who claim they can't draw. Actually, they might not be able to draw in the way they expect to draw, but they *can* draw.

Our culture stifles most people's confidence in their innate abilities to express themselves visually. A child's coloring book symbolizes adult concepts of the world. The child colors inside the lines, but they are not the child's lines. The child becomes dependent upon these lines and does not struggle for her own. Her natural inclination toward visual expression is stopped at the time when she becomes dependent on another to draw the lines for her. She can stay within the lines and color seven of the birds on the page blue, but she cannot draw her own bird soaring through the air, with a beak and tailfeathers and a large bald spot on its head.

If you clip a cocoon to help a butterfly emerge, you will cripple the butterfly. Pushing against the interior of the cocoon is an essential, organismic struggle that brings fluids into the spiny tubules that will eventually harden into wings. Without this resistance and great effort, the wings will not develop and the butterfly will not fly. Likewise, if you meet a child with nonjudgmental support at the edge of his or her struggle, that child will break through challenges into the next developmental stage in his or her own time and own unique way. Every individual longs for a cocoon of safety, for loving support and encouragement to break through the discomforts of learning in order to discover his or her unique and personal vision of self and to realize fulfillment as an individual.

Another access point to the intelligence that drives us toward exploring the creativity of self is prana. I am not referring to yoga education that begins and ends with repeating the statuelike poses of popular yoga styles; daily repetition of these routines is like coloring seven of someone else's birds blue. I am speaking about awakening prana to guide us into the corners of our body, to fill out the expanses of our flesh and bones and to round out the edges of our being. Although learning traditional yoga postures provides a vocabulary for movement, it is all too easy to substitute the learned forms for the subtler and less defined, yet richer, protean dimensions of awakened creativity. In a parallel vein to what I was discovering through emphasizing prana awareness in yoga, I was interested in learning how adults could regain access to innate creativity when given a supportive environment in which they could follow their own inner guidance, rather than depending upon someone to teach them the external skills of drawing.

The fifteen hundred pages of my analysis were now ready to present to my committee. I was working from the minority viewpoint that artistic development had its own purpose. I was arguing for "art for art's sake." My interest in the subjective nature of creativity was being dismissed by behaviorists as unquantifiable and therefore "statistically irrelevant." The behaviorists were attempting to reduce creativity in the education of a child to a series of stimulus-response patterns; visual arts education was being harnessed to enhance learning skills in other domains, such as math and language (as recognized in the instruction "color seven of the birds blue").

My dissertation was based on a study I conducted of creativity in the drawing process. In observing thousands of children from a wide cross-section of cultures and backgrounds, many researchers of early childhood development agree that all human infants go through universal developmental stages as they learn to draw. These universal stages in the morphology of forms on the way to self-portrayal indicates that there is something innate in human beings that compels us to visually locate ourselves in the world. This urge to communicate our relation to the world around us is as primal and present in the child as the instincts for purposeful movement and verbal language. These externally observable commonalities in our quest for self-representation is a mirror for the internal propulsion toward perceiving, understanding, and knowing one's self as an autonomous, unique individual.

Under the auspices of my mentor, Professor Ken Beittel, I set up a drawing laboratory for college students who had never been trained to draw. From all the students I worked with, I selected one upon which to base my final study.

Rachel came for a one-hour session each week. She sat at a drawing table supplied with paper and drawing pencils, pens, markers, charcoal, and crayons. A mirror mounted above the table allowed me to take time-lapse photographs of her process without disturbing her. Before settling, she would fidget, stare into space, or drum her fingers on the white Formica surface of the table until something came to her to start with. From there she let her drawing experiments begin to grow.

The following week I would show her the photographic record of her drawing time as it unfolded the week before. When we looked at the sequence of time-lapse photos she was able to make careful observations about her internal process, recalling specific details about what was running through her mind at the time she was drawing. I observed that the stages Rachel went through to discover her own standards of artistic satisfaction with her drawings were the same stages a child goes through. Although she had not been supported as a child to draw, she created the steps of a bridge between the stages when her drawing ability ceased as a child to the stage of proficiency she developed as an adult artist. She scribbled. She named her scribbles. Her self-portrayal progressed through images of a smiling sun with radials, then a tadpolelike body with appendages growing from the trunk, and on through all stages of naturalism. She grappled with inventing ways to portray multiple time and space realities, allowing her dreams and fantasies to appear on the drawing paper. She drew the events of her life. She was graduating, leaving the security of her friends and sorority. She was facing a new job, a new marriage to a non-Jewish husband, a new town and a whole new life. Her critics were on her heels the entire semester I was with her.

From her own self-observations and from the feedback she gave herself over the semester, Rachel taught herself to draw in a way that pleased her. Her fears, her dreams, and her strengths all came into her work. She reconnected with her innate urge and ability to visually represent herself and to express her world through drawing.

The intention I held for Rachel's self-satisfaction was fulfilled. But to satisfy the committee of advisors who would be supervising my dissertation, my work was just beginning. Initially, my investigation was classified as a "case study" by the behaviorists, meaning it was not scientific; it was personal and subjective rather than objective, and the data was anecdotal. My task for the next five years was to elevate the legitimacy of my research from the status of anecdotal to that of philosophical by analyzing the material for a theory of creativity. My real challenge was to establish the fact that Rachel taught herself to draw and that her work unfolded from aesthetic criteria that could be called art. To tackle these questions, I analyzed her drawing from the standpoint of the four major Western philosophies of aesthetics as identified by Stephan Pepper: idealism, behaviorism, pragmatism, and organicism. These hypotheses are mutually exclusive in terms of what they define as aesthetically or artistically of value. From each of the viewpoints, Rachel's work demonstrated aesthetic validity.

Because I was inventing a philosophical method that had no precedent, my committee was larger than usual. There were three professors from the graduate department of art education. One philosophy professor represented the school of aesthetics, and a consulting professor represented the school of phenomenology. One final consultant was from the educational psychology department. My committee members could not agree on any single point of overlap between their fields of expertise as presented in my study. I tottered from one meeting to another. Eventually I entered a downward spiral of dejection, thinking they might never be able to come to agreement about the validity of my study.

Penn State is located in an isolated bowl of mountains colloquially referred to as "Happy Valley." But I was not happy. One afternoon as I was leaving a particularly grim meeting I spied a familiar grin jumping out at me from a poster on a bulletin board. It was a picture of Amrit Desai advertising a Memorial Day retreat at Kripalu Ashram. Many yoga dignitaries would be present to dedicate Kripalu's new facilities in Summit Station, Pennsylvania. Like a phone call from the governor delaying an execution, I felt off the hook. The next morning I wasted no time packing my turquoise Beetle and fleeing from this valley and its dark spell over me.

I was so glad to be on vacation from the heady pressure of academia. Driving onto the ashram grounds, I felt layers of stress shedding from my shoulders. With my hands still gripping the steering wheel, I sat in the parking lot and cried. I watched people in work clothes scurrying about.

Moving at a snail's pace, I crawled out of the car and stretched. A silver-haired woman with a European accent informed me that I had arrived a day early and that final preparations of the new facilities were in progress. All the early arrivals were being asked to help. It was lunchtime and everyone on the grounds was passing me on the way to the cafeteria.

All the people I saw were alive compared to the blank faces I had grown accustomed to on the Penn State campus. I had the feeling that I had come home, that these were my people. I wanted to be one of them, a sweaty handkerchief around my neck and a look of contentment in my eyes.

I was ready for a nap after the long drive and lunch. Vandita, the woman I registered with, showed me to the "brothers'" dormitory—a converted chicken coop. Fortunately, there were no chickens. The floor was covered with hay and draped with a big orange and white parachute. It was a relaxing place for a nap.

The amount of work that was achieved in those twenty-four hours was astounding. There was no roof on the main hall on the day I arrived; by late afternoon the following day there was not only a roof but temporary carpeting, a stage with flowers, and four thrones. Here was one group of motivated people: they were invincible in their determination to be ready for the inaugural event. I helped out by hauling some concrete rocks from the perimeter of the main hall to a big ditch. My crew leader had us hold hands in a circle and chant "Om" before we started our jobs and after we finished. I loved throwing rocks in a hole. It was just the level of activity my mind needed at the time.

The setting sun reflected off a large swimming pool outside the arched windows of the main hall, creating a spectacle of dancing light on unpainted walls and an unfinished ceiling. After the accelerated pace of preparing for the ceremony, it felt soothing to finally sit still and savor the silence. The scent of lilies and roses mingled with an ever-present aroma of my favorite spicy incense, transporting me back to fond memories of Swan Lake. Every head in the room was still wet from a last-minute shower. A hush had fallen over the hall, filling the spaces between each person in the gathering. A chorus of chanters and musicians in the now-familiar white vestments took their place to the left of a tiered platform. Four thrones sat empty. They were Indian thrones from the Mogul period—richly lacquered wood with ornate painted patterns. The eyes of Swami Kripalu were staring into the crowd from larger-than-life photos mounted in arched niches on either side of the podium.

A blaring conch announced the arrival of the procession of dignitaries. Yogi Desai led the way, smiling and stopping along the aisle to receive flowers and smiles from his admirers. I was so engulfed in the mass of devotees that I could not see him up close. Following him was the famous old granddad of yoga, Swami Satchitananda, who was clowning and performing sweet antics in Yogi Desai's wake. He was giving every flower he received to the next unsuspecting pair of hands along the runway. Behind Swami Satchitananda was the Indian ambassador to the United Nations. The last to come was Rup Verma, a well-known classical Indian musician.

Amrit took his position in the center of the stage. The bowing and formal introductions went on endlessly. Each man had his turn to receive a garland of marigolds over his head. When the huff had finally been huffed and everyone had lavishly adored everyone else on the platform, the room once again became silent. The yogi led a meditation, thanking the Supreme Being and all heavenly hosts for giving us this wonderful property and the roof over our heads. The dedication had begun. Rup Verma was seated at Amrit's feet and was joined by a man with two silver drums. Bringing the sitar close to his bosom, he strummed a raga that carried me back to the Monterey Pops Festival when I had first heard Ravi Shankar play Indian music. It was a melody fit for the occasion. Through the gift of his mastery something divine came into the room.

It must have put Amrit in a mood too, because after sitting in silence for a long time after the raga ended, the yogi had the stage cleared. Just Rup Verma remained to play again. The haunting mood of his next raga moved us deeper into rapture. Then Amrit was inspired to lead a chant of his own. Out came the box organ and he sang lines to Ram and Krishna. In the stress of my graduate work of the past months, I had begun to draw more deeply into prana through the daily practice of meditation in motion. I was fully open to receiving an infusion of energy from being with Amrit.

I began to feel the prana-awakening experience during the chanting. My hands and arms were propelled by snakelike rivers of pulsation that flowed from my belly first and then into the center of my heart. The experience was reminiscent of a recurring dream I'd been having for years in which I am bitten on my hands by two snakes that move inside and become guardian totems to my heart. I drew and painted that image many times; I did not know why it held such mystery and power for me.

As I let go deeper into the movement, a strange and wonderful sensation came upon me. My heart erupted into what felt like an orgasm in my chest. Moving into my head and behind my eyes, the quivering released a stream of faces I had worn in many lifetimes. Contained in every face was a pair of eyes staring into me. I opened my physical eyes and the yogi, from his throne up on the platform, was staring at me. He stopped chanting as he continued to gaze at me. His look turned friendlier as he recognized me as the art teacher from Tampa. In a voice out of character with the mood of the moment, he said, "Welcome to Kripalu Ashram, Doctor Don Stapleton." I could not reply that I did not yet have my doctorate degree. I could not have spoken a word in that moment. I was flattered to be acknowledged and was very embarrassed to be singled out in this way.

Maintaining his focus on me, the yogi had a microphone brought over. He asked me to share what I was experiencing during the chant. My hands and arms were still pulsing. I clutched the microphone with two wet hands and looked into Yogi Desai's eyes. He must have known that words would eventually come from my mouth because he waited quite patiently. When I began to speak, the energetic experience I was having earlier began all over again. I spoke haltingly about snakes and a dream and faces of other times. As I spoke I felt the top of my head opening. From above my body I could see the entire room of people. Although my eyes were focused on the guru, from my circle vision I could see surges of protoplasmic energy moving through the room, connecting people to one another. There were many tears and heart shudders in the room as I spoke. I felt as though my body had become the ground for a lightning bolt passing through the crowd.

I cannot remember how I got from where I was standing to the front of the room, but I do remember Yogi Desai saying, "Don, come up here to me." When I got to the platform I hugged him around the neck, trying not to crush his marigold garland. When I sat on the floor at the edge of his chair I started to shed tears and then shiver. My body, my emotions, and my mind spun out of control. When I could speak again I told him about my recurring dreams of snakes. He spoke of awakened prana transforming into what the yogis refer to as serpent power, or kundalini energy. It sleeps in the base of the spine; when aroused, it moves up through the body and precipitates all kinds of phenomena. It is advisable to seek the counsel of an experienced yogi when this event occurs, to assure that the energy becomes a source of inspiration rather than of fear or confusion.

I cannot explain the experiences of that evening, nor many that occurred during the following days of the retreat. I had the feeling that this yogi was my guru. I knew that I would be moving to his ashram as soon as I could arrange my life to do so.

My sense of time and reality was noticeably altered when I returned to Penn State. I was not the heady doctoral candidate returning to the halls of academia for the final defense of his dissertation. I was a human being with an open heart. Until this week-end, I had been the caterpillar pressing against the imprisonment of my unyielding cocoon. In the drive from the ashram to State College, Pennsylvania, I felt like an exhausted butterfly crawling into the sun to stretch my wings.

So many realizations came to me during the drive. I saw that until this weekend I had been someone who was working toward goals—particularly at this juncture toward the goal of completing my doctorate degree. Being a professional student was the well-known cocoon that gave me my identity. I did not know who I would be without the labor of writing a dissertation; I could not picture my life without the struggle of proving myself. But I now realized the freedom that awaited me in completing the degree and getting on with my life. I knew where I wanted to be next in the world and my entire psyche mobilized to fulfill the transition.

I was so hungry on the drive home. I stopped three times for ice cream. When I returned to my cottage I lay down in bed and did not get up for eighteen hours. During that time, every experience of my life seemed to flash on the screen of my awareness. All the feelings I had never allowed to surface about certain events and people in my life appeared as an epiphany, precipitating one cathartic release after another. I clutched the prayer beads the yogi blessed for me on the last morning of our retreat and held on for dear life as I went through a personal tunnel of darkness.

When the world began to settle, I opened my eyes and saw my Smith Corona Electra waiting for me. I calmly began to read what I had written to date.

Carl Jung called it *synchronicity* when random events suddenly reveal a hidden relationship or pattern of meaning. The four profiles of Rachel's creative process stood oddly isolated. She looked like four different Rachels. Indulging in a hunch one morning, I put the four files in a circle. I got out my tarot deck. Invoking the presence of my wisdom guides, I asked for a reading to help me more deeply understand Rachel and her drawings. I was stunned at the clarity of insight that those cards revealed. I looked at the four Rachels and a whole person emerged in the story of the cards.

Acting on my inspiration, I wrote a final chapter to my dissertation using mysticism as the basis of a theory of aesthetic value that has the power to integrate the four mutually exclusive rational views. I told Rachel's story according to the random reading I had performed. Although I could not get all the members of my committee to accept the final chapter as a valid philosophical method, they all agreed that the material belonged in an appendix to the work. The novelty of my approach shocked my committee into agreement with one another about the validity of my study.

The hardest part of my work—getting this committee to stand behind me—was now complete. The next challenge to overcome was clearly in my vision. The aesthetics professor on my committee was rumored to have written his dissertation in less than fifty pages; he blithely convinced the other members that if I could not say what I had to say in two hundred pages, it should not be said at all.

I took his warning seriously. I cut my work down from fiftenn hundred pages to less than five hundred for the final draft.

I believe that it was my fierce determination to move forward in my life that accounted for the miracle that happened on the day of my final defense. An eerie afternoon darkness rolled in, the skies heavily clouded. As the solemn event of my presentation commenced, a massive electrical storm with bone-rattling thunder began punctuating almost every remark I made. Every window clattered. Against the backdrop of nature's percussion, I presented and defended my treatise on creativity. The storm began to pass. When their questions subsided, Dr. Beittel addressed me: "Don, you may leave the room while we make our determination."

Minutes crawled by like hours. The arched hallway had never been so still. Frozen on the edge of my bench, I studied every remaining drop of rain that rolled down the leaded-glass panes on a window in front of me. The vacuum of this timeless tunnel was broken when I heard a door opening. I was called back into the room. Everyone was standing and looking very somber. Ken Beittel moved toward me. As he shook my hand, a warm smile broke across his face. "Congratulations, Doctor Don Stapleton. You are now entitled to the rights and privileges of the doctoral degree."

There were frustrating days of getting the typist and graduate school to agree on the final format of the archival copy of my dissertation, Xeroxing, binding, questionnaires to fill out, and fees to pay. Now I had one final decision to make—which graduation robe to buy? Two colleagues were graduating with me. They were debating about whether to purchase the Madison robe or the Jefferson robe. Preparing to spend the rest of their lives in the medieval robes and hoods of academia, they were purchasing a garment to wear in all future processions in which they would be grandly escorting candidates down the same pathway they had trodden. I chose the disposable model. I did not want to spend the rest of my life in a black robe with a hood and mortarboard. I was headed to the ashram. I had chosen a path of white cotton.

From my perspective now, as I tell you this story, it strikes me as odd that I could not see that I was leaving one haven of safety for another. But it would be another fifteen years before I could see that and twenty before I could admit it and take appropriate steps to push out of that cocoon and into my next stage of metamorphosis.

I was grateful for the next year of teaching in Florida with a "Ph.D." after my name. It came as a relief to be able to joke that the post-nominal Ph.D. stood for "Piled Higher and Deeper." Although receiving the degree itself seemed anticlimactic, I now had the time to savor the journey of self-discovery that the ordeal had provided. At twenty-seven years old, my Volkswagen was turning over 100,000 miles and I had completed the final stage of my life plan as it had been written to date. The rest of my life belonged to me. I seized the freedom to live from the fresh stirrings in my heart.

I felt little remorse in seeing my treasured Queen Anne sofa and chairs of ruby-red velour on the back of someone else's truck. I sold everything that I could not pack into my Beetle. Because in a year I would be moving into an ashram and living in a dormitory space, I figured I better begin to condition myself for the austere change.

My last year in Tampa became an education in group living. I shared a house with an assortment of characters who, like myself, were following one guru or another. Eleanor had received a prana-awakening initiation through a French kiss that a guru had given her at a party. (This was bewildering to me, since Amrit was advocating sexual abstinence.) Three others were disciples of Baba Muktananda; they practiced long hours of meditation between frequent snacking. And there was the couple who enjoyed the freedom of total nudity, both in and out of their bedroom; they were inspired by the teachings of Stephen Gaskin of the Farm. On Monday nights we had a (clothing optional) house meeting at which we'd decide how the chores would be divvied up for the week. On Sunday mornings we collectively hosted a gathering of ten to twenty people at our house on 20th Street for Sufi dancing, yoga, meditation, and storytelling. It was during these Sunday gatherings that I began to take notice of Jan, an exceptionally attractive undergraduate who was also taking my yoga classes at the university.

During the year before moving to Kripalu, I sponsored another of Amrit's visits to Tampa. This time he stayed at our house on 20th Street. Of various events during his visit the one I remember best was receiving my new name. This meant I would officially be his disciple. When he first said the name, it sounded Italian: Samadarshan. My parents back in Texas were already mortified that their son the professor (and only recently the doctor) was moving into an ashram. Yoga was of the devil. Amrit was a false prophet. And Donnie had gone off the very deep end! I knew they would be totally convinced of this fact when they heard my new name, so I wasted no time flaunting it. My fervor knew no bounds.

After the yogi's second visit, Jan, who was later to be given the name Amba, came to the Sunday events on 20th Street faithfully. She came to all of the evening events and meditations that had anything to do with Amrit or Kripalu.

A growing number of people was interested in moving to Kripalu, though lingering doubts tempered my certainty about making such a wholesale life change. Rather than resigning my position from the University of South Florida in Tampa, I took a leave of absence for a year. Before finalizing my move to Pennsylvania I secured a position at the Philadelphia College of Art, teaching and supervising the graduate program in art education. This arrangement allowed me to keep one foot in the familiar academic world and another in ashram life.

Three days a week I drove into Philadelphia from the original Sumneytown campus of Kripalu. On the other days I immersed myself in my ashram job, writing copy and designing ads and brochures for Kripalu activities. I had always looked down on commercial art and would never have pictured myself in such a job to earn a living. But my yoga practice was now expanding to include surrender. I was willing to do whatever was requested in my new practice of learning to say "yes" to life.

I spent my first year of ashram life saying "yes" to everything. Saying "yes" meant participating in all of the structured experiences of group life: dish crews, laundry crews, breakfast crews, and ashram-wide housecleaning. The hardest thing to say "yes" to was the overly regimented and uninspiring morning yoga practice, which included synchronized jogging in laps. There were attendance sheets and checklists to verify that we were doing each prescribed yoga posture every day. There was next to no instruction or facilitation in learning prana-flow yoga, the meditation in motion that was Amrit's signature style. In the overly controlled schedule there was no personal time to explore one's own meditation in motion or to integrate the steady stream of new experiences. Especially difficult was the regiment of keeping time sheets to track every 15-minute block of time. These were tallied at the end of the week and submitted to your "coordinator," who was responsible for helping you to stay on task.

Amrit was not present for the 4:00 A.M. yoga sessions. My source of inspiration came after yoga in the mornings, when Amrit often joined us for *satsanga*—chanting sessions and a discourse. He also joined us for longer periods of satsanga in the evenings. Being with Amrit in these times was magical. He was able to stimulate insight and inspiration during his discourses by drawing wisdom directly from his heart. Satsanga was also a time to share our experiences with the "family" and to receive guidance from Amrit on the issues that emerged in our ashram life. For those who ventured to resist or complain about the compulsory celibacy, the long working hours, or the structured morning yoga practice, he always had clever and convincing ways to turn negativity into a challenge to surrender. His chanting often precipitated the group catharsis and prana awakenings I had first witnessed at Swan Lake, but such access to prana had very little to do with the physical yoga practice being promoted at the ashram.

Had it not been for the opportunity to contribute my educational skills to the yoga instruction program, I could not have stayed at Kripalu. My knowledge of the subject of adult education became obvious when I was asked to write and design a brochure advertising Kripalu Yoga teacher training. My research for the project began by observing the course as it was being offered. The teachers were afraid of losing control and the students were afraid of making a mistake. From my first session with the

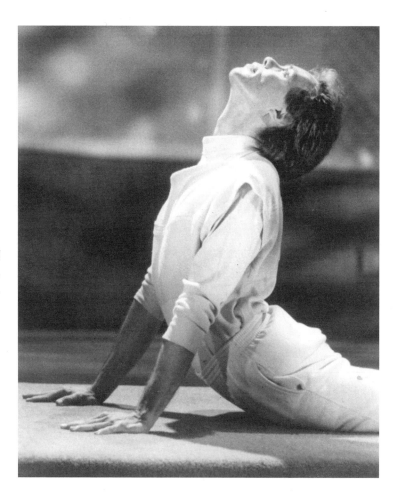

Don teaching prana flow yoga, 1989.

teachers, I was welcomed enthusiastically. Without a model of a more open-ended learning process in their own backgrounds, the teachers felt relieved to be offered an option for a livelier and more personally fulfilling approach to teaching yoga. It was clear that yoga, especially the philosophy of this guru's posture flow, would be more effectively transmitted as an experiential learning process rather than as a set of authoritarian guidelines.

I structured our first training sessions using clay as the medium to illustrate the principles of creativity that are implicit in experiential learning. Making imaginary objects while blindfolded provided an opportunity to illustrate the differences between perceptions that arise from an internal felt sense and those that arise from an expectation to make something look like it "should" look. The students were asked to work together, without speaking, to make something as tall as they could, something inside something else, and something delicious to eat. Their hands began working together to follow the promptings of whatever emerged through their mutual interaction with the clay. The clay began to take on a life of its own as the teams drew from their intuitions to bring their creations forth. They were able to break through the self-conscious expectations of doing it "right" or making it look good and shift into the joy of interacting with the clay from a direct sensorial inquiry. The idea of learning through the body from the inside out became an obvious possibility. But especially liberating was the opportunity everyone now had to play.

The yoga postures the students invented while blindfolded provided an opportunity to notice how it felt to lead a yoga posture using the language of sensation to shape the experience. As the environment loosened up, each person was willing to look at the experience of yoga education with less seriousness and fewer preconceptions than before. The intention was to arrive at a place in which each learner would be empowered to value the innate wisdom within him- or herself and to follow the impulses and intuitions that come from his or her personal experience of being in a body. Through this early teaching process we articulated the awareness that one's internal experience is the doorway to attuning to and awakening the flow of prana.

At this point, yoga education at Kripalu underwent fast and dramatic changes. Attuning to prana through meditation in motion became a part of every class. Amrit encouraged me to continue nurturing an attitude of openness and experimentation in retraining the yoga staff. The experiential learning process took permanent root in the pedagogy of Kripalu Yoga when the focus shifted toward discovery and as each teacher was empowered to draw from direct experience as the source of authority.

From that time on I was responsible for creating the curriculum for Kripalu Yoga education, training the teachers and designing and directing a wide variety of yoga programs that embodied the experiential learning process. I was named the director for Kripalu Yoga teacher training. As the guest programs rapidly grew, bringing hundreds and then thousands of participants to Kripalu, my role expanded to meet the need for refining the program manuals, producing instructional audio- and videotapes, and mentoring new program directors who could deliver the unique approach of prana-awakening yoga through their own creativity. Just as quickly as Kripalu Ashram became a magnet for those who wanted to learn to teach Kripalu Yoga and to have an in-depth residential experience, Kripalu began to expand into the bigger world as well. I developed and taught many outreach programs that disseminated the Kripalu experience throughout the United States and abroad. For several years I traveled as much as I taught on the Kripalu campuses. As long as I continued saying "yes" to Amrit's authority and returning the credit to him, I enjoyed unlimited freedom for developing my own approach to yoga.

To his great credit, this was a period of time in which Amrit himself was open to learning from teachers from a wide variety of disciplines. He embraced each contemporary idea with great enthusiasm and was known for "cutting and pasting" elements from many sources to enhance the Kripalu approach. Amrit was ecstatic about the expansion of Kripalu's profile in the public eye. Although he rarely attended my program sessions, I received his unequivocal support. Amrit continually assured me that the results of my approach to teaching were reflected in the attitude of self-confidence and openness in the groups I taught. When the groups I taught attended his lectures, he was impressed with their understanding of Kripalu Yoga and grasp of the subtleties of applying the yogic principles to their personal lives. In my secret fantasy, Amrit had become more than my guru—he was actually becoming a good friend. It seemed to me that because he trusted my work with yoga education at Kripalu, he became freer to pursue his own continued growth as a yogi.

It took me a while to realize that some Kripalu residents were living in an ashram not because they shared a love for hatha yoga; many seemed to be there for the sense of self-confidence they were receiving through Amrit. I garnered tremendous doses of Amrit's praise and attention, gifts that fulfilled needs I had for recognition and feeling important in the world, but I had other motivations in my life as well. I had a life before Kripalu that had been richly fulfilling, although incomplete. I enjoyed the sense of self that had come through my art, my professional career, the journey I had been through in proving myself to the doctoral committee, and a feeling of self-confidence that came from being successful in the world. And I was continuing my development as a professional educator in my role at Kripalu.

But some residents were at Kripalu because it was a place for them to gain a sense of self in the world. Without previous professions, relationships, or successful careers, many of the younger residents were looking to Kripalu to fulfill their life purpose as individuals. Kripalu could provide this to some extent, but to live and serve at Kripalu would always mean prioritizing the goals of Kripalu above one's own personal development and individuation. It would also mean that Amrit received the credit for whatever work you did on yourself. Your growth and success was the result of his inspiration. All personal goals that fell beyond the acceptable norms of the Kripalu culture were suppressed, or fulfilled outside the sanction of group scrutiny. In this climate it became automatic to trade off one's quest for self-fulfillment and individuation for the feelings of being loved and accepted by Amrit and those who loved him. The biggest inhibition to unlimited self-development and spiritual growth for the residential community at Kripalu was the position of ultimate authority that Amrit insisted on maintaining.

Amrit secretly gave me a piece of advice early in my residency. He took me aside and advised me to train others to do everything that I was doing so that I would be free to continue to work with him directly and thereby continue growing under his personal guidance. He encouraged me neither to get caught up in the role of yoga educator nor to be identified with the results. In this way, I could be using the work

I was doing as an aspect of my own yoga practice and spiritual growth. In yogic terms this is called karma yoga, the yoga of action with nonattachment to the results. Amrit implied that my spiritual growth would be greatly accelerated because the results of my good karma were in service to the guru, who had transcendent access to knowing what was best for me.

By accepting this formula for self-development, I relinquished personal ownership for any original thinking or creativity that I put into the hundreds of programs I designed and directed for Kripalu. Teachers were presented to the public as interchangeable units. Our names were rarely listed alongside the programs we were directing. A guest would register for a particular program but not for a particular teacher who might thereby develop a following. When a Kripalu teacher gained too much attention, power, or recognition for his or her ability to inspire others, Amrit and Krishna Priya would intervene with a change of jobs, change of role in the ashram hierarchical structure, or even a change of locations from one campus to another. No one was allowed to attract a following or notoriety in any form that Amrit perceived as undermining his authority.

Amrit began to change. And Kripalu changed as a reflection of his interests. Although he continued to teach about Kripalu yoga, he stopped practicing the yoga himself. I imagined that his interests in other approaches to yoga and self-development became so expansive that he lost the sense of power and simplicity in the essence of his unique approach.

Amrit began to set his sights on the bigger world around him. Although it was unclear what he was looking for or in what way he wanted to redirect the Kripalu focus, he began to demand unquestioning support for implementing each new idea that passed his screen. His vision grew to enormous proportions and started to hit the limits of the resources we had available as an organization.

For years Amrit had drawn support and inspiration from close disciples, like myself, who were able and willing to practice his teachings and to honor him with our gratitude by supporting his direction. In these new times, those of us who had been very close to him were sensing that he was inviting a more authentic level of relationship, one in which he desired feedback about the limitations we experienced in our personal relationships with him. In a few situations it seemed as though our intuition and our efforts were accurate. He was curious about our feedback and interested in altering his behavior to improve his effectiveness as our guide. He began to explore himself and to reveal certain levels of insecurity. But as the process invariably cycled back to his need, in his role as guru, to retain ultimate authority, his willingness to face his personal limitations returned to the shadows. He began to view our new levels of authentic relationship as a challenge to his immanent authority and became punitive and vindictive to those who dared go too far.

It was inevitable that the moment would come when Amrit would ask me to let go of my way of directing the yoga trainings. I had placed my emphasis on teaching methods that evoked the awakening of prana. The approach that I represented for twelve years required personal ownership of the material and individual expression of the principles involved. From Amrit's perspective, students who found their inspiration from inside their own experience were less willing to simply follow his guidance. His position as the ultimate authority would be challenged.

Early one Monday morning, Amrit called to ask me to bring the senior yoga teachers to his house for a meeting. He announced that he was going to assume the role of structuring and standardizing the yoga curriculum. Over the previous weekend, he had experienced a yoga class from a new resident that he wanted to use as his new paradigm for all classes. Gripped in the shock of heart-stabbing pain, I let go. I had fallen into the ego trap of identifying with the yoga as mine. And Amrit was asking me to give back to him what was already his, in his role as guru.

For the first few days following his pronouncement, I dissociated from the pain by attempting to use this opportunity of great suffering as an opening to deepen my personal commitment to yoga, to nonattachment, and to surrender. But as I began to withdraw from teaching, the pain was inescapable. The further I got from being a teacher, the more clearly I was able to see that the direction in which Amrit was headed no longer held integrity for me personally.

In taking on a new role, my pain seemed to resolve. I became an administrator and stepped aside to allow a new generation of teachers to work with Amrit to help him manifest his vision. The practice of surrender to the guru, however, had now become a source of internal turmoil.

In reaction to the open-ended approach to teaching that I had developed, Amrit became fixated on standardizing the yoga content to a series of postures taught in a rigid way. He dictated the sequence, the verbal descriptions, and even the way the classroom was to be set up. He insisted upon precise rows, with the teacher positioned up front. His goal was to reduce his yoga to a formula that would be predictably the same from one teacher to the next and from one class to the next. He held no regard for the varying levels of experience in any given class or for the physical differences and limitations that are always present in any given group. If you were in one of these classes and could not do one of the postures in the way it was being guided, you were instructed to watch. His position became so intractable that he required the residents of Kripalu to attend these new-style classes or leave the community.

Had I foreseen the direction in which Amrit wanted to steer the yoga curriculum, I would have left Kripalu much sooner. But the course of events was slow and the dissolution of prana-oriented yoga was jagged, veering from one superficial approach to another. At first Amrit attempted to use a technique that had been effective with method dance training called the "press point" system. When the results were not uniform and not instantly gratifying to him, he brought in Bikram Choudhury and his style of repetitive forced stretching in a heated room. Amrit retained the idea of forced stretching associated with sweat yoga but dropped the heated room. Predictably, this formula resulted in numerous injuries and so was doomed to failure.

One system after another, Amrit forged his way toward a goal that became more and more splintered as he went along. He did not know what he wanted. He was motivated by the desire for recognition as a worldwide yoga personality and by greed for numbers. He wanted to reduce his yoga to a formula that everyone could teach and that could be performed without thinking. Although his desire to control escalated, his actual influence on the organization began to diminish.

In my administrative role I became the director for the Kripalu programs division; the division was titled "Transformation Development and Delivery." I sat on all the planning councils, which conducted the activities of the multimillion dollar enterprise. Serving on the board of trustees, I represented the division that produced the major sources of Kripalu revenue and activity.

Kripalu's success as a financial entity had become a trap for the senior-resident population. Eighty-five members of the 350-member community had been residents for fifteen or more years. We had built the organization from our early days with Amrit. It was this group that had run the day-to-day operations and kept the work growing. More importantly, this core group of disciples had nurtured the spiritual essence of Kripalu and offered guidance and instruction in the Kripalu lifestyle. Facing the natural developmental need to evolve into greater responsibility and maturity in the path of service, senior members of the community were aching for self-expression. It was the time in my life to learn another important lesson about being in human relationships.

Something was off in the world of Kripalu. Because we did not have the ground for authenticity in our relationship with the guru we were not able to be true with one another. We could not say "no" to Amrit. In the model of surrender to the guru, you always say "yes." When the guru is wrong and you know it, you say "yes" anyway because a higher value is placed on surrender than on the truth as it appears to you in the moment. If you see the world differently, it is because you are blind to the bigger picture that the guru, in his transcendent wisdom, can perceive. You are trained to mistrust your own instincts, your own truth barometer, and your ability to know what is right for you. You are separated from your evolutionary impulse to create forms that embody your connection to the source of spirit.

It came as a powerful lesson to realize that until I could say "no" to Amrit, my "yes" had no real meaning. I learned to say "no" to him as I sat through hours of the usual meetings and began to pay closer attention to his body language. I noticed that although he was smiling, there was a clenching in Amrit's jaw when he did not like the decision being made. He would never freely admit to having "negative" feelings such as fear, anger, jealousy, or insecurity; by his definition, an evolved soul such as himself would be above these baser human emotions. In his attempt to appear nonattached to the results, Amrit would speak abstractly through parables or spiritualized principles to influence decisions. But when he was in disagreement, he would not express his true feelings.

In one of these meetings we were discussing some residents who had not worked a full schedule for several months. These senior residents had given their hearts to Kripalu and been a major force in the organization's leadership. Some had developed chronic fatigue syndrome and other severe health issues; some were undergoing psychotherapy. Amrit wanted the administrators to ask these residents to either start working full time or to leave. He was clearly out of touch with the multidimensional reality we were being asked to address as the leaders of our spiritual community.

The atmosphere in the meeting was stifling. I was suppressing my reactions to the calmness in his voice, which contrasted so intensely to the insensitivity of his demand. I realized that most of the administrators in the room were silently in agreement with me, but over the period of a few minutes Amrit had managed to convince almost all in the room that something terrible was going to happen if we did not take action by making examples out of these residents.

I agitatedly asked Amrit, "Are you afraid of the results of supporting these leaders in finding a niche that is supportive to their growth at this time?" He was obviously upset about being asked if he was afraid. He denied having any fear at all. His jaw twitched and his eyes glassed over. I asked him about what he imagined would happen if we allowed the residents to stay. He painted a very negative prediction. I said that I didn't see it that way. "I have a different picture. I'm responsible for the consequences because I'm their administrator. I do not have any fear about the outcome. I can work with them." Other administrators began to share their perspectives, some of which were in alignment with mine, others with Amrit's. It came down to the simple fact that we disagreed.

For two days Amrit made phone calls to others in the meeting asking them to support his viewpoint and to pressure me to relent. I spoke to Amrit many more times and continued to say no. He let the issue go. The residents stayed. But he was silently furious with me.

I began to say no to him on all issues about which I disagreed. In one evening satsanga during that time I was sitting in my assigned front row center seat. Amrit looked over my head as he spoke to the community about how he was being misunderstood and mistreated by the administration. He indirectly referred to me several times; he taught about the ego and how sometimes it won't let go when a disciple has not matured into the responsibilities a guru gives him. Afterward many upset members of the community stopped me in the hallways or left angry phone messages asking why I was mistreating the guru. His unspoken threat in much of his communication during this time was that if he didn't get his way, he would leave.

As the issues of individuation and autonomy became more critical and I represented a different position than he assumed, Amrit publicly attempted to shame, cajole, and manipulate his will into action. His lectures became political diatribes; he lost his ability to inspire his followers on the spiritual purposes for maintaining community life together. It became obvious that he was operating from fear. He knew that he had lost control of the community. Many who knew him closely began to feel that he had lost his personal vision and, perhaps, had even lost his own connection to the wisdom of prana.

It was during this period that my conflict with Amrit intensified to the level of affecting my physical health. For the first time since taking yoga on as a lifelong practice, I allowed my responsibilities at Kripalu to interfere with my personal practice of yoga. The buildup of tension culminated in an injury that caused a severe scoliosis of my spine. Yoga had come easily to me when I had a physical body that was relatively free from pain. Facing a lifetime of chronic pain, I was now challenged to reach further inside to find another level of self-responsibility.

During a workshop presented by Rishiji Prabhakar, one of many visiting yoga gurus from India, I fell onto my shoulders and neck in the midst of a Sufi spinning exercise. One of my partners released his grip and I stumbled backward. I was knocked unconscious for several minutes and then minimized the severity of the shock by neglecting immediate treatment for the injury. I could not focus on myself because I felt responsible to honor my role as moderator for the public debates that were escalating between Amrit and Rishiji. I willed myself to be present for what turned out to be nasty interchanges in which both yogis were attempting to pull the audience to his own point of view.

Although I felt it was my role to bridge the gap between these two teachers whom I admired and respected, I had to finally accept that these men might never come to understand each other. At the end of all attempts at reason and civility with the two of them behind closed doors, I found my angry voice. In fact, I was angrier than I have ever been, not just at the two of them, but at myself as well. They both wanted something and expected that the other would openheartedly provide it with no expectations in return. Each was trying to con the other, and I was enabling their dynamic.

In hindsight, I was in shock. I was not okay. I was not in a state of mind to be able to assess my condition. I did not realize at the time how my fall had been a message from my body that I had thoroughly embodied the spinning differences of these two yoga experts who were in disagreement about the spiritual path. My body was screaming for me to confront a personality pattern that had motivated me from early childhood—the need to be a peacekeeper at all costs to my own personal well-being.

Not surprisingly, my spine was growing more torqued by the day as a result of the injury and my denial of its severity. I couldn't sit, walk, or stand without pain and discomfort. Thirteen days later, when I sat in a chiropractor's office to view the full spinal X-ray, I was sickened to actually see the seriousness of my injury—a full S-shaped scoliosis. I was bent out of shape. The adjustments and treatment on a vibrating table with thermal heat bags made the condition worse. Here I was again at the mercy of yet another expert.

At the advice of a close friend I consulted a network chiropractor. There were no back-cracking adjustments, no X-rays. Michael had me lie on my side; he put cushions under my head and between my knees and then left me alone for several minutes. Michael placed a fingertip on the sole of my foot upon his return. Feeling the gentle nature of his contact, I curled into the fetal position and began to sob. There were no questions, no explanations, no further treatments other than letting my body begin to release some of the trauma—not only from the injury, but from the escalating tensions gripping me at Kripalu and from the aggressive therapy the first chiropractor administered.

Over the next few sessions, I began to own back the responsibility for listening to what my body had been trying to tell me for months. Michael supported my healing process by letting me listen to the wisdom of my own body. In the turnaround at that early stage of my healing process I began to realize the indispensable process of self-inquiry as the fundamental basis for accepting myself as I am and for restoring balance.

Reaching back in time, I recalled my original experiences in Tampa when I first began allowing prana to move my body, when I was not following someone else's instructions and was not in a yoga class with other people. The power of yoga came to me as an awakening to my inner self, when I was alone and when I allowed my body to be moved through its own intelligence. It's not that I didn't receive benefits from practicing yoga in a room full of other people, following someone else's instructions. In some group class situations I enter into explorations of the bodymind that would not emerge if I were not with others. I get ideas and learn subtleties of various postures and movements by watching how prana moves other people. But when it comes to settling into the core of my being, there is no substitute for the relationship I have with myself.

Exploring the bodily sensations of scoliosis was now my teacher. Working with this condition began to open the doorway to discovering other memories hidden in my body. In the world of internal self-development, prana unwinds its mysteries in a zigzag pattern.

In one phase of movement inquiry I discovered patterns that have been present since birth. Noticing the way my head is positioned over my shoulders, I recalled vague references my mother had made about my being blue and bruised at birth. Looking for clues to deeper understanding of my body, I asked her for all the details she could remember. I learned that the doctor used forceps to deliver me, the umbilicus wrapped around my neck. That inquiry led to a story about a time my grandmother accidentally dropped me on my head when I was eighteen months old. Knee scrapes, bicycle falls, sprained ankles—every bodily experience is written in the body's memory and can be accessed by allowing prana to work its way into deeper layers of awareness. Recalling information associated with a particular injury or condition can be helpful in releasing trauma from the body. But such understanding is not a shield from ongoing life and the confrontations that arise in each new situation, as I was soon to learn.

As one of many among my fellow residents who were feeling the effects of conflicting values at the core of Kripalu our entire community was being propelled into a period of upheaval and change. Finally, a tumultuous event occurred in which the logjam of power at the top began to shift. A long-range strategic planning council authorized by the board of trustees confronted Krishna Priya about her unwillingness to empower the senior administrators to make desperately needed changes in our future directions. She resigned her role as CEO on the spot. Following a brief time of filling the role on an interim basis, the board elected me to the position of CEO and proceeded to initiate an organizational plan that restructured the power and assets of Kripalu. Rather than basing our future on the authority of the guru's control, the plan was based on authentic relationship and shared power. I called myself the "C E Zero" because I was determined to see that the role itself was dissolved in favor of a relationship-based approach to making decisions.

As the board was just about to finalize and implement our new plan, terrible stories were revealed about an illicit sexual relationship between Amrit and Krishna Priya that had spanned much of the history of Kripalu's existence. Others came forward to divulge stories about being coerced into sexual relations with Amrit under the rubric of being given special initiations. The community entered a meltdown as Amrit refused to assume appropriate responsibility for his actions or to express remorse over presenting himself and his teachings in one light while secretly living a different life in his private affairs. The responsibility fell upon the board to confront Amrit and to ask for his resignation.

As the pressure was mounting toward imminent change at Kripalu, and as my own questioning of personal integrity was building in me, another shift was taking place in my being. I was allowing myself to fall in love with the woman I'd been admiring for more than twenty years.

Two years after I first moved to Kripalu, Amba, the undergraduate student who would often attend our Sunday morning gatherings at the house on 20th Street, became a resident. At the ashram, men and women—or "brothers" and "sisters," as we were called—were discouraged from socializing or forming relationships in support of the practice of celibacy, so I spent little time with Amba during her first four years of residency. I remember her as one of the few consistent early-comers who did pranayama while waiting for Amrit to arrive for his evening lecture. I chatted with her when I went to the office to reserve a car for an occasional trip to town or would see her at the reception desk when I came for a meeting with my coordinator. Occasionally we would reminisce about the good old days in Tampa.

Over the next four years it became obvious that Amba was a highly skilled yoga teacher; with her interest and skill in interacting with people, she became a key instructor for the programs department. I met with the teachers to schedule various program activities and yoga classes for the guests. It was not until I had this opportunity to work with her more closely that I began to sense my attraction to her.

During a break one morning while sitting on the rooftop outside my room, I was questioning my commitment to remaining single for the rest of my life. It was dawning on me that I loved Amba. The guests adored her because she always brought joy wherever she went and because she had a talent for piercing the pall of seriousness that often hangs over a yoga class. I began to look for her in satsanga, just to see where she was sitting and what she was doing. I found it refreshing that she refused to wear a sari, as Amrit had requested of all sisters, because she wanted the freedom to dance in the back of the hall when Amrit was chanting. That morning on the rooftop I was filled with the feeling that if I could marry Amba I would laugh for the rest of my life.

I did not reveal my love to Amba. After two more years at Kripalu she was ready to graduate into a bigger world. Upon leaving Kripalu, Amba taught yoga in fitness centers, opened her own yoga studio, and created yoga travel retreats to Costa Rica. Once settled in southern California, she invented a new form of yoga that combined yoga, movement, and bodywork to produce a state of deep, relaxed awareness in her clients. Her reputation among the inner circles of celebrity spread and she was able to bring the power of prana-awakening movement into the lives of highly creative artists.

In 1992, ten years after Amba's departure, I was returning from a five-month tour of India with Rishiji Prabhakar. I had been sent by Amrit to receive training to direct the

Siddha Samadhi Yoga meditation course that Rishiji had developed. A number of Rishiji's disciples and teachers-in-training were married. One of the many eye-opening experiences during this intensive training was the modeling I received about the many ways in which marriage and teaching yoga could be a dynamic combination for growth.

On returning to the States, I passed through Los Angeles to visit a mutual friend of Amba's and mine. Knowing that I was coming, Carl invited Amba to drive over for the day. Carl was called away in the afternoon, leaving Amba and I alone. After an awkward start, our conversation quickly gravitated toward telling our stories about our feelings for one another.

Amba began by revealing that she had become infatuated with me at the first yoga class she took with me at the University of South Florida. In that class she felt energy move up her spine and flood into her heart. That experience left her with the realization that yoga was an answer to her search for inner awakening. Now, fifteen years later, I was shocked to learn that she had had been drawn to me since that day and I had never suspected it. I told Amba my story, beginning with the time when we worked together at Kripalu and I realized that I was falling in love with her.

Sitting face to face and sharing heart to heart with Amba, I was reevaluating Amrit's advice to me. A few years earlier, upon hearing my interest in giving up celibacy for marriage, Amrit first expressed delight that I wanted to open my heart more deeply; he then went on to advise that if I could open my heart fully to one person, I could magnify my love by opening my heart to multitudes—that is, if I could manage to avoid getting stuck in the cultural form of marriage. Now I questioned my choice of allowing his guidance to override my instincts. The couples in India had modeled mutually empowering marriages. I began to imagine what a relationship with Amba could bring into my life.

That significant day of sharing our stories with one another began to alter my sense of the future. It was not until two years later, when Amba came to Kripalu on her way to Costa Rica, that I had the courage to be honest with myself and to let my love for Amba guide my steps.

It was the summer of 1994 when Amba traveled to Kripalu to say good-bye to her longtime friends. She had received funding for her project of opening a yoga retreat center in Nosara, Costa Rica. On her annual trips to Kripalu over the many years since she had left, she would always seek me out to share her experiences of yoga and her teaching adventures in the world. On this final visit she came to me for suggestions and advice on her business plan. She was so alive with enthusiasm that I knew her retreat center would be an unquestionable success. Busier than usual, I had only enough time to hear her ideas and to register my unconditional support for her venture. But underneath the exterior of my support, I was feeling the secret treasure of our mutually shared passion slipping away.

On this farewell visit, Amba was staying with friends living near Kripalu. Our friends invited me for a good-bye dinner in her honor on Saturday night. I arrived a little early to find Amba not quite ready. As I sat waiting, I watched three white-tailed deer casually grazing in the piney woods beyond the deck of their living room. A door opened from off to the side of a massive stone fireplace. Before I could actually see her coming around the corner, I heard Amba giggling about how early I was. I immediately noticed the softness of her long white cotton dress as she slowly came into view. With luminous eyes and a glowing smile she moved toward me.

I cannot tell you what I ate for dinner or at what moment our friends disappeared, leaving Amba and I alone in front of the fireplace. We connected physically for the first time. Affectionately cradling and massaging each other's feet, we began to communicate through the language of touch. There was far more silence than words. I kept slipping into stillness, mesmerized by the strength coming through Amba's hands and into my body. From the depths of her enthusiasm she began to describe the exotic place by the ocean where she would be creating her dream retreat. We talked late into the evening. After our final embrace, I found my way through the door and into my car for the drive back to Kripalu.

My feet burned all night long! I called Amba early the next morning. "What did you do to my feet?" I asked. She laughed to hear of her fantastic powers that had caused such a response. Our laughing together on the phone was the dream I had pictured on the rooftop years earlier. I was now on fire with the realization of how I wanted to live for the rest of my life. With that phone call we understood that our love was going to lead us somewhere we both wanted to go. I spent the next day with Amba. The more I heard about Costa Rica and the preparations Amba had made to bring her clients to a jungle retreat by the ocean, the more I began to see my own future taking shape.

By Monday I was plotting ways to conceal myself as a stowaway, but on Tuesday reality set in. I was leaving for Texas for a visit with family and Amba was on her way to Florida to see her family before moving to Costa Rica.

Once in Texas, my mother listened to my story of twenty years of unspoken love and coached me to never doubt Amba's love for me. "She has loved you for a long time and she will love you forever." Jubilant for me, it was my mother who insisted that I get on the plane to Florida before Amba left for Costa Rica. In response to my concerns about my ability to be a father to Jonathan, Amba's five-year-old son, my mother offered this parting advice: "Don't try to be Jonathan's dad. Don't try to be a role model. Don't even think about trying to be anyone other than yourself. Amba loves you both. Her love will bring you together."

Amba picked me up at the Miami airport. We had eight days to make nachos and fill each other in on twenty years of life history. I proposed to Amba on August 8, 1994, in a corner booth at Dos Amigos restaurant in Marathon Key, Florida. I learned an important lesson in that moment: never propose marriage to someone who has a bite of burrito in her mouth. Amba's eyes said yes, but I had to wait an eternity to hear the word fall from her mouth. The giddiness I felt is the stuff that romantic love stories are made of.

Eight days later, charged with the determination to resolve my commitments and begin the process of leaving, I returned to Kripalu to broadcast the news. "I am announcing my plans to marry Amba. I will be moving to Costa Rica with Amba and her son, Jonathan, to open a yoga retreat on the Pacific Coast. I am committed to following through with the implementation of our new strategic plan. I will remain in my position as CEO and chairman of the board of trustees until we are all satisfied that the new leadership has the support it requires to move Kripalu into the world of authentic relationship."

Many of my closest friends understood how my quest had guided me to the doorstep of this opportunity for an important new beginning in life. They were sad to lose me but overjoyed at my transformation. Others felt abandoned and fearful of what would become of our new strategic plan and the community without my lifetime commitment to back up the transition into a new Kripalu.

What delusion had I been under for all of these years that I didn't recognize how oblivious I was to my need for personal love? I had the impersonal love of a guru. I had the shared company of an ashram community. But for the fulfillment of my deepest longing to know myself, I needed intimate and genuine love.

It was in that very week after returning to Kripalu from my days of bliss in Florida that the first revelations of Amrit's sexual misconduct first surfaced. Our journey as a community coming to terms with the devastating reality about Amrit's covert sexuality was nightmarish. My transition was not going to be as easy as I had hoped.

For the next several months I watched the community I loved disintegrate before my eyes. Even though we had lived our lives with a harmony of purpose for so many years, without the guru the basis of our relationships began to shift radically. The shock of being thrown into sudden responsibility for creating a new future for Kripalu was overwhelming. In a climate of trauma and self-protection, the administrators closed ranks to safeguard the assets, which were perceived as security for the continuation of Kripalu. Legal suits were in the works against Kripalu's assets. Our long-awaited support for implementing a new vision for Kripalu disappeared, along with the possibility for starting any new projects. Drawing from their past experiences of running Kripalu, the administrators returned to the safety of earlier authoritarian forms of leadership.

It became obvious that we could not turn back the prevailing tide of fear that was swallowing our vision of participatory decision making and authentic relationship, a vision that included graduating senior members with dignity and acknowledging the value of their service by supporting them to create smaller, more diversified yoga centers. I remained in leadership until the organization stabilized, traveling back and forth between Kripalu and Costa Rica, but because I was engaged in opening a new yoga center in Costa Rica I was perceived as "the competition" by some members of the Kripalu board. It would take the next few years for the vortex at play in Kripalu to settle and I was graduating into my new life.

In this period of introspection into the events of my life, I came to see how I had benefited from the privileges I uniquely received through my various positions at Kripalu. Along with my closest colleagues, I recruited and supported many new generations of residents to give their lives to Kripalu. We had aided Amrit, albeit unconsciously, to carry out his misuse of power and authority. We had not honestly faced our own dysfunctions soon enough; we had not acted to seize our collective power to protect others from experiencing what we ourselves had experienced. However remorseful I felt for these losses, I returned again and again to accepting the way in which I had come to learn these lessons in life.

On the constructive side, I saw how I had personally applied my talents to influence the creation of a major positive force for healing in the world. I had been a voice for innovation and creativity. I had spent years at Kripalu exploring the interface between willful yoga practice and prana-flow yoga, meditation-in-motion.

Nevertheless, it was a time of great pain. I grieved the loss for many years. Were it not for my kindhearted companion, our incredible son, and the embracing power of nature in Costa Rica, I think I would have died. Spending hours walking alongside the roaring Pacific Ocean, letting the reverberations of these events unwind through my nightmares, I rode through peaks and valleys of recovery, anger, and understanding, eventually emerging into forgiveness.

Never had I drawn so deeply from the counsel of prana as my source of inner wisdom. My commitment to a daily yoga practice consisted of getting out of bed whenever I awoke in the night or the wee hours of early morning as the compelling force of prana began moving my body. Deep in the jungle, often under the canopy of stars, I was guided to the open-air yoga pavilion. The sounds and fragrances unique to the jungle at night were partners to the primal resonance that animated my being. I came home to myself with every shudder of leaves when the wind moved the trees. Every song of a bird or pulse of an insect's wings that circled around me were as strands of connection that drew me home in the center of myself.

I felt the quickening of prana flowing through my hands as I cradled muscles and joints that longed for deeper sensorial awareness. I surrendered the weight of my body into gravity by hanging upside down from the inversion swing and gradually began to restore the natural curves in my spine from the effects of scoliosis. Reversing the polarities of my body this way gave me a new way to stand in life. I began to develop a more grounded relationship to earth and her gravitational pull.

I began developing the ability to differentiate sensations that correspond to the different ways that prana moves inside the body. As my practice deepened, I began to discriminate among various dimensions of my awakening self and embarked on research into the ways yogis have experienced and articulated the *koshas*, the multiple dimensions of being.

In this period of heightened curiosity about following the wisdom of prana, my body was being guided through the developmental stages that a newborn experiences when first encountering the sensorial phenomenon of being in a body. These developmental stages formed the basis for the sequence of inquiries that I began to refine and to share with others in our yoga teacher-training programs. I realized that the developmental sequence of inquiries provided a missing link for yoga practitioners who were searching for a way to transition from structured yoga practices into a deeper relationship to awakened prana as their inner guide. When combined with instruction in traditional yoga postures, I found ways to support beginners to draw confidence and support from the technical knowledge of yoga and to simultaneously respond to the wisdom of prana as an internal reference and guide in their practice. It became clear to me that the developmental sequence of inquiries offered an important interface between willful practice and surrender to prana.

Any remnant of doubt about the intelligence of awakened prana as the source of evolutionary consciousness was subsumed into the miracles of physical, mental, and emotional transformations occurring from within my cocoon of being.

Now, in the generosity of the Great Mother, Nature, I was given the time it took to receive and be nurtured. I was given the permission to be on the planet just as I am. I was given the grace to accept myself in relation to the unfolding of all the dynamics that give shape to who I am.

From my distant vantage point in the jungle, I stayed informed about the goings on at Kripalu and found great comfort that new life and fresh talent began to arise from the ashes of the bygone era. I accepted invitations to return as a teacher, to codirect the yoga teacher's conference, and to pursue my writing as a scholar-in-residence. As new styles of leadership emerged Kripalu was able to birth into the vibrant and healthy organization that it is today.

By the fruits of this journey I was given the opportunity to articulate the guiding principles of Self-Awakening Yoga, which I am grateful to share with you in all of the next chapters of this book.

2 "Who Am I?": Self-Awakening Yoga Methodology

SELF-AWAKENING YOGA IS BASED ON THE FUNDAMENTAL INQUIRY "Who am I?" The insights that unfold as a result of this inquiry into your inner experience are gifts from your teacher within.

In the inquiries of Self-Awakening Yoga, you are invited to witness the actual experiences that arise when you let go of attempting to control your experience. From many interesting perspectives of self, each of the inquiries presents an opportunity for cultivating your receptivity to the mystery of the unknown. In this way, Self-Awakening Yoga can be a perpetual source of inspiration for evolving into ways of being that are not the results of your past. You are the being endowed with infinite capacity to birth yourself into new forms in response to a continuously unfolding universe.

The structural details of any yoga practice or spiritual system can be alluring; it's easy to mistake external techniques for consciousness. But a practice comes alive with creativity when you commune with your body's sensations, as you live in the question of what is unfolding from the inside of your physical world. The principles of Self-Awakening Yoga can help you learn how to use your yoga practice—regardless of its form—for inventing explorations that provide personal access codes to the wisdom being of your body.

Being true to the intelligence of the body requires leaving the known as a jumping-off point and venturing into unknown territory to allow prana to truly guide you. Taking your yoga learning to this level of personal ownership frees you from the illusion that "truth" exists outside of you—in techniques, in the authority of an expert or teacher, or even in achieving your future ideals. Open-ended movement inquiries give us access to our evolutionary potential and open possibilities for progressing to a level of integration that goes beyond any previously experienced. The doorway to this alignment of self is located in the here and now, with observing and interacting with what is present in our bodies and communicating at the level of sensation.

The energy that animates the body is prana. According to yogic philosophy, this creative energy that flows through you is the same intelligent life force that animates the entire universe; the individual self, then, is seen as a multilayered field of condensed energy within this larger field of prana. By attuning your mental awareness to the workings of prana in your body, you access your ability to interact with the quality, purpose, and direction of your life, and thereby affect the world in which you live. From the early yoga shamans to innovators in modern times, yogis have left a trail of diverse methods for gaining access to this mysterious force—what has come to be understood as a primary goal of yoga.

The great sage Yogi Patanjali begins his famous discourse on yoga with the word *now*:

Atha-yoganusasanam: "Now the discipline of yoga."

With this one word Yogi Patanjali introduces the purpose, the practice, and the results of yoga. The barrage of forces that compete for attention in our lives make it difficult to enter the present moment—gathering body, mind, and spirit into the same "field" runs counter to the ongoing action demanded by the many projects that consume our focus on any given day. "Being" can seem luxurious, at best; many of us struggle with the thought that stepping into now, this one moment, with all parts of our being means leaving more "important" work behind. Even when we take time to practice yoga we can succumb to the effects of bilocation—the body can be on the yoga mat while the mind is at the office, picking up the kids, or rehearsing a conversation we're avoiding. The practice of attuning to sensation provides us with speed bumps for noticing when we have zoomed out of the present moment into the past or future and teaches us how to build pathways into the pranic field of creative energy available to us in each and every moment.

Who Is the "Self" of Self-Awakening Yoga?

Awakening to the self is a journey in which the individual, or personal, self expands consciousness to include the layered dimensions of experience that are interconnected with universal consciousness. Ignorance of the unity inherent within all existence is called illusion, or *maya*, and results in *duhkha*, or suffering; awakening to this unity produces the state of bliss, *ananda*.

The journey of awakening into expanded consciousness begins when we ask ourselves the classic yogic question: "Who am I?" The first thing we notice in answering that question is that we each live in a self-contained physical body, separate from others. Like a peanut in the center of a chocolate-coated M&M, the physical body is the most dense, solid form of energy. Consisting of the material elements of earth, water, fire, and air, the *anna-maya-kosha,* or physical body, is "home base" for the other, subtler, layers of the self.

But the physical body is more than a sum of its essential material elements. The body is animated by prana, or the *prana-maya-kosha* in yoga philosophy. Accessing the workings of prana happens by connecting our mental awareness to the tides of sensation as they ebb and flow through various regions of the body. In observing sensations as they pulse through the body, the life force within our physical organism registers on the screen of our mental awareness. This level of the self, the *mano-maya-kosha* or "ego-mind," arises out of the sense of "I" as a separate self that is responsible for fulfilling the biological imperative of securing the survival needs of the organism. By comparing this moment, this "now," with all past moments for information, the ego-mind learns how and when to move toward life-sustaining experiences and when and how to avoid pain, injury, illness, or death.

An axiom in yoga states that where the mind goes, prana flows. The ego-mind maintains its role by directing prana to act through the body to fulfill the body's survival imperatives. Beliefs about the goodness of one experience over another give rise to our perceived reality—our interpretations of how the world works and our place within it. Emotions arise from the ego-mind as well—the feelings we experience around getting or not getting, being included or not included, feeling secure or threatened are all energetic responses that we sense and feel in the body in reaction to events in the world in and around the individual self. Our feelings and emotions motivate us to take appropriate action to satisfy the needs of our personalities.

None of us could survive without a healthily functioning ego-mind. Try to cross a street without being able to judge how fast a truck is coming toward you and you will appreciate the way the ego-mind protects your survival by constantly monitoring your environment for safety. Apply for a job with a healthy salary attached and you will appreciate the skills and experience that are represented in your resume. We need the healthy ego to create a foundation for further expansion of consciousness. However, there is more to the self than a good job and a healthy body.

Discrimination Generates Witness Consciousness

How does consciousness expand beyond perceiving the world through the ego-mind, which experiences the moment dualistically, protects our autonomy, and operates out of the fear of losing its identity? Another dimension of the self, the *vijnana-maya-kosha*, arises when we make the discriminating observation that there is more to life than wanting, getting, and having. One ice-cream cone is pleasurable. Two ice-cream cones are even more pleasurable. But upon eating three or more ice-cream cones, the original pleasure turns to pain. To the ego-mind, the moment of "now" appears to present a need for choosing between polar opposites—such as pleasure and pain. But from the perspective of the entire universal field of consciousness, all human experience is interconnected within the whole. What appear to the ego-mind as mutually exclusive choices, with mutually exclusive cause-effect outcomes, are in reality mirror images of a unified phenomenon—two sides of the same coin.

Discriminative wisdom begins to develop when we notice that the outcomes of our choices do not always yield the pleasurable or desirable effects that we once experienced from making that same choice. Examining our life experiences with such discrimination develops a mental "muscle" that begins to slow the reflex to act on every desire that surfaces in the moment. In slowing down to discern the possible outcomes of a given choice, we can suspend the reflex to fulfill that desire immediately. Placing this speed bump in the highway between between stimulus and response allows the time and space to notice that there are deeper levels to our desires. I may notice that I don't really want the second or third ice-cream cone and that what I really want is to sit down and get started on that project I've been avoiding. Applying discrimination in this way allows us to see ourselves more deeply and to make better informed choices in the future as to how to best care for and nurture ourselves.

This muscle that we develop to see ourselves more expansively matures into witness consciousness. When the witness is present, we no longer judge ourselves for the choices we have made through the ego-mind. Witnessing allows us to compassionately accept the ego-mind and its actions by recognizing that it is performing a good job of doing exactly what it is designed to do—split the moment and make a decision for or against the seeming opposites. Compassion, forgiveness, and acceptance of ourselves is fundamental to releasing prana from its limited functioning through the ego-mind, opening the flow of prana toward discovering hidden potentials and expanding consciousness into greater dimensions of the self.

In the inquiries of Self-Awakening Yoga, we begin "growing in" our capacity for witness consciousness at a most fundamental level—by training our awareness to focus on sensations that arise when we slow down and move in the relaxed way the body is designed to move. Other thoughts and feelings are present when you enter into a movement inquiry, but they begin to recede to the background as we focus awareness on the rise and fall, the ebb and flow of movement at a deeply cellular, moment-by-moment level.

A physician once told me a story that illustrates the interrelationship between body, prana, ego-mind, and witness. An elderly gentleman came for an office consultation prior to scheduling surgery. The cantankerous old fellow was hard of hearing. His body was so stiff that he could not isolate the movements of his torso from his head, neck, and shoulders. Later, when the gentleman went under anesthesia, his body became so pliable that it took several husky orderlies to move him from the gurney to the operating table. After the operation, the doctor observed his patient coming out from under the anesthesia. At first he resembled a sleeping baby, his whole body moving in response to his breath. But as the fellow began to regain consciousness and to remember who he was, the doctor watched his body contort back into the shape of a stiff old man. What the doctor noticed was that muscles and bones can return to their natural, flexible shapes and functional relationships when the ego-mind, the personality, is not present. But when the ego-mind resumes control over the body, the body shape-shifts to fulfill our identity.

How does the ego-mind lose contact with the intelligence of the body? Ordinarily the ego-mind is guiding prana to shape and direct the body to accomplish its tasks and goals. All thoughts, images, feelings, and experiences are related to the project of the moment, which is in service to maintaining our self-identity. For example, when you are sitting in front of your computer writing a letter, your attention is focused on the screen in front of you. You are thinking about the person to whom you are writing. You are thinking about what you want to say. You are thinking about doing a good job so the recipient regards you more highly. Everything that is important to your ego-mind is channeled into writing that letter. You forget to notice that your shoulders start to creep up toward your ears. You do not notice that you move your head closer and closer to the screen as you become more concentrated. Because you want to finish the letter today, you lose track of the time. You forget to take a break. You are so absorbed in that letter that it becomes the singular reality.

Suddenly the phone rings. You jump out of your seat. Reluctantly, you tear yourself away from the letter to answer the phone. When you reach for the phone, you notice that your shoulders are tight and your mouth is dry. You look at your watch. Where did those three hours go?

In this example, attention is directed toward particular, thoughts about the letter, but you lose awareness of your body in the process. Witness consciousness allows us to remain involved in whatever project absorbs our attention at the moment while simultaneously maintaining awareness of the workings of prana in the body. Developing witness consciousness can be as simple as deliberately slowing down.

Pausing briefly for stretch breaks, drinking water, readjusting the height of your chair are little ways of checking in with your body to notice where tensions begin to accumulate. In listening to what the body is saying during these little pauses, you may notice other ideas or insights that can inform and enhance what you are communicating in your letter. In this way you attend to the task at hand while also creating the condition for prana to move toward fulfilling the evolutionary potential of the self in the same moment.

Self-Awakening Yoga helps develop discriminative wisdom by introducing yoga-movement inquiries that originate from internal sensory conversations. All systems of hatha yoga begin with attention to the body through the physical practices of postures and pranayama, but most do not provide transitional steps for turning to the wisdom of prana for entering into our creative, evolutionary capacities, which lie beyond the form of a rote practice. It is helpful to leave a few minutes at the end of a yoga practice to allow your body to be moved by prana, as a way to receive the benefits of the practice at a deeper level of self. But merely providing the time is not sufficient for bridging the modes of practice. I have repeatedly observed that yoga practitioners who are comfortable and familiar within a structured sequence of practices have a difficult time when asked to enter into a spontaneous flow of movement guided by inner promptings. Oftentimes the response is to simply repeat the same familiar routine.

The inquiries of Self-Awakening Yoga offer an experiential bridge designed to guide the practitioner through the developmental stages that are encoded within the body's memory from birth. While inquiring into the body's primal movement patterning and focusing awareness on the inherent sensations that arise in moving, the practitioner has the opportunity to access the flow of prana that animates the body. The sequence of movement inquiries offered in this book reveals fundamental insights into issues of structural alignment, mobility, balancing flexibility with strength, differentiating functional movements, and energizing core strength. I have noticed that combining familiar postures with regular exploration into these inquiries can open a whole new dimension to one's practice. Observing the nuances hidden within our unconscious body habits can provide practical avenues to greater freedom of movement. In developing witness consciousness, you train your awareness to focus on particular sensations for the purpose of developing concentration. At this deeper level of concentration, your thought waves and the sensation begin to synchronize. Awareness actually amplifies the sensation. As prana is released from the constraints of the ego-mind, it is free to bring the physical body back into its more relaxed, harmonious state of being.

Self-Awakening Yoga is based on the intention of opening channels of communication between the mind and body for the purpose of learning what the body has to teach us about the workings of prana, and to ultimately turn to the wisdom of prana as our trusted friend and inner guide.

Entering Body Time

Harnessing the ego-mind to focus on actual bodily sensations can feel like pulling the plug on a VCR in the middle of a video. Interrupting the flow of mental activity must occur in order for the ego-mind to turn its direction inward and begin a process of tracking the subtleties of physical sensations. Why would anyone deliberately want to cause an interruption in the flow of mental activity? Unfortunately, oftentimes a physical accident, trauma, or illness can trigger the desire to look more closely at the way we are living our lives and the influences of our choices on our physical health and emotional well-being. Acute physical or emotional pain can be received as a wake-up call, getting us more interested in caring for ourselves and inquiring into the origin of the pain. But you do not have to wait for some crisis or catastrophe to begin this process. In fact, you can look back on any particular event in your life in which important changes emerged as the result of hard times. Learning from these experiences can be enough motivation to begin to reclaim your power and self-responsibility before disaster recurs.

As prana awareness awakens, the body is prompted to move in unexpected and novel ways, urging you into deeper and deeper experimentation—beyond the exercises in this book and beyond any yoga instruction you will receive from an outside source. Developing the ability to scan your body for sensations can provide another dimension to the yoga or physical activities you are currently practicing. Staying present to your experience will enhance the benefits of any activity you perform and will give you the ability to enjoy it more fully and to avoid injury.

To capture the attention of your ego-mind and to draw it back to the sensations in your body, you need to provide something interesting and worthwhile for the mind to observe. The key to enjoying the journey is to give the ego-mind fascinating assignments in small enough increments so that the benefits of scanning for sensations become obvious. The mind needs a job to do. So you give it the job of watching the sensations in your body. To do this, your ego-mind begins to slow down and anchor on the bodily sensations. Awareness of these bodily sensations becomes a bridge between your ego-mind and body.

Tracking sensation is the mental process that allows us to bring the body's subcortical patterning to the screen of conscious awareness. Physiologists call this ability to sense ourselves from the inside out our kinesthetic sense. If I asked you to close your eyes and bring your finger to touch your nose, you would be using your kinesthetic sense to perform the action. The kinesthetic sense is the part of our physical intelligence that monitors movement in space from an internalized sensitivity; kinesis involves a complex set of sensations that are monitored by the sensorimotor nervous system through a network of specialized nerve cells called proprioceptors. The terms *kinesthetic sense* and *proprioception* are often used interchangeably.

At first you might feel a little silly when you pause and ask your body about the sensations you experience. If the body seems mute, it might feel as though it is much easier to ask an expert, book, teacher, therapist, minister, or psychotherapist to analyze what you need. But your body knows more than you think it does. The self-awakening approach to yoga offers a way to get very interested in what the body is saying and in the way that the body is saying it. You are not responsible for analyzing what your body needs. You are not responsible for fixing the problems you perceive through your pain and your discomfort. You *are* responsible for getting to know your body and for establishing a relationship with yourself in which it is enough to be interested in your body as it is in this moment. Each moment is different. Your body is the expert. Your body is doing the best it can to maintain its integrity, its efficiency, and its survival imperatives.

Earlier, I shared that my enthusiasm for yoga was shifted to a deeper level as a result of a rather serious spinal injury. At first, I wanted to use yoga to heal myself from the scoliosis in my spine. But in witnessing my experience, I came to realize that I might have to live with the condition of scoliosis for the rest of my life. The doctors agreed that this would be so. The yoga that I practiced was the yoga of entering into deeper relationship with myself through my body to get to know the sensations of the condition. The more I accepted the conditions and sensations as they manifested, the more my body first began to find its way back to its original state of balance and flexibility and then to evolve into greater levels of freedom and flexibility than I have ever known before.

I am not saying that deepening your awareness of sensation in your body will heal your injuries or strengthen your weaknesses. I am saying that if you are to be in relationship to yourself you must begin with where you are. In this state of self-acceptance, prana is freed from the habitual and often unconscious patterning in your body and is released, activating hidden potentials and new capacities. Awakened prana is a healing and integrating intelligence. Something in your being will shift. It will not be something you plan, wish for, or cause to happen through your will and actions. What happens will be the result of witness consciousness and self-acceptance.

Using the "As Is" Principle to Enter Body Time

The most consequential skill you can develop for the purpose of bringing your ego-mind into a more curious and interested relationship with your body is scanning. Scanning directs your awareness inward, focusing the ego-mind to interact with the body. This simple yet profound practice establishes a fascinated and friendly relationship between ego-mind and body. By harnessing the power of your mental awareness to witness the spectrum of sensations that arise within your viscera, you are both initiating emotional and somatic equilibrium in your life and building a foundation for fulfilling your ultimate creativity.

Scanning works like this. Imagine that you could swallow a microscopic video camera that travels anywhere throughout your viscera you desire to go, exploring the innermost surfaces and textures of the tissues, organs, and glands. If you're a person who does not readily visualize, you can use an ultrasonic microphone to listen in instead, similar to the way dolphins use sonar in their communication. If you aren't visually or aurally attuned, you get specially outfitted sensitivity probes that let you touch your body from the inside out.

Every human being has the somatic capacity to sense her or his internal experience. You may need to get a bit imaginative in the beginning to discover the sensory data that registers in your awareness, but it is well worth your efforts to discover the world inside your own body walls. When you do not actually sense an area of your body, you can jump-start the process by imagining what an internal area in your body would look, feel, or sound like. Imagination is a helpful medium for developing self-awareness.

Here is a simple way to help you remember both the purpose and the process of scanning. I call it the "As Is" principle: Awareness of Sensation through Internal Scanning. The principle of accepting yourself and your experience as you are is fundamental to developing witness consciousness, the state of nonjudgmental self-awareness.

To take a journey of any kind you must begin from where you are. Accepting the moment as it is requires that you begin with an accurate visceral sense of your body in current time and space, without imposing judgment or analysis on what you observe. In this process we are more interested in the differences that arise from one sensation to another, from one part of the body to another, than in fixing or changing anything what we notice. The simple act of nonjudgmental self-awareness signals to the body that we are interested in approaching ourselves to learn from our observations.

The body has many reasons not to trust our good intentions. How many exercise programs, diet fads, yoga classes, or health regimes have you initiated with the intention of changing your body, losing weight, aligning your posture according to some idealized notion, or awakening kundalini? To accept the body as it is precipitates a radical intervention in our ordinary relationship to the body.

Recall the axiom "where the mind goes, prana flows." Whatever sensation you focus upon precipitates the flow of a river of energy from the wellspring of your organism. Sensations that we notice in this manner intensify. Focusing your awareness on sensation is like turning up the volume to particular parts of your experience. When you notice a particular sensation without judging it or expecting something to happen as the result of your observation—like magic, something does happen! Your organism receives

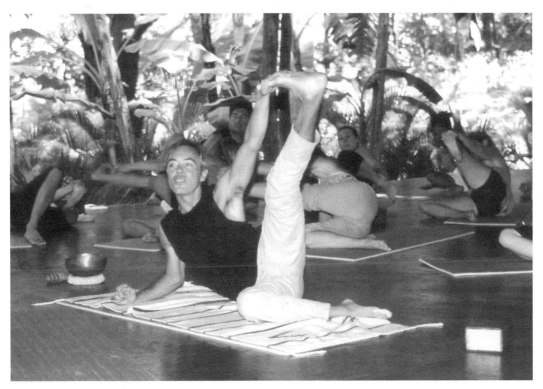

Don leading a Self-Awakening Yoga inquiry at Nosara Yoga Institute, 2002.

feedback through the nervous system and conscious mind about the state of affairs in that region. You are bringing that aspect of your being, that part of your body, out of amnesia. If you automatically engage your ego-mind to attempt to fix what you observe, you preempt the opportunity for your organism to make its own adjustments toward balance and more efficient functioning. The "As Is" principle holds that you are not responsible for doing anything at all about what you observe. You are assuming appropriate responsibility simply by witnessing your experience.

Without an intention to witness yourself in this way, repetitive exercise and even yoga can deaden sensitivity, suppressing your ability to be aware of sensation. It is possible to turn yoga into a habit or routine in which you do not have to remain present to the actual experiences that are occurring in your body. You can be following directions, either from a teacher or a conditioned set of postures, while your ego-mind is in a totally different domain of experience. By not witnessing the intelligent movement of prana, you are likely to miss the subtle effects of the postures, because your ego-mind is absent to the workings of prana throughout the body. The effects of prana are unpredictable; they can be overlooked by a mental headset that is fixated on a predetermined goal.

The Five Functions of Prana

Prana, the vital life force, operates in our bodies in five different ways. The interactions of these various forms of prana comprise the *prana-maya-kosha*, the prana body. The Self-Awakening Yoga inquiries are designed to enhance the functions of prana by drawing your awareness to their associated sensations. With many of the inquiries you will experience sensations of pulsing, streaming, or tingling as prana moves into various parts of your body. As you differentiate the sensations associated with these pranic movements, the overall intelligence of your organism increases.

The word *prana* as it is commonly used refers to five energies and their functions in the body. *Apana* is the downward movement of energy through the body that is most noticeable as the sensation of heaviness in response to the force of gravity. Releasing into the pull of gravity stimulates and activates all bodily functions having to do with elimination, such as releasing sexual fluids, menstrual blood, urine, and feces. The sense of being rooted in the earth, steady and secure, results from the groundedness that occurs through body awareness of apana.

Apana is counterbalanced by *prana*. In this functional context, *prana* refers to the upward movement of energy through the body that occurs as a natural rebound from sinking roots into the earth. The more grounded and stable the body, the greater the sensation of balance, mobility, and buoyancy. Apana and prana interact to create the "double stretch" in yoga postures that produces a natural elongation of the spine and the sense of effortless extension. Prana enters the body through the lungs and flows into the heart, activating two of the vital pulses in the body—what we sense as the breath and the heartbeat. When all five pranas in the body are strengthened and intensified, they converge in this upward-moving prana and awaken the *chakras*, the energy centers located along the spine. As prana flows into the chakras the self receives information as to its unfolding life lessons, ranging from survival to sexuality, individuation, relationship, self-expression, life purpose, and evolutionary potentials.

Samana is the firey energy of digestion and absorption. The experience of being nurtured in the womb through the umbilicus provides a basis for digesting and absorbing nutrients throughout life. On an emotional level, samana provides the impulse to digest the experiences of our life and the courage to enter the unknown. The belly center is also the body's energy battery, where vital force is produced, stored, and transformed into action whenever needed.

Udana is the energy of voice, speech, and communication. When communication develops internally through interaction of body, mind, and spirit, it is natural to expand our relationship to the world around us, expressing the insights that arise along the journey. Udana provides the impulse to balance the inner world with the outer world through relationship and communication. Strengthening the energy of udana increases our ability to contain the paradox of polar opposites and to harness their interaction into creative expression.

Vyana is the network or distribution system through which all of the pranas are directed to the precise locations within the organism for performing the synchronized functions that are required by the nervous, muscular, skeletal, reproductive, and endocrine systems. In its expanded functions, vyana activates thoughts and thinking, imagination, intuition, and intentionality, penetrating every dimension of our being to energize, enliven, or awaken and inform that area of experience as to its interconnected relationship within the whole. Vyana activates our sense of time and temporality, allowing us to travel through time and to project awareness into different times in different places.

Together these five pranas comprise the intelligence referred to in Self-Awakening Yoga as the wisdom of the organism. Awareness of these energies is developed by witnessing the multitude of sensations that emerge through the body in any given circumstance or experience. In the inquiries you will be guided to notice the most obvious sensations that are associated with pranic functions.

The state of bliss, *ananda-maya-kosha,* emerges when we recognize that prana infuses every part of our experience, synchronizing all of the *koshas* within the whole of our being. The body will continue being the body. The ego-mind will continue doing its job of surviving and nurturing the emotional and physical needs of the organism. But the witness now has the capacity to redirect the flow of prana from its previously monopolized assignment of survival, instead beginning to use the ultimate creative powers of intuition and intentionality to evolve new circumstances that were not possible before. The body is more than simply a vehicle for the ego-mind to maintain; the body has the power to transform and evolve new capacities. Drawing from the bliss of having intuited and then realized the union of all aspects of the self within the whole, the witness now draws from the power of unlimited consciousness for manifesting new circumstances that support evolution of the self.

Differentiating Sensations Stimulates Bodily Intelligence

To anchor the attention of the ego-mind on the subtleties of internal experience and to enhance communication between the mind and body, the inquiries in this book employ a variety of methods that increase points of reference through differentiation. Based on the five functions of prana as described above, the inquiry methods draw from various combinations of the actions that prana is continuously orchestrating.

When you ask your body to enter a new experience, the body must invent a novel response to the unfamiliar situation. According to the theory of world-renowned brain researcher Karl Pribram, a person's overall intelligence can be measured by the number of connections between the dendrites, the branching fibers at the end of neurons. These nerve endings communicate with one another in answering the novel request. That communication results in actual growth in the dendrites—they lengthen, branching outward to gather more information to assist in their processing.

By paying attention to sensations that arise in various body parts during the inquiries, you are training your awareness to watch for the subtle messages that arise in your body and setting up multiple pathways for various parts of the body to be in direct communication with one another. You may begin to notice that parts of the body may not want to move readily or easily; you may also notice that, in order to move one part of your body, you need to move other parts as well. For example, try spreading your toes wide apart. Now see whether that movement is easier to accomplish by spreading your fingers apart too; open your palms while you spread your toes. Using your hands in this way helps the toes to get the message that they, too, can spread. Eventually you'll be able to spread your toes fully without needing assistance from your fingers.

Making a before-and-after comparison allows you to establish a frame of reference to compare how you feel during a movement and how you feel after completing the movement. You may be in for some surprises. Sometimes the after effect is felt more strongly in a part of the body that seemingly had nothing to do with the movement you just completed. Other times the effect will be localized where you expected it to be. And sometimes there is no perceivable effect at all. By pausing to observe in this way, you are allowing the new pattern to interact with other areas in your body.

Similarly, making right-and-left comparisons supports your ability to differentiate sensations that arise in movement. Some inquiries begin with movement on one side of the body and then ask you to pause to experience the sensorial difference between the two sides of the body. This comparison helps to register the effects more dramatically in your perception. Often, the leg or arm that is moved first will seem heavier, longer, or more relaxed on the ground than the one waiting for its turn to move. In pausing before going to the second side, you are giving your ego-mind a commercial announcement for the future; in noticing the effects you are saying to yourself, "Look at the difference that occurs after doing something so simple." Establishing a deeper relationship with your body through awareness is not hard work. On the day you don't feel like getting on the floor to move around, you will have built in this little future-dated message that it doesn't take a lot of time or effort to do something that can make a big difference. So go ahead: get out of bed and see what happens!

The more focused and specific your awareness becomes in observing sensations, the more your mind is willing to remain engaged in an experience. Following sensation becomes hypnotic, and it is pleasurable to focus on sensations that are obvious. Every day your body and your experience will be different from the day before. We are always in the state of dynamic interaction with the forces of our lives. Differentiating specific sensations can begin to seem as important as reading the daily newspaper: in this case the news is your body and how it is doing today. It is worth the time to get interested and involved.

Learning through Experiential Language

Much of our learning through the body occurs as coaching about good posture, studying in a gym or studio, or under pressure to achieve some kind of predetermined goal. Many of the authoritarian directives used in situations in which we learn have become internalized in the voice we use to speak to ourselves from the inside. "Belly in, chest out! Drop your shoulders! Do this; don't do that." No one wants to be told what to do, but in order to learn something new we temporarily give over our authority to a coach, teacher, or videotape in the hopes that what is presented will help us in some way. This is a natural stage in the learning process. But it is essential to bring the locus of authority back inside your own world to reality check: Is what I'm hearing true for me? Does this work for me? What is missing here?

The inquiries of Self-Awakening Yoga could also be used to reinforce such reliance on external authority and to separate yourself from receiving bodily wisdom. For this reason, the inquires are written in experiential language, framed in such a way as to reflect back to you that the source of your learning is occurring in your own relationship to yourself. Experiential language does not occur as a demand from someone outside yourself. It occurs as though you are listening to the inner voice of your own body speaking from inside yourself. For example:

> Become aware of the sensations in your right arm and shoulder. What is your shoulder saying to you? Without straining or forcing, exhale. On the next inhaling breath, allow your arm to be lifted from the little finger side of your hand. Let go of the sense of doing anything at all. Simply watch how the movement is happening through you. Breathe as you need to. Slow the movement down. Allow the arm to continue stretching until it finds its way all the way above your head, reaching up through the ceiling. Inhale through the entire right side of your body. When you are ready to release, allow the arm to float back down through the space around you until you feel your arm hanging at your side once again. Feel the space you have created inside for your shoulder to expand. Feel the difference between your two arms.

In this example, notice the use of phrases such as "allow," "be aware of," "release," "when you are ready," and so forth. With practice, shifting the way you talk to yourself internally in experiential, nonjudgmental, nonauthoritarian language becomes natural and habitual. You will notice the difference inside yourself when you shift the locus of responsibility back into the experiential domain of self-learning.

Verbal cues not only affect the regard we have for our inner self but can also affect the physical qualities and efficiency of the movement. Movements are encoded in the brain as neural patterns that respond to sensorial images. These images contain the operating instructions for how that movement is to be performed. Using functional images that enhance the body's intelligent response for initiating a movement is a way to increase the intelligent communication between all of the coordinated actions that are engaged in a movement. Can you sense the bodily difference these two different instructions would make in the quality of your internal experience? "Lift your arm above your head." Or, "Reach for an imaginary cluster of grapes hanging two feet above your head." Functional imagery can be auditory, visual, kinesthetic—even tasty or aromatic. "Notice how your body wants to let go into this long, warm stretch." "Feel your head hovering above like a helium-filled balloon." "Allow your body to melt down to the ground." "Glide your palms along the carpet. Feel the texture of the ground." "Bring up a delicious stretch." In each of these examples, notice how your body's visceral response stimulates the movement of prana by engaging the senses.

Expanding Consciousness through the Body's Wisdom

All along my yoga journey, I have drawn inspiration from the legends of those who have blazed the trail ahead. Listening to Amrit's stories of the way he learned from Bapuji (Swami Kripalu) in his early days gave me insight in how to learn from a yoga teacher in an external way. There were the obvious customs, such as studying his teachings and following his instructions for practice. But the less obvious insights about the relationship came through the quality of love and respect that Amrit held for Bapuji, an ocean of gratitude that Amrit experienced for the opening that occurred inside himself. Although Amrit followed Bapuji's instructions to a certain degree, his own external practice of yoga took a very different form than that of his teacher. He followed and continues to follow his inner guidance for the practices he offers to the new generations of his students.

Through my love for Amrit, I was able to follow his direction, trusting that the results would lead me ultimately back to my own inner guidance. Although the events leading up to my eventual separation from him were difficult and complex, I will always be grateful to him for his inspiration to inquire more deeply into myself. The form of yoga I now practice is related to his influence but is guided from the connection I have made with my internal teacher.

The great yogi Krishnamacharya taught four students who, in following their own inner guidance, have developed very different forms of practice that are touching millions of yoga students today—Indra Devi, Iyengar, Patabhi Jois, and Desikachar.

The essential message underlying the difference in forms is that the journey to self-awakening is ultimately guided by wisdom that comes from within. The value of following a teacher or a structured set of practices is to receive inspiration, confidence, and courage to make the inner journey. In making a gradual transition of withdrawing authority from the external teacher or prescribed yoga practice to the internal teacher, we are learning to discriminate the difference between the techniques of a practice and consciousness. As consciousness unfolds, the techniques we have used naturally recede in importance to the background.

With respect to the forms of your current or future yoga practice, I sincerely intend that the methodology presented to you in the inquiries of Self-Awakening Yoga will provide support for receiving the fullness of inner wisdom that you are nurturing through your practice. As you go deeper into the meditative state, you will discover that your ability to know yourself at every level is limitless.

You may have noticed throughout that I have not referred to yogis as awakened or enlightened souls but as seekers engaged in the infinite inquiry of self-awakening. When *yoga* is perceived as a verb, our inquiry provides inexhaustible access to the mystery of the unknown. We each embody the capacity for continuous expansion of consciousness and infinite degrees of awakening to the nature of our multidimensional selves.

Wouldn't it be fascinating to be able to transport ourselves as observers to the forests of ancient India as the early shamanic yogis engaged in their solitary explorations into states of consciousness through energetic practices of every description? Can you imagine the conversation that transpired when a solitary yogi stumbled upon another, sharing their stories and corroborating their findings? Their experiences of the path were different. How else would they ever come to know or understand the experience of the other without first questioning the differences in worldviews that did not overlap? Are we to assume that the shamanic yogis agreed about their experiences and methods? Our birthright as human beings is to use the intelligence that continues to evolve within us to expand our consciousness through our own connection to the universe as it is revealed in the wisdom of our body. We are each original yogis, expanding consciousness from where we begin in this moment.

3 Initiating Your Self-Awakening Yoga Journey: Using the Inquiries

THE INTENTION OF THE SELF-AWAKENING YOGA INQUIRIES is to cultivate awareness of the actual sensations that arise through movement, as a way to reawaken your capacity to learn directly from and through the body. The inquiries are organized by chapter to follow a progression of movements that parallel the developmental learning processes that your body undergoes from early infancy into adulthood. Your movement capacities are as individual to you as your fingerprints or your DNA structure. Some of the inquiries may feel familiar to you; others may feel foreign. The spontaneous variations that arise in each of the inquiries are gifts from your inner wisdom guiding you to experiment, making each experience your own. Follow your hunches for inventing new inquiries and variations in response to your needs and interests.

Although the inquiries are arranged in a sequence that follows one profile of growth, your own felt sense of order is the best way to sequence your inquiries. There are many ways to begin working with the inquiries. One way is to thumb through the chapters, noticing what feels immediately inviting to you. What would feel good to your body today? What looks like fun? Beginning where your interests are drawn is a good way to develop confidence in your own learning process and trust in your ability to access the wisdom of your body directly.

If you are practicing on your own, there are several options for becoming familiar with the movements that will facilitate a greater connection to your internal kinesthetic intelligence. You may want to read the directions in advance, looking at the photographs in order to mark out the basic steps. Then close the book and go inside, doing the movements according to how your body remembers the inquiry. Remember: there is no right way to do the movements. Noticing that you skip a part or consciously add a new variation will tell you that you are well on your way to taking ownership of your learning process.

Some people find it helpful to read the directions out loud. Giving voice to the inquiries in this way engages more of your body and breath. If you are going to read the directions aloud, go ahead and make an audiotape so you can follow your own voice, with your own sense of timing. Listening to the inquiries on the CD that accompanies this book can help you develop a sense of pace and timing. A more comprehensive set of recorded inquiries is available in the "Yoga As Is" series, listed in the resources section at the end of the book. But truly there is no substitute for attuning to your own inner voice for entering movement inquiries such as these.

Another way to use the material is to work with a friend, taking turns reading and guiding the inquiries. Witnessing the experience of another is a good way to expand your sense of what is possible. Using the inquiries of Self-Awakening Yoga with another person can add greater focus to both of your intentions and aid in creating a committed time and place for practice. In whatever combination of strategies you devise, the benefits of mobilizing your inner wisdom will provide a lasting source for empowering yourself with the ability to learn directly through your own body.

The inquiries begin by acknowledging the ego-mind as the first layer, or *kosha,* of conscious experience that comes into play during each exploration. The recurring directive to "make a suggestion to your logical mind" addresses the ego-mind or personality. At the level of ego-mind, or normal waking consciousness, brain wave activity is geared toward linear thinking, planning, analyzing, and problem solving: this is called the beta state. In the state of witness consciousness, the relaxed awareness associated with intuition, visualization, and attunement to and entrainment with bodily sensations and kinesthetic awareness, the brain waves enter the alpha state. Sleep and dream activity occur in the deeper states of delta and theta.

In the inquiry process, we are inviting the ego-mind to participate in the experience by suspending its controlling and critiquing functions to allow for relaxation to occur. By acknowledging the important role that the logical mind has to play throughout an inquiry, you are giving it permission to watch the experiences that arise during the deeper alpha state. Engaging the logical mind in this way allows you to remember the effects of a movement inquiry and thereby recognize the value of spending time in this way. It's like getting the boss on your side so that you acquire the resources to do your job. When you drift to sleep in the delta and theta states during an inquiry, you experience deep relaxation but without the ability to witness your experience.

If the term *logical mind* creates pause or confusion as you progress through the inquiries, shift to a term that you can better relate to: *ego-mind, personality,* or *conscious mind* are a few options.

Another recurring directive that appears at the end of each inquiry states, "Now begin your return . . ." Many experiential events occur while you are in the state of deep relaxation that is often induced during an inquiry. Some of the events are easy to recall because they are more familiar and understandable to your logical mind. But events that are unfamiliar and do not have a ready frame of reference for logical explanation can go unnoticed and slip away. The phase of an inquiry during which you return from relaxation is the time in which the logical mind can remember the events so they can be scrutinized more closely. It is the job of the logical mind to protect the organism from harm. If something strange or unusual occurred during an inquiry, the logical mind can suppress the memory and cancel out the beneficial effects of a new experience before understanding and valuing what is occurring. By thinking to yourself, "Now I am beginning my return," you are asking your logical mind to resume the important role it has to play in supporting your continued growth through the inquiries by recalling and replaying the effects throughout your organism.

Gathering your awareness in order to transition back to a normal state of alertness is an important for allowing you to go about your next activity without feeling foggy. By clearly marking the time boundaries of an inquiry exercise, you are establishing a functional relationship with your logical mind in creating various kinds of time for various kinds of mental activity in your life. Bodily time, which arises during an inquiry, can feel eternal to an impatient logical mind that has so much important work to do. When trust arises that the experience will end with alertness and greater vitality than when you started, your logical mind will prioritize your time for inquiry.

Entering the moment is not a linear process. We are always in the middle of many overlapping and shifting contexts that open doorways into the unknown, informing dimensions of our consciousness with insights from unexpected sources. In the natural flow of life, self-awakening occurs in the rising and falling of the peaks and valleys of discovery. The inquiries of Self-Awakening Yoga do not produce a steady state of "being awakened." An individual who is self-awakening will never be limited by the achievements of the past, but rather, has the ability to respond to the moment with infinite capacity to continue expanding awareness. It is natural and inevitable that we all enter periods in our lives that call for a renewal in enthusiasm and inspiration for the journey by providing some ways to rejuvenate our ability to take a step back to witness. The inquiries offered to you here are tools for self-nurturance, explorations for deepening direct communication with your body, and helpmates in the lifelong process of awakening to the wisdom that lives inside. May you journey well.

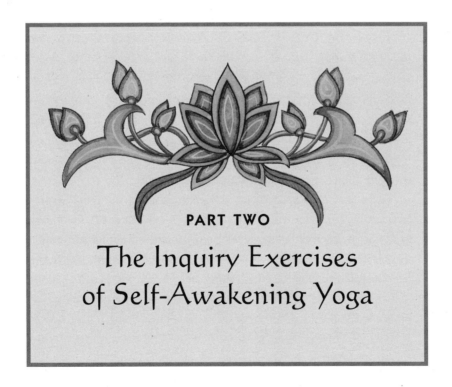

PART TWO

The Inquiry Exercises
of Self-Awakening Yoga

4 Releasing into the Embrace of Gravity, Growing into the Light

How do we begin to cultivate awareness of the inborn wisdom in our bodies and use it for expanding consciousness?

OUR UPRIGHT POSTURE IS A CROWNING developmental achievement resulting from an interplay of responses to two primary, existential phenomena—the first being the all-pervasive presence and shaping force of gravity and the second being the biological imperative to move toward light. We start by asking this question: Why *do* we feel the urge to push up off our bellies and pull ourselves to standing, and then to continue stretching, reaching, and growing toward light?

On a phylogenetic level, our migration toward the light began in the brine—amoebic life-forms moving via the undulation of their cellular membranes. Successive forms begat locomotion by developing flagella, cilia, fins and tails, and eventually legs, each form bringing us progressively closer to the sun's light. Aided by the electron microscope, which explores subatomic structures, and with advanced capacities to assay minute cellular secretions, biologists over the past twenty years have made profound discoveries confirming the long-held theory that evolution is driven by tropism, a physiological urge to move from darkness toward light. The earliest single-celled creatures in the dark ocean depths developed photosensitive spots, which enabled increasingly complex organisms to perceive the sun's light and adapt to living ever closer to that light. Gradually these rudimentary organs evolved into eyes.

Although advanced species, such as mammals, developed and refined the capacity to receive images through eyes, human beings also retained the primal capacity to perceive and respond to light through a photosensitive gland that is more ancient than our eyes. Called the pineal gland, this organic structure is so powerful in human beings that it allows the fetus to perceive light and dark while in the womb, long before the eyes develop. There is evidence to support the theory that the entire endocrine system—including the pituitary, thyroid, and thymus glands—is formed by the embryonic migration of tissue originating from the pineal gland. The same rosette pattern that exists in the retinal tissues of the eyes also exists in the cells of the pineal gland, leading researchers to assert this embryological migration of pineal gland tissue to the eyes during fetal development and providing a physiological basis for what ancient legends describe as a "third eye." The pineal gland, located just below the soft spot in the baby's crown, retains its photosensitivity to light and dark throughout a person's life.

The photosensitivity of the pineal gland is an important element in all aspects of human growth and maturation and is the underlying process governing physical health, emotional adjustment, ideational development, and spiritual well-being. Discoveries over the past twenty years have revealed that the pineal gland remains active throughout all life cycles from conception to death, determining growth and maturation, behavioral patterns, reproductive cycles, and even skin coloration and hair growth. The discovery of the pineal secretion melatonin has opened a doorway to unlocking and understanding our sensitivity and capacity to adapt, via circadian rhythms, to environmental phenomena such as temperature fluctuations, geomagnetism, and electromagnetic fields, as well as stimulating a variety of psychological states ranging from bliss to depression and bipolar schizophrenia.

The important role played by this small gland was acknowledged historically as far back as early yogis, who determined that the pineal body was the master gland associated with the expansion of consciousness into states of enlightenment. The ancient Greeks called the pineal body the "seat of the soul." Because of its physical location in the middle of the crown, Descartes hypothesized that the pineal body was the primary center where the immortal soul could incarnate into bodily flesh. In the early part of the twentieth century, Edgar Cayce entered into trance states and intuited vast and detailed information about the role that the pineal gland has played throughout evolution and how its functions interact with other glandular secretions that affect the development of the personality. Until the latter part of the twentieth century, the depth of Cayce's scientific insight had been lumped with all previous metaphysical theories and legends about the pineal gland. Not until the 1980s did the scientific community begin to realize that the pineal gland really was more than an irrelevant vestigial remain from earlier evolutionary forms.

From the beginning of yogic exploration, yogis claimed experiences of an inner light of consciousness. The stories of some of the early yogis that have been passed down through the ages suggest that working with the phenomenon of illumination can lead to a state of enlightenment. Scientists discovered the presence of the photosensitive compound phosphorus in the pineal gland in the early 1970s; when exposed to electrochemical stimulation, phosphorus actually glows in the dark. If you have ever witnessed phosphorescent tides along the ocean's edge, you will forever be astonished by the bright and sparkling glow of light emitted from simple organisms that amass phosphorus. Cayce determined that the physiological basis for experiencing inner light is implicit in the bioelectrical activity of the central nervous system. Through advanced brain imagining it can now be observed that entering deep states of meditative awareness stimulates this bioelectrical activity, activating not only the photosensitivity, the "illumination," of the pineal gland but also activating the secretion of serotonin, the psychoactive hormone that produces euphoria.

In response to our question as to *why* we feel an innate urge to move from darkness into light, given what we now know about the pineal gland and its photosensitivity we can say that the human body—our very organism—is encoded with the evolutionary impulse to grow toward light. Yet the urge to move toward light is tempered by the reality of gravity in the physical environment. As early land creatures moved out of the darkness of the ocean depths and crawled into daylight, another phenomenon—the shaping force of gravity—impacted their development. No longer free to wriggle and float about in the water, emergence onto land limited these early creatures to living on their bellies; with the intensified force of gravity affecting the body, amphibians had to remain in or near water during the early stages of maturation. Under the new stress of body mass and weight impacting and impeding mobility, the imperatives for safety and sustainability demanded new experimentation and physiological adaptations. With ever–increasing levels of efficiency in slithering, pushing, pulling, and crawling toward their goals, all land creatures, under the compelling force of gravity, have evolved bodies that fulfill the inborn imperative to continue expanding into greater complexity, intelligence, and awareness.

The inquiries of this chapter provide an opportunity to access the early learning events that began to shape your experience of being in your body. Just as early organisms emerged from water onto land, the human fetus also shifts from a sense of weightlessness and from gill-breathing in the uterus to lung-breathing and a sense of density in the gravitational field. By becoming aware of and releasing into the effects of gravity on your body, which your infant body innately knew how to do, a paradoxical lightness of being emerges that allows you to notice deeper levels of your experience of self. Making friends with gravity opens the doorway for attuning to the wisdom of your evolutionary body, which is guiding your development and expansion of consciousness.

The first inquiry, Heavy Body, Effortless Awareness, allows you to get acquainted with your body in a new way by learning to recognize the observable effects of gravity on your physical being. Learning to feel the balancing forces that act upon your body, you also begin to notice the places where you hold tension, the places in the body that do not allow for even distribution of the force of gravity. Such tension can be an effect of chronic stress. Becoming aware of and acknowledging these effects of chronic stress stimulates a natural movement of prana where it is most needed in the body.

The second inquiry supports communication between your mind and body by connecting with your breath. Traveling to the Origin of the Breath brings expanded awareness to your breath as a way to experience greater depth in your daily world by reminding your organism of its primal transition from the womb to taking the original breath of life in Earth's atmosphere. You will notice that the way you breathe has a profound effect on the quality of your life. Bringing awareness to the patterns of your breathing is a direct bridge from your mind to your body.

Just as the infant shifts from the security of an ever-present rhythm of the mother's heartbeat to discovering a pulse in the center of her own belly, our basic organismic trust in our belongingness to the benevolence of life is restored as we follow the third inquiry, Attuning to the Pulse of Being. Here you will learn how to recognize "body time"—sensate awareness shows us that cellular communication occurs in its own temporal dimension. The attention you give to sensing your inner wholeness by working with the pulses in this inquiry provides access to penetrating subtler dimensions of your own physiology, the precursor to working toward enlightenment through the body.

Rather than feeling victimized by the gravity of circumstances that you face on a daily basis, you can use the inquiries in this chapter to return to a state of effortless awareness. All inquiries of this chapter provide ways to access the evolutionary potential of your body, as encoded in the breath, the pineal gland, and the cells' knowing of gravity. As you deepen into sensate awareness, you step into the journey of releasing sensory overload in your nervous system, processing the memories held within the cells and expanding your capacity for deepening communication between body and mind.

Heavy Body, Effortless Awareness

Inquiry: How does it feel to surrender to an unobstructed flow of gravity throughout the body?

Bringing awareness to the way in which your body aligns itself in response to gravity can dramatically influence your health, behavior, and consciousness. A harmonious relationship with gravity is a strong foundation for balance, both physical and emotional.

When the force of gravity isn't evenly distributed throughout your body you can feel heavy; you may feel emotionally drained and struggle with a life that feels beyond your control. Muscles and organs that bear unequal forces create internal pressures that prevent you from receiving oxygen and nutrients. These blocks can cause congestion in the flow of circulation and the processes of digestion, respiration, and elimination, leaving toxic deposits in the recesses of your organism. Vital information that flows along the network of nerves can get distorted as a result of restrictions in the nervous system.

By lying horizontally and attuning to the sensation of gravity acting upon your body, you give your body an opportunity to relax around its restrictions, allowing this fundamental physical force to shape and align your body. In the gravity scan of Reclining Mountain pose you are allowing the innate wisdom of your body to bring you back into balance. Lying in your bed for five to eight hours each night doesn't fulfill your body's need to be horizontal. A bed is soft and does not provide the same feedback as a solid surface that is truly horizontal. And when you are sleeping you are not focusing your awareness on the sensations occurring in your body; gravity is, of course, doing its magical work, but your awareness is not engaged. To create a harmonious relationship between body and mind, your conscious awareness needs to be present. Giving yourself a few minutes to get horizontal and use your awareness to scan your body is a simple and yet powerful way to let gravity begin the work of balancing and rebalancing the body. All you have to do is remain present to your experience by watching, sensing, and allowing.

Every individual develops habits that result in muscles that may be too loose or too tight. These often unconscious muscular habits cause the skeleton to tilt or compress as a result. Have you ever watched a potter forming a bowl on her rapidly turning wheel? If the clay is not centered from the beginning, the bowl will spin wildly out of control. Becoming aware of the force of gravity acting on your body is a way of noticing how the opposing physical and emotional energies of your life are interacting to shape your body in this moment. At first when your body enters into stillness, you may notice that your thoughts and emotions begin to speed up. A backlog of concerns and worries can grab your attention and hijack your mental awareness toward solving problems or resolving emotional conflicts. Acknowledging the presence and importance of these issues at the beginning of your inquiry is a way of saying to yourself that you will address these thoughts and emotions in due time but that the time you are about to spend has a different purpose. This inquiry time is for the purpose of slowing down to notice the effects of gravity on your body and to allow other dimensions of your experience to surface, dimensions that are not so obvious in everyday life. In this way you acknowledge the mental and emotional priorities that your body works to fulfill on an ongoing basis, and you expand your awareness to include physical sensations, which can only be recognized by attuning to your body. Expanding your consciousness to include the body's language of sensation as one of your modes of self-knowing broadens the scope of your overall self-awareness and frees the intelligent energy of prana to restore balance not only to the physical body but to the mind and the emotions as well.

By allowing your body to lie flat on the ground for a few minutes each day in the Reclining Mountain pose prior to doing any other movement, be it yoga, sports, or walking, you give your body the opportunity to organize itself toward an even distribution of forces. As your consciousness expands to receive the balancing redistribution of energies, you will be more likely to align your attention toward listening to and fulfilling the deeper purposes of your life.

The inquiries in this chapter are best read into a tape recorder and played back to yourself. Make sure to leave space between each instruction to sink into the experience. After you finish the inquiry, experiment with coming into Standing Mountain pose. Notice how comfortable you feel while holding the posture for a longer time than you usually hold it. Observe how effortlessly you can be in the posture without jumping in to the next activity of your day.

Exploration: Reclining Mountain Pose

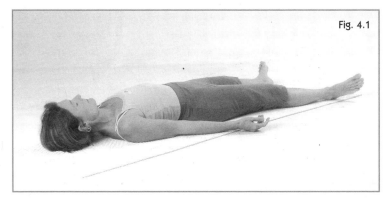

Fig. 4.1

1. Begin by lying on the ground (**fig. 4.1**). Suggest to your logical mind that this is a time for slowing down and attuning to the world of sensations and experiences that arise within your body. Do you notice any expectations of yourself as you prepare to enter the state of relaxed awareness? Let them go; create an intention for yourself to allow your experience to unfold without attempting to make anything happen.

2. As you begin to notice the contact your body makes with the ground, make any adjustments that help you feel settled.

3. What is the shape of the impression your body makes on the ground? Are there any areas that seem to resist the pull of gravity or that hold on in some way? Allow any resistance to be, precisely as you are experiencing it. Suggest to your logical mind that there is nothing to change or to fix in what you observe. Simply notice what you notice.

4. How heavy are your bones? Can you feel your bones begin to glide downward through layers of muscle and tissue in response to the pull of gravity?

5. Draw awareness to the sensations in your feet. What do you notice about your toes and ankles? Notice how heavy your feet become as you release them toward the ground. Are your feet the same temperature, or is one foot warmer or cooler than the other? Do you notice any pulsing or tingling sensations beginning to arise?

6. How heavy are your shinbones? What shapes do your calf muscles make as they contact the ground? Sense how your calves begin to hang as you release them toward the ground. As your calves relax, can you sense energy flowing through the muscles?

7. Can you feel how your kneecaps are sitting on top of the knee joints? Imagine that your kneecaps are becoming very heavy; as they melt downward, feel how the backsides of your knees begin to sink toward the ground. As your knees and kneecaps become heavier, can you feel sensations circling through your knees?

8. Now bring awareness to the long thighbones. How do they fit into your hip sockets? Picture the way the quadriceps muscles on the topsides of your thighs begin to spread and hang across the top of the thighbones. Can you feel the hamstring muscles hanging heavy from underneath the thighbones? As the muscles and bones of your thighs get heavier and heavier, can you feel the weight of your lower legs letting go into the ground? What sensations do you notice in your thighs and lower legs?

9. What is happening in your lower belly? Can you feel how the lower abdomen expands like a balloon when you inhale and relaxes toward the ground as you exhale? Imagine someone placing a round, smooth stone on your lower belly. Do you notice any changes in the speed and depth of your breathing as you respond to the weight of the stone?

10. Sense how the organs and glands of your lower belly are being massaged by the pull of gravity. Can you sense how energy is moving in the lower belly as your breath fills and bathes the tissues and cells? Notice any pulsing or gurgling sensations.

11. Imagine a spiral of energy entering through your navel and traveling directly into the solar plexus. Imagine how this spiral of energy enters through the front side of your body and exits through your backside down into the ground. Notice any sensations such as warmth or pulsing as your belly releases into the pull of gravity.

12. Can you sense how your upper chest is moving in response to your breathing? Imagine that a warm, smooth stone is riding the swells and dips of your chest as the breath flows in and out. Allow your ribs to hang as they become softer. Notice how your breastbone sinks downward in response to gravity, melting down into the core of the chest. Feel the rhythm of your heartbeat and the expanding and releasing of your lungs. The chambers of your lungs are constantly absorbing oxygen and releasing carbon dioxide as your heart steadily pumps rivers of fluid nutrients throughout your entire organism. How does your mood shift as you witness the strong, silent power of your organism in action?

13. Imagine how the round, interlocking bones of your spine are organized in the center of your torso. Can you sense the wavelike movement of your spine in response to the breath? Picture how the plump pillows of the discs are cushioning the spaces between each vertebrae. Imagine the flow of nerve impulses traveling through the spinal cord and branching out to communicate with every cell in your body. Notice how the undulations of the spine give shape and support to your entire structure. Sense how the muscles surrounding and cradling the spine begin to relax, allowing your whole spine to become even more mobile and heavy.

14. How heavy are your hands, arms, and shoulders? As you notice how your hands are resting on the ground, sense what surfaces of your wrists and fingers make contact with the ground. Is one hand more open or more closed than the other? What wants to let go in your hands? Do you notice any pulsing in the center of the palms? Are the shoulders and arms on the ground in the same way, or is one shoulder and arm heavier? Release the weight of your hands, arms, and shoulders down into the ground.

15. Draw your awareness to your throat and neck and jawbone. Listen to the sound of your breath as it passes through the back of your throat. Can you sense how the bones and muscles of your throat and neck are softening and relaxing into the pull of gravity? Notice how your body feels as your attention is drawn to the internal sound of your breath. How heavy is your jawbone when it is hanging freely?

16. As your awareness travels to the sensation of heaviness along the backside of your head, can you sense the actual weight of your head? Imagine that the weight of your head is sinking down into a bowl that is exquisitely shaped to receive the capsule of your cranium. Let the weight of the organ and the glands that fill the cranium release into that bowl. As the weight of your head begins to let go into infinite degrees of relaxation, observe how energy begins to flow down through your neck and spine.

17. Sense the folds in the muscles between your eyebrows. Suggest to your logical mind that now is the time to relax the worry muscles of your brow. Imagine the folds parting, as if opening the curtains of a theater stage. What do you notice when the muscles of your forehead are relaxing?

18. Can you sense the shape and size of your eyeballs resting in their sockets? How heavy are your eyes? Imagine your eyes sinking back into your head, like two stones dropping into a clear blue lake. Let your eyes become heavy. Release the weight of your eyes down into infinite space. How does it feel to allow all expressions in your eyes and face to melt down into the ground? What is the look on your face

when all the roles and masks dissolve into deep relaxation?

19. Now, becoming aware of the organ of your brain, notice the size and weight of your brain floating in your skull. Can you sense the muscle of your mind, the pulsing of your thoughts and thinking? Allow all thoughts and thinking to dissolve into pure sensation. Let the energies of that sensation flow down your neck and into your spine like a waterfall. Suggest to yourself that now is the time to enter an even deeper state of relaxed awareness: knowing without thinking. Release your whole being down into the ground. Attune to the pulse of your whole being. Notice how your body looks and feels when you are relaxed and at home in your center. Listen as the wisdom of your organism receives from every dimension of your experience. Suggest to your logical mind that it is safe, desirable, and pleasurable to expand awareness to include all layers of your experience.

20. As you begin to prepare for your return to wakeful consciousness, suggest to your logical mind that you will be returning with the feeling of having had the right amount of relaxing, rejuvenating, healthy sleep, feeling wide awake and fully alert.

21. Begin your return by rocking your ankles from the inner anklebones to the outer anklebones. Roll your wrists from the inner wrist bones to the outer wrist bones. Roll your head from ear to ear.

22. Deepen your breath as you bring up a good stretch. Let sounds arise spontaneously as you stretch. Curl your knees into your chest, rock to your side, and roll up into a sitting position. When you open your eyes and come to standing, pause to notice the effects of having been in deep communication with your internal experiences. How does your body feel when it is rooted on the earth while opening to the infinite space above and around you?

Traveling to the Origin of the Breath

Inquiry: From where do the impulses to inhale and to exhale arise?

Awareness of the breath calms the mind and relaxes the body. Yogis discovered that following the breath to its origins creates a bridge between the body and the mind. Undisturbed breathing quickly induces a meditative state in which the mind becomes absorbed in the sound of the breath and the pleasurable sensations of breathing. Conscious use of the breath in yoga *(pranayama)* allows you to synchronize your breath and movements, inducing a trancelike state of increased awareness, sensitivity, and concentration. By elongating the length of inhaling and exhaling breaths while in motion, the actual elasticity of muscles increases. The increased concentration that comes from being drawn into the moment induces balance between strength and relaxation, effort and effortlessness. *Pranayama*, which translates as "control of the life force," is the way yoga allows you to access the life force and put it to work for you.

Life begins with your first breath in and ends with your last breath out. Breath is life. Although people can survive for many days without food and water, we can sur-

Use Breath Awareness to Break through Cultural Hypnosis

If health and happiness were as simple as breath awareness, why wouldn't breath awareness be part of our early childhood education? Why wouldn't we be teaching breath awareness in hospitals and clinics instead of waiting for the symptoms of stress to claim ever greater portions of our life's strength? It is as though there is a conspiracy in culture that separates us from the wisdom we carry inside.

Every human being on the planet has the choice to listen to the instinctual knowledge that is continuously being offered by the miraculous mechanisms within our own bodies. But it takes courage to break our connection with the hypnosis that everything that is important occurs outside of us. We would have to close our eyes and ears to the outside world long enough to notice what is going on inside our skin. We would temporarily lose the sense of connection to the world of social and cultural stimuli outside of ourselves and risk the possibility that we might discover nothing inside but emptiness and aloneness. To begin an experiment as simple as watching the breath requires a radical and courageous break with the cultural beliefs and norms that govern our personal existence.

vive for only a few minutes without oxygen. The way you breathe has a profound effect on the quality of your life. The act of breathing is usually automatic and unconscious; this breath inquiry will help you to bring conscious awareness to the patterns of breathing that connect your mind with your body. Bringing awareness to your breathing is the most direct bridge between body and mind.

Under ordinary circumstances a person's breathing is fairly shallow, involving only the upper part of the lungs and using only a small percentage of the lungs' five- to seven-quart capacity. Over the long term, shallow and superficial breathing deprives the body of oxygen and does not give the lungs an opportunity to empty the stagnant, residual air that remains deeper in the lungs. Lowered immune-system responses are a direct result of shallow breathing.

Even more hazardous to good health is the habit of mouth-breathing. The sinus passageways of the nostrils close down in response to stress. When this form of stress becomes chronic, we grow increasingly unconscious that we are breathing in this manner. Yet the body is designed to inspire through the nostrils. Nostril-breathing filters impurities from the incoming air. The mechanism built into the nostrils also adjusts the temperature and humidity of the inhalation by either heating or cooling the air. Shallow mouth-breathing combined with poor postural alignment can turn your lungs into a toxic-waste dump.

Have you ever become stiff or sore after a good physical workout? Muscle fatigue and soreness are direct results of shallow breathing. Bringing awareness to your breathing enables you to expand your overall lung capacity. Keeping a steady flow of deep breaths going while you exercise will aerate the blood, helping to reduce the buildup of lactic acid in the muscles. When you incorporate this breath scan into your daily routine, over time you will notice your general health beginning to improve. As your breathing becomes more efficient, your lungs will expel germs and environmental toxins more readily. The results: fewer colds and common ailments to drag you down. You can even use this breath inquiry to help you break the cycle of craving experiences or substances or self-defeating habits that rob you of your vitality.

Perhaps the most observable effect of developing awareness of the breath is that you will likely begin noticing that you breathe more often throughout the day. It is fascinating to watch how breath is connected to your simplest work habits. Deep concentration slows the breath. Worry can cause us to hold the breath for long periods of time. You might find yourself observing how thoughts and emotions are connected to your breath patterns. When the mind becomes scattered and confused, the breath pattern is usually simultaneously chaotic. By noticing connections between breath patterns and mental states, you begin developing a tool for changing your moods and mental states. Becoming aware of your breath brings about mental clarity and steadiness in the areas of your life that deserve your best attention.

As with the gravity scan Reclining Mountain Pose, this inquiry is also best read into a tape recorder and played back for yourself. Leave ample time between each question or instruction to deepen into your experience. After finishing the exploration, choose a yoga posture that is particularly challenging for you. Begin by drawing awareness to your breath and observe how remaining in contact with your breath as you enter the posture allows you to experience the challenge with greater comfort and steadiness.

Exploration: Self-Balancing Breath

1. Lie on the ground, taking the time you need to make any adjustments that allow you to settle into your body **(fig. 4.2)**. Recall the sensations of becoming heavy, as in the previous inquiry. Scan your body and allow gravity to work on your bones; feel them glide downward through the layers of muscle and tissue.

2. Are there any areas in your body that are resisting the pull of gravity in this moment? Allow any resistance or discomfort to be present precisely as you experience it.

3. As you become aware of your mind, notice the speed of your thoughts, the pulse of your thinking. Are any particular thoughts arising in this moment? Allow whatever thoughts that are present to simply be.

4. Invite your logical mind to remain present to help you witness the dimensions of your experience. The body lives in a dimension that is much slower than mental time. You cross a time boundary to enter the temporal dimension in which the body

actually lives. Suggest to yourself that you begin crossing this time boundary now.

5. What is your internal mood in this moment? Are particular feelings or emotions present? Suggest to your logical mind that it is safe, desirable, and pleasurable to expand awareness to include all of the thoughts, feelings, and emotions arising in every level of your being.

6. As you give permission for all parts of your experience to be present, notice how quickly and effortlessly your body settles into relaxation. Observe how deeply your mind begins to slow down to attune to the sensations that are arising in your body. Where does your awareness travel as your body relaxes and your mind slows down?

7. Beginning now to enter an even deeper state of relaxed awareness, notice the sensations of breathing in and breathing out. Without attempting to change or alter your breath in any way, simply notice the way your body is breathing in this moment. What sound does your breath make as it enters and leaves your nostrils? How far down in your torso can you feel the movement of your breath: to your collarbones? to your ribs? to your upper belly? to your lower belly?

8. Travel to the place in your being where the impulse to inhale arises. Let go of any attempt to control or direct your breathing in any way—simply notice where in your being the impulse to inhale arises.

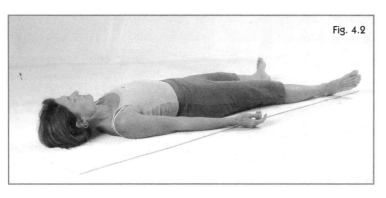

Fig. 4.2

9. Where does the impulse to exhale arise? Travel to the place in your being where the impulse to exhale arises. Let go of any attempt to control or direct your breathing in any way. Where in your being does the impulse to exhale arise?

10. Notice how many layers of your experience begin to unfold as you travel to the origin of the impulse to inhale and to exhale. Allow all the time it takes to travel to the origin of your breathing.

11. How does your body feel when you are listening to the sound of your breath and traveling to the place in your being where the impulse to inhale and to exhale arises? Can you feel infinite degrees of release as you relax control over your breath and breathing? Who is breathing your body in this moment? Who is being breathed?

12. Notice how your awareness is expanding to include the pulsing sensations that stream through your entire organism. Listen to any messages that are coming to you through the wisdom of your organism. Let go into the pulse of your own being.

13. In this place of deep, relaxed awareness, notice how you feel when you are at home in the center of your being, receiving from the wisdom of your organism. Notice any changes that have occurred in your breathing since you began.

14. Suggest to your logical mind that you will be returning to wakeful consciousness with knowledge and wisdom from your organism. You will be returning with the feeling of having had a healthy, rejuvenating sleep. You'll be returning wide awake, fully alert, and ready to move on to the next events of your day.

15. Slowly begin your return, rocking your ankles from the inner anklebones to the outer anklebones. Roll your wrists from the inside to the outside. Roll your head from ear to ear.

16. Deepening your breath, bring up a good stretch, allowing any sound to emerge as you move.

17. Curl your knees to your chest and rock from side to side. Roll to your side and slowly lift up to a sitting position, letting the head be the last part of the body to come to vertical.

18. Notice the speed of your thinking. Notice your mood. When you open your eyes, notice whether your vision has altered in any way. Do colors appear brighter? duller? Are shapes appearing with greater clarity, or are they more diffuse than usual?

19. As you transition to your next activity, carry with you the awareness of your breathing.

Attuning to the Pulse of Being

Inquiry: How does the sense of inner wholeness arise from noticing polarities in experience?

Many different kinds of pulses occur simultaneously in the body. We have already observed the most obvious one—the flow of the breath in and the breath out. That is a pulse. Another pulse is the rhythm of the heartbeat. Pulses convey the movements of digestion and peristalsis and the undulating movement of our intestines. Every sense organ has its unique means of excitation, the stimulus getting transmitted to the brain in impulses. The speed of our brain's activities create the rhythm of our thoughts and thinking. *Alpha, beta, delta,* and *theta*—these terms refer to the frequency of chemical and electromagnetic waves emitted by the brain in various states of awareness. The waves of our moods, emotions, and feelings—these are body rhythms made up of more pulses.

Many Oriental forms of medicine are based upon pulses associated with the energetic processes in the body, but you do not need to know the details of the meridians or be versed in a specific tradition to begin to enhance your bodily functions by attuning to your pulses. In fact, the discovery of the ancient healing modalities associated with acupuncture, auyurveda, shiatsu, and yoga emerged from the same inquiry you are about to undertake.

All shamanic and energetic systems of natural healing have come from practitioners who were fascinated with the miraculous pulse of their own beings. By following an inquiry into the pulse of being, early yogis entered deep states of awareness that allowed them to penetrate the subtler dimensions of their own physiology. As you go deeper into the meditative state, you will discover that your ability to know yourself at every level is limitless.

What generates a pulsation that we can sense within our bodies? Simply speaking, the body, like a battery, is polarized into positive and negative charges. A pulsation is generated by the subtle electromagnetic charges that are emitted and the chemical reactions that are stimulated within the organs and glands of your body. Similar to an electromagnetic generator, your body contains positive and negative electrical and chemical charges that are constantly being switched on and off by the triggering of nervous impulses.

Scanning your body for the sensations of pulsing actually improves the efficiency of the pulsing currents that operate in the various systems—this phenomenon is related to the way in which an ordinary bar of iron gets turned into a magnet. I remember my seventh grade science teacher demonstrating the process of making a magnet. From the pockets of her official laboratory apron she fished out two iron bars. She put them together and pulled them apart. She asked one of the students to do the same thing and to report what they observed. "Nothing," was the response.

She then took out a large magnet and began stroking one of the iron bars slowly and systematically with the magnet. After several minutes, she brought the two original iron bars back together. We were shocked to find that the bar she had been stroking had become a magnet! That was very cool. We tested the two bars with other bars. It was a fact: one of the original bars was the same, but one had become a magnet.

How did this happen? She showed us diagrams of the molecules of a nonmagnetized iron bar that depicted unorganized masses of positively and negatively charged molecules working in all directions. The diagram of a magnetized bar showed molecules arranged in symmetrical patterns, all working in the same direction to create a force field.

The principle underlying this phenomenon is that you can organize a field of molecules by bringing it into contact with an already organized field. In this case, the molecules in the nonmagnetized bar get reorganized for efficient magnetic polarization. In the same way, the force fields surrounding and interpenetrating our bodies are relatively chaotic, pulling us in every direction by attractions calling our attention through the senses. When you lie down on the ground and begin to scan your body for sensations of pulsation, your awareness serves as a magnet, sweeping through the disorganized and chaotic field and realigning the flow of energies into a harmonious balance between the positive and negative charges.

Try reading these instructions into a tape recorder and playing them back for yourself. With practice, this pulse scan will begin to produce a pleasurable sensation that may feel like an electric current passing through your body. Can you recall the sensations of pulsing, streaming, or tingling during the gravity or breath inquiries above? Your body will very quickly begin to pulse when you bring awareness to any particular sensation for observation.

Exploration: Synchronizing with the Abdominal Pulse

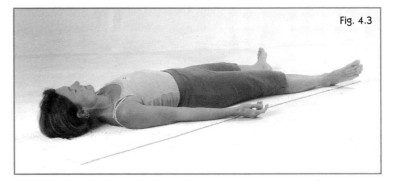

Fig. 4.3

1. Lie down on the ground, taking the time you need to make any adjustments and readjustments that allow you to settle into your body (**fig. 4.3**). Recall the sensations of becoming heavy, as in the first inquiry. Scan your body and notice the effects of gravity relaxing your bones downward through layers of tissue.

2. Are there any areas in your body that are resisting the pull of gravity in this moment? Allow any resistance or discomfort to be present precisely as you are experiencing it.

3. Notice the speed and momentum of your thoughts and thinking. Do you notice any particular thoughts arising in this moment? Allow any thoughts to simply be.

4. Invite your logical mind to remain present to witness the dimensions of your experience precisely as is. There is nothing to change about any dimension of your experience. The body lives in a time that is much slower than mental time. We are asked to slow down to listen to the communications coming from our cells. Notice how you begin to cross over a time boundary to enter the time in which the body actually lives.

5. As you give permission for all parts of your experience to be present, notice how quickly and effortlessly your body settles into relaxation. Observe your mind beginning to slow down to attune to the sensations that are arising in your body. Where does your awareness travel as your body relaxes and your mind slows down?

6. Now travel into the deep core of your belly. What is your internal mood in this moment? Do you notice the presence of any particular feelings or emotions? Suggest to your logical mind that it is safe, desirable, and pleasurable to expand awareness to include all of the thoughts and emotions arising in this moment.

7. Using the power of your awareness, sense the pulsing in your belly. If you do not sense this pulse, imagine a pulsing in your belly.

8. Imagine that you are connected to the warmth of the sun through an imaginary umbilical cord. As you breathe in, inhale warm, glowing sunlight into the core of your belly. Sense the pulse in your belly growing stronger and warmer. As the heat in your belly expands, imagine this glowing energy streaming down the hollow tubes of your legs, filling your feet and toes.

9. Can you feel or imagine a pulse in the soles of your feet? When you sense the pulsation in the soles of your feet, allow it to synchronize with the pulsing in your belly.

10. Send the warm, glowing pulse from your belly up through the hollow core of your torso and imagine your arms, hands, and fingers filling with expanding energy. Can you feel or imagine a strong, steady pulse in the center of your palms? When you have the sensation of pulsation in the palms, allow the pulsing in your palms to synchronize with the pulsing in your belly.

11. From the pulsing center in the core of your belly, send warm, glowing energy upward through the neck to fill the inner sphere of your skull. How strongly can you feel the pulsing in the center of your forehead as your whole head fills with glowing energy? When you feel the pulsing sensation in your forehead, allow that pulsing to synchronize with the pulse in your belly.

12. Expand your awareness to include the pulsing in the soles of your feet, the pulsing

in your palms, and the pulsing in your forehead. Allow all of these pulses to synchronize with the pulsing in your belly.

13. Notice how the entire interior space of your body is filled with warm, glowing energy pulsing to the rhythm of your belly center. Imagine the glowing sensation becoming so concentrated that liquid warmth begins to stream through the pores of your skin, radiating through the body wall to envelop all of the space around you. Allow your whole being to bathe in the pulsing energy of prana streaming through every cell of your physical body.

14. Gradually bring your awareness back to the surface of your body. Allow the energy to return to the interior of your physical body, increasing in potency.

15. Now sense the energy returning with ever-increasing potency to the center of your being. How does your body look and feel from the inside out when you have the potency of prana nurturing every dimension of your being? Notice how you are connected to the universe surrounding you yet rooted in the center of your own being. Receive through the wisdom of your body in this moment.

16. Let go into the pulse of your own being. In this place of deep, relaxed awareness, notice how you feel when you are at home in the center of your being, receiving from the wisdom of your organism. Notice any changes or effects that have occurred in your breathing since you began.

17. Suggest to your logical mind that you will be returning with the knowledge and wisdom generated by your organism. You will be returning with the feeling of having had a healthy, rejuvenating sleep. You'll be returning wide awake, fully alert and ready to move on to the next events of your day.

18. Slowly begin your return, rocking your ankles from the inner anklebones to the outer anklebones. Roll your wrists from the inner wrist bones to the outer wrist bones. Roll your head from ear to ear.

19. Deepening your breath, bring up a good stretch, allowing any sound to emerge as you move.

20. Curl your knees into your chest and rock from side to side. Roll to your side and up into a sitting position.

21. Notice the speed and momentum of your thoughts and thinking. Notice your mood. When you open your eyes, notice whether your vision has altered in any way: are colors brighter or duller? shapes clearer or fuzzier? As you transition to your next activity, carry with you an awareness of being in harmony with the pulse of your own being.

Before Moving On . . .

How do we hear messages from the wisdom of the organism? We hear those messages through the language of sensation. This chapter began by recognizing the central theme of Self-Awakening Yoga as being the possibility for harnessing our awareness to establish direct communication between the mind and the body. The human body is encoded with evolutionary intelligence. In order to decode that knowledge into a usable source of guiding wisdom, we need to listen to the language of the body as it communicates to us through sensation.

The biological origins of the evolutionary impulse to move toward light, as encoded in the pineal gland, is one of the shaping influences that motivate our physical journey from infancy to maturity, from being belly-bound to standing. However, our development as multidimensional human beings is not limited to the physical; the pineal gland also stimulates development of mental and emotional intelligence that can eventually become so compelling that the language of the body is eclipsed and the wisdom of the body forgotten. In acknowledging that both physical and mental dimensions of human development have a common origin in the pineal gland, we recognize the importance of attending to the communications that emerge when we become quiet enough to let the body speak and focused enough to listen and respond to its messages.

The other shaping influence on our physical bodies, the presence of gravity, is more tangible to the senses than tropism and is therefore more readily accessible for using as an anchor in becoming aware of sensations. Therefore, the first inquiry, Reclining Mountain, began with noticing the effects of gravity as it interacts with the body in a relaxed position on the ground. In returning to the origins of the impulse to inhale and to exhale in the inquiry Self-Balancing Breath, we discovered another way to deepen the communication between mind and body by noticing how becoming aware of the sensation of breathing can be a way to slow and calm the mind and to relax the body. When the mind is calm and the body relaxed, the ordinary thoughts and feelings that occupy our awareness recede to the background, allowing a deeper level of awareness of sensations to surface along with a concomitant feeling of well-being. In the inquiry Synchronizing with the Abdominal Pulse, the subtler sensations of pulsing in different parts of the body are drawn into a harmonious communication with the central pulse in your body, the abdominal pulse, allowing for a free flow of relaxation and revitalization throughout all of the bodily systems.

All of these inquiries offer ways to strengthen the bridge of communication between mind and body. As you begin to recognize and respond to the language of your body through these inquiries, it is natural and desirable that you notice corresponding beliefs, self-concepts, and emotions that are held within your body and that shape your life experiences. In order to support the expansion of your consciousness to include the wisdom that is coming through your body, it is helpful to consider that the story of your life is written within your body—your body is a walking repository of every experience you have had in this lifetime. To the extent that you were fully present to experience the joy or the sadness or the anger generated by specific events, to that degree the experiences leave only the imprints of a memory. Some experiences that were originally overwhelming to your conscious mind may be tucked away in the memory of your muscles, organs, and glands, waiting for an opportunity to resurface—to be experienced and then released.

As you slow down and begin to draw your awareness to bodily sensations that are occurring in the present moment, you may recall some unsettling experiences from the past. Fortunately, past experiences do not have to be recalled with the same details and intensity that they occurred in order to be released from the nervous system. Self-Awakening Yoga inquiries will most often leave you feeling physically relaxed and mentally alert, with the sensation of coming home to your center. Your sense of safety and trust in the journey of your own self-awakening will grow in an inner environment that respects and honors your bodily sensations along with your mental and emotional intelligence. As you progress through the inquiries in this book, you will notice how trust in the intelligence of your body develops. Sometimes the simplest insight will come through noticing a subtle sensation, and that insight will shift a mountain of your personal history.

Building on the bodily awareness of the effects of gravity, breath, and abdominal pulsation in this chapter, the next chapter guides you into some of the earliest movements you encountered as an infant responding to the internal impulse to move your head and limbs. These explorations are the basic building blocks that empower the body to continue its journey of movement toward the light.

5 Rooted in the Earth, Open to the Heavens

How does releasing into gravity make it easier to experience natural alignment in the standing postures?

HAVE YOU EVER WATCHED A YOUNG CHILD standing or walking like one of her parents? Sometimes we can catch a momentary glimpse of a youngster actually trying on a posture to imitate a person he admires. When trying on clothes in front of a department store mirror do you shift your posture to understand how the clothing was designed to be worn? Do you tilt your head or position your hips at different angles to take on an attitude that the outfit could communicate?

Our standing posture reveals many of the choices we have made that shape our personalities and attitudes toward life. When I was an art teacher I took students on a field trip to the mall to study and sketch how people carried their bodies as they strolled by. Often you can sense what mood a person might be in by the way she holds her body. You can imagine life experiences and roles people have held by the idiosyncratic signature of their carriage. The gate and pace of a person's walk can reveal levels of comfort with movement and how that person feels about time.

Hurried, leisurely, burdened, carefree, deliberate—these qualities are easily recognized by observing how a person carries his or her head. When the head leads the body in space it seems as though that person is hurrying to get somewhere in the future. Conversely, when you see someone's gaze unhurriedly traveling around the visual field you sense a feeling of freedom to explore and to enjoy the environment. The way in which a person carries a load of packages can reveal facility and comfort with balance and organization. Athletic training, work habits, office and home furniture, past injuries, emotional wounding—these are some of the many and varied sources that interact to give our bodies their shapes.

Our postural patterns also reflect the beliefs and attitudes we hold about ourselves. Many people take up a yoga practice in order to begin interacting with patterns of posture and movement that they know produce stress and discomfort. The standing yoga postures seem to be an obvious beginning place to interact with one's postural dynamics, yet working with the details of alignment in such poses as Mountain, Triangle, Warrior, and Chair may not access the deep, intrinsic muscles that actually give shape to our stance. These classic postures do encourage tone, strength, and balance in the larger, more superficial muscles of the physical structure. The classic standing and balancing yoga postures, such as Tree, Eagle, King of Dancers, and Heron, do produce concentration and mental clarity. But to gain access to the place in our being where our inner self is creating our core stance, we must slow down and notice the subtle sensations and messages that arise when we enter into a supported, meditative inquiry into our internal experiences of grounding and balance.

The deepest structural muscles, which are also often the tightest and strongest muscles of the body, are the short muscles that connect and coordinate the intricate movements between the vertebrae of the spinal column. Called the "antigravity muscles," these small, strong bundles of muscle fiber enable us to defy gravity's urge, allowing us to maintain a vertical spine in standing. The classic standing and balancing yoga postures do not necessarily affect these deeper, structural muscles; it is difficult to sense the movement of these muscles from a standing position. However, when you lie down with the intention of noticing how your body makes contact with the ground, you release the weight of the body and allow the body to be supported by gravity rather than work against gravity.

In this chapter we begin our movement inquiries from a supine position in order to let gravity begin to communicate more directly with the kinesthetic intelligence in the small, strong antigravity muscles. The intention of the following explorations is to begin accessing our natural state of alignment and flexibility without doing any effortful work. When you approach your body with the attitude of no effort, you begin to discover that steadiness comes not from a rigid position but from the ability to balance and change in response to new situations in each moment. After experiencing the effects of these inquiries you may notice shifts taking place in your basic sense of groundedness, your postural alignment, and in your ability to perform any work, exercise, and movement—especially your yoga.

Using Gravity to Realign Your Body

Inquiry: What is my body ready to release that will allow greater freedom and relaxation in practicing standing postures?

Have you ever noticed how the responsibilities you carry in life begin to accumulate as tension in your neck and shoulders? Like Atlas, the mythological Titan who holds the heavens on his shoulders, it is a common human experience to feel that we shoulder the burdens of our life. It is easy to become unconscious of the habitual holding of the muscles in our head, neck, and shoulders. Giving someone the "cold shoulder" or "carrying a chip on the shoulder" are common expressions that foretell some of the emotional patterns we commonly bear in the body that begin to restrict our freedom of movement.

Here is an opportunity to release the "shoulds" that are sometimes held in the shoulders. Explorations 1 and 2 of this inquiry provide an opportunity for noticing how effortless it can feel to allow the natural movements of your head, shoulders, and arms to emerge when you are not fighting gravity in a standing position. By giving the weight of your body to gravity you can sense how the bones and muscles move in

Notice the Effects of Natural Alignment on Lifestyle Choices

Moving with expanded flexibility, coordination, and range of motion may feel unfamiliar at first—instead of being drained by unconscious holding patterns and inefficient alignment, you will be opening a reservoir of energy, making that energy available for greater creativity and self-expression. How would you like to redirect your life choices? Your lifestyle habits may begin to seem a little odd. Your easy chair may not feel as easy as it did before. You may notice that your office furniture doesn't provide the support you desire for staying balanced while working. Your shoes may not feel like such a good fit anymore.

In fact, you may begin to notice that the simple things in life, like your shoes, your chairs, your mattress, and even your clothes, are not designed with the actual shape of your body in mind. You may notice that you are less willing to slip into the cultural images that shape your body, and that you are awakening greater interest in the natural design and architecture of your own evolving body. Go on a treasure hunt and search for a pair of shoes that are shaped to support your feet or a chair that supports your natural alignment.

relationship to one another when they are participating with gravity. Any yoga posture that requires you to extend your arms above your head, such as Extended Mountain, Warrior, Yoga Mudra, Chair, or Crescent Moon, will happen with greater awareness when you return to them after these inquiries.

In Exploration 3 of this inquiry the energy you have awakened by freeing the head, neck, shoulders, and arms gets drawn down into your hips, legs, and feet, kinesthetically connecting the large segments of your body. The intelligent energy of prana is invited to flow in an unobstructed stream from head to toe, restoring your physical structure to a natural state of balance. When you return to your standing and balancing postures, such as the Mountain or Warrior, you will notice the beneficial effects of these inquiries.

Exploration 1: Head Roll—Letting Go of the Weight of the World

1. Lie down on the ground **(fig. 5.1)**. This is a time for slowing down and attuning to the sensations that arise within your body. Begin to notice the contact your body makes with the ground. Make any adjustments that help you settle into gravity.

2. Imagine the impression your body makes on the ground. Scan your body to observe the areas that seem to resist the pull of gravity or are holding on in some way. Breathe. Let any resistance be as it is. There is no need to alter or to change any aspect of the sensations you observe as you enter deeper levels of awareness.

3. Begin to sense the weight of your bones gliding downward through layers of muscle and tissue in response to the pull of gravity. As you notice the weight of your bones, can you envision how the tubular structures of your bones contain fluids and soft tissues that are also being drawn by gravity?

4. Now draw your awareness to the sensation of heaviness in the back of your head. Notice how dense and solid your head feels. How heavy is your head? Is it as heavy as a bowling ball? a watermelon? Can you sense the weight of your brain suspended in the fluid capsule of the skull? How heavy are your eyes in their sockets? Can you sense the expansion and contraction of the pressures in your head as you allow the breath to flow upward into the bowl of your head?

5. Imagine the back of your head sinking down into a bowl that is exquisitely shaped to receive your cranium. As your head begins to release, notice how you can relax your jaw and tongue. Encourage your practiced expressions to melt away from your facial muscles. Release all roles, all responsibilities, and enter into the sensations of heaviness in the back of your head.

6. This hollow bowl in the ground is perfectly shaped to receive the full weight of your head. Invite the weight of your head to release down into the bowl in incremental

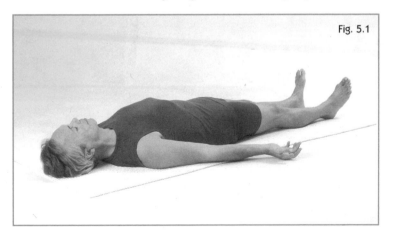

Fig. 5.1

degrees. Find what is full release for you at this moment.

7. Now the bowl begins to glide slowly upward from the back of your head to the crown (**fig. 5.2**). What sensations arise in the back of your neck as the upward-gliding bowl moves to the crown of your head? Take an internal picture of the way your body looks and feels when the weight of your head is received into this perfectly shaped bowl that continuously glides upward to your crown. Notice any pulsing, streaming, or tingling sensations that may begin to occur.

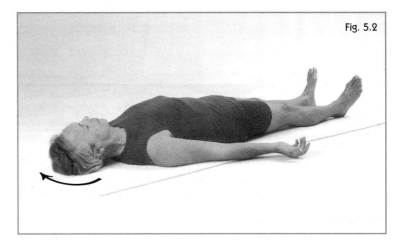
Fig. 5.2

Exploration 2: Shoulder Release

1. Lie down on the ground. Bring your awareness to your breath and your breathing. Without attempting to change or alter your breath in any way, notice how far down the spine you can feel your breath moving.

2. Notice the weight of your shoulders and arms on the ground. Can you sense whether one shoulder and arm seem more relaxed or heavier on the ground?

3. Slowly begin to roll your head from side to side. Let the movement start slowly. Can you sense the fluids inside your head moving as you move? Notice your breathing: is it easier to hold your breath or is it easier to breathe with the movement? Breathe in the way that is most pleasurable to you.

4. Without using effort, let the movement of rolling your head from side to side gradually get larger. Do you notice any difference in temperature from one side to the other? Can you sense any differences in mood between sides? Does rolling to one side feel easier or more fluid or more familiar than rolling to the other side?

5. Where does the movement stop on each side? What stops the movement? Do you notice that your chin bumps into your shoulder on one or both sides?

6. As you roll your head to the right, reach the right shoulder, arm, and wrist away from your chin and down toward your right ankle (**fig. 5.3**). Let your arm stay heavy. Notice the friction as your heavy arm slides along the ground.

7. As you roll your head to the left, slide the left shoulder, arm, and wrist down toward your left ankle.

8. Continue rolling your head from side to side. Inhale as you roll the head to one side

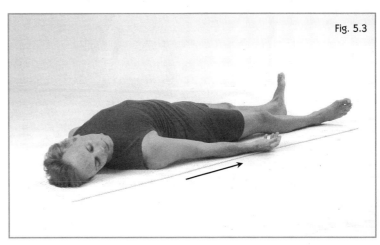
Fig. 5.3

and reach the shoulder and arm toward the ankle; exhale as you roll the head through center; inhale as you roll to the new side.

9. Is it more pleasurable to breathe with the movement in this way? Do you notice that reaching the shoulder and arm away from the chin creates more space for the head to roll? Do you notice how much more deeply you can breathe when the shoulder and arm are released down toward the feet? Can you sense how your shoulder blades move down the backside of your rib cage when the shoulders release toward the feet?

10. Let the momentum of your movement build until you feel your head rolling from ear to ear, bringing each ear near to the ground or touching the ground on each side. Let your head roll without controlling the speed of your movement. Can you sense how your whole body wants to move in response to releasing your head? Experi-ence what happens when you let the body do the movement without any inhibition or instructions from your mind.

11. Now slow the movement until your head returns to the neutral position. As you bring your body into stillness, do you notice any sensations continuing to play through your nerves and muscles? Do the muscles along the backside of your body feel any warmer than when you began? Do your shoulders and arms feel any heavier on the ground than when you began? How far down your spine can you feel your breath moving?

12. Create an image of the way your body looks and feels when the weight of your head is rolling from ear to ear and your shoulders and arms are reaching down and away from your chin. One last time, roll your head from side to side and compare the quality of the movement and your sen-sations to when you first began.

Exploration 3: Hip Release

1. Lie down on the ground. Notice the weight of your hips and legs. Can you sense whether one hip and leg seems more relaxed or heavier on the ground, or if one side is more held against the pull of gravity?

2. Slowly begin to roll your head from side to side. Can you sense the fluids inside your head moving as you move? Notice your breathing as you move. Is it easier to hold your breath or is it easier to breathe with the movement?

3. Without using force or effort, begin rolling your head from ear to ear, as in the previous exploration. As you roll your head to the right, reach the shoulder, arm, and hand down toward your ankle.

4. Use your kinesthetic sense to feel your right heel. Begin to reach your right heel, hip, and leg along the ground away from your right pelvic joint (**fig. 5.4**). How does it feel to have the whole right side of your body reach-ing away from your chin?

5. Use your kinesthetic sense to feel your left heel and leg. As you roll your head to the left,

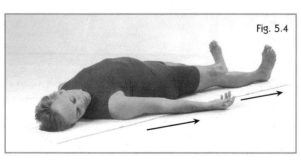

Fig. 5.4

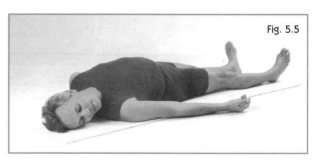

Fig. 5.5

reach the length of your left arm down toward your ankle as you simultaneously reach your left leg away from your pelvic joint. Your arm and leg are both stretching along the ground down away from your chin.

6. Continue moving in this side-to-side way a few times. How are you breathing? Can you inhale as you roll your chin to the side and exhale as you come back to the midline? Find a way to coordinate your breath with the movement.

7. Does reaching the limbs away from the chin create more space for the head to roll? Do you notice how much more deeply you can breathe when you release the whole side of your body downward, away from the head? Let the movement build until you feel your head rolling from ear to ear, bringing each ear close to the ground (or touching the ground) on each side (**fig. 5.5**). Experi-

ence what wants to happen as you let go of your control over the movement. What happens when you let the intelligence of your body take over the movement?

8. Slow the movement down until your head returns to the neutral position (**fig. 5.6**).

9. As you bring your body into stillness, do the sensations born of the movements continue to play through your nerves and muscles? Is your body pulsing or tingling? Do your hips and legs feel any heavier on the ground than when you first began? What changes do you notice in the way your low back or shoulders now contact the ground? Notice your mood.

10. Allow your awareness to dissolve into the steady stream of sensations that arise from your organism in this moment. Suggest to your logical mind that your body is a source of wisdom. Allow the wisdom

Windshield Wiper Ankles

In standing, the weight of your entire structure passes through your ankle joints, transferring gravity downward into your feet. Here is a simple way to discover how you can move the weight of your whole leg effortlessly by rotating your ankles.

Lie on the ground and bring awareness to your ankles. Can you get a kinesthetic sense of the inner and outer anklebones of each foot? Notice the arch underneath your ankles. Is one foot more turned out than the other? Now rotate your ankles from side to side in a windshield wiper motion (**fig. 5.8**). The more you release the weight of your legs to be rolled by the ankles, the more effortless the movement becomes.

Explore rotating both of the heels to the right, then to the left. Can you vary the pattern and rotate both of the big toes in toward the midline, then rotate the little toes down to the ground? Experiment with as many movement patterns as you can invent. Can you feel how rotating the whole leg by focusing on your ankles actually encourages the movement to travel all the way up into your hip sockets?

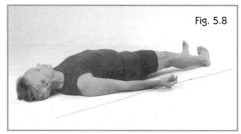

Fig. 5.8

When you stand, notice how your ankles are connected to your feet. Do you feel more grounded? For fun, try doing the Tree pose, standing on one foot. Do you notice any more stability in the ankles than before?

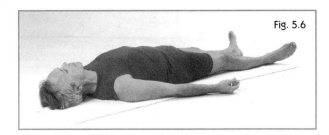

Fig. 5.6

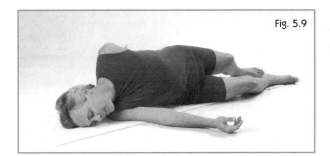

Fig. 5.7

of your organism to provide you with a sense of security and comfort.

11. Begin your return by rocking your ankles from the inner anklebones to the outer anklebones. Roll your wrists from the inner wrist bones to the outer wrist bones. Now roll your head from ear to ear.

12. Bring up a good stretch. Allow your breath to deepen and let emerge any sounds that happen spontaneously as you stretch **(fig. 5.7)**.

13. Curl your knees into your chest, rock from side to side, and roll up into a sitting position.

14. When you feel ready, allow the windows of your eyes to open and receive the world from the fresh perspective of this movement experience.

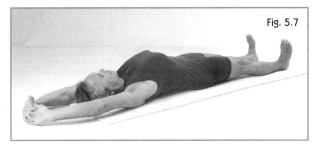

Fig. 5.9

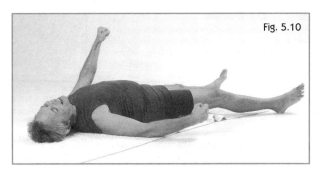

Fig. 5.10

Integration: Whole-Body Release

1. Begin by rolling the head from side to side. Let the movement build to allow the shoulder to release away from the chin. Then add the hip release to your movements by releasing the legs and heels away from the pelvis. Now you have the whole body engaged in the movement **(fig. 5.9)**.

2. If you had permission to have a tantrum or to throw a little fit in this moment, how much more control could you release over your movement that would allow your whole body to expel any compressed or pent-up energies? Your body is supported on the ground. Suggest to your logical mind that it is safe and desirable to allow any release that wants to happen through your voice and your movements in this moment **(fig. 5.10)**. Releasing control in this way may feel unfamiliar at first, but as you relax into the fun of the drama you may be surprised at how energized you feel afterward. No one is watching you. You can trust your body's wisdom to follow this experience through to deep relaxation on the other side.

3. When you feel ready, allow your movements and sounds to subside. What energetic effects do you notice taking place in your physical body, in your mood, and in your self-perceptions at this time? Are there any surprises? Allow yourself to receive messages from the wisdom of your organism from every dimension of your experience.

4. Slowly begin your return. In your own time, return to sitting. If you notice any lingering insights that call attention, this would be a good opportunity to write in your journal.

The "Yes" Movement

Inquiry: How does it feel to have the freedom to say "yes" with my whole body?

Our heads are designed to move freely, independent of our shoulders. When this freedom is restricted, we may find simple movements, such as turning to look over the shoulder, effortful or limited. Sometimes even the simple movement of nodding the head in a "yes" or "no" direction feels more like a "maybe" because the shoulders come along for the ride.

Whenever the head moves, the shoulders may think they need to be working too. When I'm tired I notice that my shoulders tense up, making it difficult to back out of my long driveway. Placing my arm across the back of the driver's seat and twisting to look backward reveals the reluctance of my head to move independent of my shoulders.

When muscles don't know that they are holding on or overworking, slowing down allows us to notice the subtle patterns that confine our freedom. In the first exploration below you will have an opportunity to notice how the bones and muscles of the shoulder girdle can move efficiently and effortlessly in relationship to one another. Oftentimes when work is requested of the body the shoulders engage first, either to initiate the movement or to assist other parts of the body. Reaching from the shoulders to pick up a heavy load—a movement pattern that many of us default to—eventually strains the muscles of the neck and low back. In the following inquiries you will locate the center of gravity as the origin for all arm-lifting movements. By allowing your head, neck, and shoulders to remain relaxed and open you can draw the strength to lift and hold your arms from the central core of your body.

After working with this exploration you may begin to notice that your arms seem heavy and resistant to remaining extended in the standing yoga postures that require lifting your arms above your head. Perhaps it is because of our sense of bearing or "shouldering" responsibility that the shoulders think they need to work even when they would be of best help by remaining relaxed, as is the case when holding the arms overhead. The Shoulder Thump exploration provides information about what it feels like when the deep shoulder muscles of the rotator cuff are not needed and can be "turned off"; these muscles are the subscapularis, infraspinatus, and teres minor. Also affected are larger, more superficial muscles of the back and trunk, including the latissimus dorsi, the upper trapezius, and both the pectoralis major and minor muscles. In the Side-to-Side Shoulder Release we explore how the head can be activated to move independent of the shoulders. This series of movements differentiates the action of the upper-body segments and produces a deep release that encourages prana to flow into the higher centers of communication and self-expression.

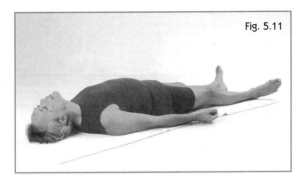

Fig. 5.11

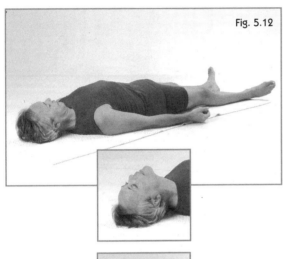

Fig. 5.12

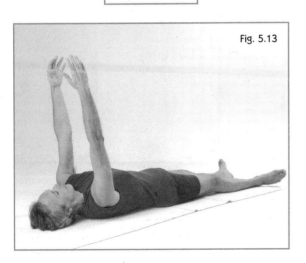

Fig. 5.13

Exploration 1: Shoulder Thump

1. Lie down on the ground. Suggest to your mind that this is a time for slowing down and attuning to the sensations that arise within your body. Make any adjustments that help you settle into your body.

2. Begin to notice the contact your body makes with the ground as it settles. Scan your body to find the areas that seem to resist the pull of gravity or hold on in some way. Let any resistance be as it is.

3. Moving to a deeper level of awareness, begin to sense your bones gliding down through layers of muscle and tissue in response to the pull of gravity.

4. When you feel the sensation of heaviness throughout your whole body, experiment with rocking your head in a "yes" movement (**figs. 5.11 and 5.12**). The back of your head stays in contact with the ground as your head rocks with the movement. Notice how the scalene muscles (at the cervical spine) and the trapezius muscles (at the upper back and shoulders) want to get involved in the movement by elevating the shoulders or hyper-extending the neck. Now let your head return to neutral for a moment and notice the internal sensations that arise from making the "yes" movement with your head

5. Open your eyes and find a point on the ceiling at the level of the horizon. Take a visual impression of this point; this is your visual "anchor." Now let your eyes soften as you maintain a steady gaze on that point. Do you notice any tendency for your eyes to grab for the point?

6. Close your eyes and let them rest for a moment. Allow your eyeballs to become very heavy. Can you feel your eyes dropping back into your head, like two pebbles dropping into a clear lake?

7. Open your eyes again, allowing the eyeballs to remain weighted. Imagine that your eyes are windows and that you are seeing through them. Rather than moving your eyes toward the point on the ceiling, allow the point to move toward you while your eyes remain relaxed in their sockets. Receive the image through the sense organ of your eyes. Inhale as you take the image all the way down into your belly.

8. Notice how it is possible to remain inside yourself while receiving through the window of your eyes. Exhale and rest, then open the window of your eyes once again.

9. Now lift your hands and arms off the ground and let your fingers reach toward your visual reference point on the ceiling (**fig. 5.13**). With every breath in, let your fingers grow toward the point like the tendrils of a plant. Notice the way your shoulders and arms feel as they stretch toward that point with each inhale.

10. Release your arms to the ground. Notice the sensation of heaviness in your arms and shoulders.

11. Once again let your breath move your fingers, hands, and arms toward the visual "anchor" on the ceiling. Notice whether your shoulders lift off the ground; bring them back to the floor while still keeping your arms and fingers upright, moving toward the point. Your arms reach as your shoulders remain relaxed on the ground.

12. Now lift the right shoulder off the ground, arm and fingers moving toward the point on the ceiling (**fig. 5.14**). Maintain a soft gaze on the point. On an exhale let the shoulder thump to the ground while the arm and fingers remain upright. Imagine

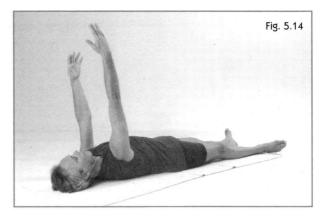

Fig. 5.14

the whole shoulder capsule is heavy, like a sack of potatoes. Let the bones and muscles of the right shoulder be as heavy as they actually are.

13. For the next six or seven breaths, lift the right shoulder on an inhaling breath, then let the shoulder thump to the ground on the exhale. Listen each time for the sound and quality of the thump.

Finding an Effortless Gaze in Yoga Postures

In many yoga postures the directive to find a visual reference point, a *drishti,* is a means of deepening concentration and engaging more of the nervous system in becoming conscious of the movement of prana. Here is a way to relax your eyes and notice your ability to receive information through your eyes without getting drawn outside of yourself to see. This is a good way to keep prana flowing through your eyes, allowing for a deep sense of contentment to arise from knowing your relationship to the world around you.

Imagine that you receive visual information through the window of your eyes. As you inhale, receive the image down into your belly. Imagine drinking in the image through your eyes into your belly.

Whenever you notice your eyes grabbing at the visual world around you, take a moment to close your eyes and let them rest. Suggest to yourself that you have the power to receive images; you do not need to move outside of your center to receive images through the windows of your eyes. When practicing your standing and balancing postures during yoga practice, notice how much deeper you can relax into your experience when you soften your gaze and remain at home in the center of your being.

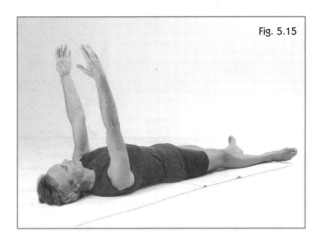

Fig. 5.15

14. Lower both arms to the floor. Close your eyes. Notice the difference between the two shoulders on the ground. Notice any pulsing, streaming, or tingling sensations that arise.

15. Open your eyes again and receive the visual reference point down into your belly. Let both arms and hands come off the floor, fingers growing toward the point. Switching awareness to the left shoulder, lift it off the ground and then let it thump down. Repeat this lift six or seven times, listening for the sound and quality of the thump. When you lift to extend the shoulder you are giving the muscles of your shoulder girdle the message, "This is what it feels like to switch on"; when the shoulder thumps to the ground, the message becomes "this is what it feels like to switch off."

16. Inhale on the last lift of your left shoulder. Hold the lift, keep holding the breath, and then let the shoulder thump. Now float both arms down to the ground.

17. Pause for a moment and do an internal scan to notice the effects of the Shoulder Thump.

18. One last time, open your eyes and softly gaze at the reference point, then inhale and extend both arms and fingers toward the point (**fig. 5.15**). Experiment with the sensation of lifting your arms from the center of gravity in your belly. Do you notice a difference in the sensation when the lifting movement originates from your center of gravity? Now alternately lift one shoulder on an inhaling breath and let it thump on the exhale; follow with the same movement with the other shoulder. Continue with alternate shoulder thumping, staying slow enough to feel the sensation of heaviness each time the shoulder releases toward the ground.

19. Release both arms to the floor. Make the "yes" movement with your head and observe any differences in the way this movement now feels as compared to when you began. Do you sense pulsing, streaming, or tingling sensations?

20. In this state of relaxed awareness, recall the sensation of receiving the world through the window of your eyes. Recall the sensation of lifting your arms while remaining connected to your center of gravity. Imagine what it might feel like to be standing in Mountain pose and allowing your arms to be lifted from your center of gravity. As the arms float up, energy moves down into your belly and legs, grounding you into the earth.

Exploration 2: Side-to-Side Shoulder Release

1. Continuing your exploration from the position on your back as above, bend your right knee, sliding your foot along the ground until the foot is standing a comfortable distance from your right hip (**fig 5.16**). Notice the contact your foot makes with the floor. Imagine that you are standing on this foot.

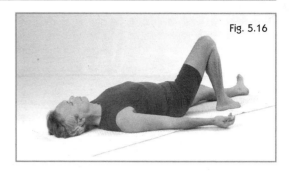

Fig. 5.16

2. Now bend your left knee, sliding your left foot along the ground until it is standing (**fig 5.17**). Feel the contact both feet now make with the ground. How much space is there between your low back and the floor? Has the curve lengthened out, bringing your low back closer the floor? Notice that when your knees are bent your low back lengthens along the ground.

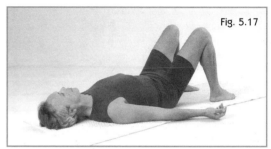

Fig. 5.17

3. With the awareness of originating the movement from your center of gravity, lift your arms over your torso and bend your elbows, adjusting your hands so that each hand grasps the opposite elbow (**fig. 5.18**). Notice how the shoulders come toward the ground as you hold your elbows upright toward the ceiling.

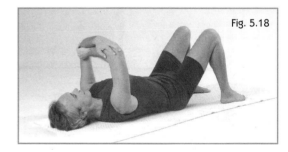

Fig. 5.18

4. Open your eyes and find a point on the ceiling. Receive this visual reference point through the window of your eyes down into your belly. This is your visual anchor. Holding on to your elbows and with your eyes focused on this point, lower your elbows over to the right side (**fig 5.19**). Without using force or effort, see how far the elbows go toward the ground on your right side without losing sight of the visual reference point on the ceiling.

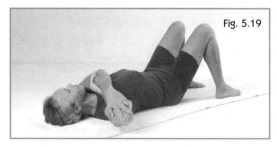

Fig. 5.19

5. Bring the elbows back up to the midline over your torso and then lower them again to your right side; repeat this sequence four or five times. Inhale and exhale with the movement. Notice the action in your left shoulder blade as you lower the elbows to the right. Each time you lower your elbows to the right imagine that your left shoulder blade wings out, gliding from the center to the left side of your back rib cage.

6. Release your elbows and lower your arms to the ground (**fig 5.20**). As you close your eyes, do you notice one shoulder feeling heavier than the other?

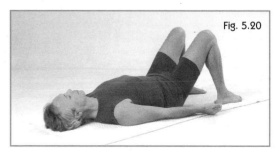

Fig. 5.20

7. Open your eyes and receive your visual reference point. Now take hold of your elbows and repeat this same movement on the left side. Imagine the right shoulder blade winging out as you lower the elbows toward the left, all the while maintaining a soft focus on your visual reference point. Repeat the sequence a few times, inhaling and exhaling with the movement.

8. Release your elbows, lower your arms to the ground, and close your eyes. Notice the contact your shoulders now make

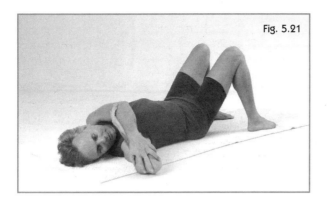

Fig. 5.21

with the ground. Use your kinesthetic sense to observe the internal effects of the movement.

9. Open your eyes, grasp your elbows, and lower them again to the right side. This time let your eyes follow your right elbow as it moves down toward the floor on the right side (**fig 5.21**). Notice how your head rolls in response to the eyes looking at your right elbow. As you follow the movement of your right elbow with your gaze, slow down to notice that your eyes are initiating the movement of turning your head to the right. Do your elbows come closer to the ground when you let your eyes and head

follow the movement of the elbows?

10. Continue this movement three or four times to the right side only. How far down your spine you can feel your breath moving as you continue the sequence?

11. Come to rest in the center, then repeat the movement, this time lowering the elbows to your left side. Watch your left elbow reach toward the floor and allow your head to roll, following the lead of your eyes. Continue this movement to the left side three or four times, then pause. What effects do you notice from your movements?

12. Now you are ready to let the elbows travel from one side to the other, following the movement with your eyes and your head. Remind yourself to breathe with the movement. Repeat this side-to-side movement seven or eight times, allowing the movement to become familiar and comfortable.

13. Release the elbows and lower your arms down to the ground. Close your eyes and experience the effects of the movement.

Integration: Head, Neck, and Shoulder Release

1. This movement series builds on the previous explorations; it will help free the head, allowing the head to move independent of the shoulders. Once again, open your eyes and take hold of your elbows. Begin the previous pattern, lowering your elbows to one side and then the other as your eyes and head follow.

2. Now leave the elbows on the right side. Keeping the elbows where they are, slowly begin to let your gaze look toward your left, with your head following the movement of your eyes (**fig. 5.22**). See how far you can look to the left until your chin bumps into

your left shoulder. Reach your left shoulder down toward your ankle and see if the head can roll a little farther.

3. Let your eyes look to the place on the floor where you imagine your left ear would touch. Hold this position for a few deep breaths. Notice how far down your spine you can feel your breath moving. Before releasing the position, gently nod your head in the "yes" movement, allowing the back of your neck to release. The "yes" movement releases the sternocleidomastoid muscles, the long, cable-like muscles that connect the head to the torso. These

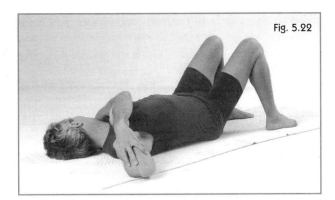

Fig. 5.22

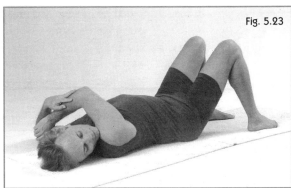

Fig. 5.23

muscles are often unwittingly switched "on" on one side of the neck and "off" on the other side. Conscious and exploratory "yes" movements restore the natural balance of these muscles.

4. Now lead with your vision back to the right and roll your head along until you are gazing at your right elbow once again.

5. Reverse sides by lowering your elbows over to the left, eyes and head following the elbows. Holding your elbows to the left, let your gaze slowly turn to the right, looking toward the place on the floor where you imagine your right ear would touch (**fig. 5.23**). Holding this position for a moment, reach your right shoulder and arm toward your right foot to create space for your head to roll a little farther. Look to the place on the floor where you imagine your right ear would touch. Take a few deep breaths. Make the "yes" movement with your head, releasing the back of your neck.

6. Bring your elbows back to the midline of your body, then begin lowering your elbows in one direction as your gaze and your head turn in the opposite direction. Slow down and let the pattern form. It is natural to get confused at first. That is a natural stage in learning a new pattern. Allow the confusion.

7. Repeat until you have the pattern of elbows going in one direction, eyes and head looking to the opposite side at the

place where you imagine your ear would touch the floor. Breathe into the movement. Go back and forth several times until you experience a rhythm in your movement.

8. Keep the movement going a few times and see if you can notice the precise moment that the eyes and the elbows cross at the midline of your body.

9. Now let go of the elbows and lower your arms to the ground. Stretch your legs long on the ground. Close your eyes and experience the effects of the movement. Notice any pulsing, streaming, or tingling sensations that may begin to occur.

10. Notice any internal shifts that occur as you lie on the ground. Particularly notice the curves beneath your neck and low back. Are they closer to the ground than when you began? Suggest to your logical mind that your body has released the muscles of your neck and low back to work in harmony.

11. How does it feel to have the freedom to roll your head in the opposite direction from your elbows, arms, and shoulders? Imagine how your head, neck, and shoulders might work together in a seated spinal twist posture after completing this inquiry.

12. Begin your return by rocking your ankles from the inner anklebones to the outer anklebones. Roll your wrists from the inner wrist bones to the outer wrist bones. Roll your head from ear to ear.

13. Bring up a good stretch. Allow your

breath to deepen and let any sounds come out that happen spontaneously as you stretch.

14. Curl your knees into your chest, rock from side to side, and roll up into a sitting position. Open your eyes and notice if your vision or sense of hearing has altered in any way.

15. Slowly come up to standing. Do you feel any taller? How do your shoulders hang? Does your head feel like it is more centered over your body? Take a few steps and notice the way your feet contact the ground. Notice the way your hips and pelvis move as you walk.

Before Moving On . . .

The inquiries of this chapter can help you to become familiar with ways to release your body into gravity and so experience natural alignment in standing. You may have begun to notice that as your body changes so does your emotional stance in life. Are there any areas of your body that seem to hold more tension than others? What changes are you noticing in these areas? Becoming conscious of releasing some of the chronic tension in your body is a starting point for discovering greater resourcefulness and openness in situations that might habitually bring forth feelings of frustration, resistance, and reactivity. By taking a little time to reflect on the personal effects of these inquiries, or by recording in your journal the changes you are observing, you may discover ideas for applying your learning to daily life.

The inquiries in the following chapter focus more specifically on releasing the cervical and lumbar spine, where the deepest patterns of chronic stress are often hiding. The muscles in these particular areas of the body are the first responders to the "fight or flight" scenarios that arise throughout life. Balancing the effects of gravity in these areas of your body can begin to restore greater balance and peace of mind to your life.

6 Restoring Natural Alignment by Balancing the Cervical and Lumbar Curves

How does releasing the "fight or flight" patterns of muscular stress from the neck and pelvis bring the spine into equilibrium?

THE THREE SHOCK-ABSORBING CURVES OF THE SPINE allow us the freedom to move, walk, and run without jarring or damaging the internal organs housed in our trunk and held gently in place by muscles and connective tissue. Imagine what would happen if the spine were straight and rigid, like a broom handle. Even the simple action of walking would continuously jolt the delicate organs.

The cervical curve of the neck, the thoracic curve of the middle back, and the lumbar curve of the low back are delicately counterbalanced in an S shape to prevent injury. Along these spinal curves lie dense nerve networks that are the "hardwiring" for the human being's first-response, or survival, mechanisms—our instinctual reflexes for responding to the threat of danger. With the rapid evolution of human beings in a social context, this survival mechanism, known as the fight or flight response, has expanded from environmentally driven scenarios—do I have enough food in my body? is that predator going to take me down?—to situations where the perceived danger may not be an actual threat to physical existence at all. These perceived threats are based on psychosocial factors and revolve around questions of whether we are loved and approved of and whether we'll receive the material things that we believe to be necessary to our survival. The continual perception of threat and lack of safety, no matter what the origin, leads to chronic fear or anxiety that gets lodged in the muscles of the cervical and lumbar curves of the spine.

Centering over the Feet by
Balancing the Natural Spinal Curves

One of our greatest developmental challenges is to learn to interact with gravity in a way that allows us to stand on our own two feet. In comparison to the height and weight of the entire body mass when you are standing, the feet are relatively small, especially considering that they must support the looming structure of the upright body. By releasing into the natural curves of the cervical and lumbar spine, you aid the body in distributing the weight of your head and torso for achieving more efficient balance over your feet.

To illustrate how the inquiries from a supine position affect your standing posture, come into a standing position. As in Head Roll, imagine the weight of your head moving backward into a bowl. Exaggerate by moving the backside of your head backward until you feel the entire weight of your body moving onto your heels (**fig. 6.1**). If you go too far, your toes lift off the floor and you will begin to fall backward. Move your head as far backward as you can *without falling* and notice how this backward movement of your head straightens out the curve in back of your neck (**fig. 6.2**). This exaggeration of the backward positioning of the head is often described as the "military neck."

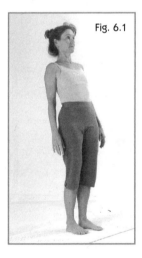
Fig. 6.1

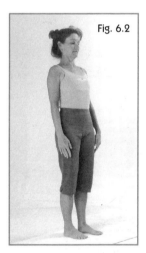
Fig. 6.2

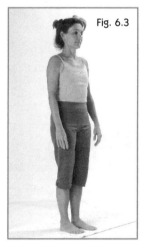
Fig. 6.3

In Head Roll, the directions begin with allowing the head to move backward into a bowl, then the bowl glides upward onto the crown. Use that same image of allowing the bowl to glide upward to the crown and experience how the curve of your neck is restored, centering your head over your spine (**fig. 6.3**). Can you sense how releasing the cervical curve allows the lumbar curve to release and how your whole torso comes to a natural balance, supported by your feet?

Play with the same images and inquiries in this chapter from a standing to notice how you have more options available for participating with gravity while standing.

When you think about (or encounter) a terrifying situation, do your shoulders tense up around your ears? do you clench your jaw? does your breathing become shallow and all of your senses go on hyperalert? To this list of physiological responses to fear add the stress you might hold around speaking up for yourself or communicating your needs and you begin to get a picture of why the cervical curve holds so much tension. "Swallow my words," "bite my tongue," "running off at the mouth," "choking under pressure"—these are just a few of the ways we commonly describe the experience of a disruption in the free flow of energy through the neck and throat.

Another first responder to stress is the low back. Physical responses to fear cause the belly to constrict, shifting the center of gravity high into the thoracic cavity to mobilize the organism for rapid flight. The fight or flight reaction to stress is biologically instinctual. In many dangerous situations we do not have to think about how to protect ourselves; the instinctual wisdom of the organism takes over. Yet in circumstances where a person has experienced repeated threats or brutal physical, sexual, or psychological traumas, the instinct for self-protection can become suppressed to the extent that immobilization becomes habitual even in the most life-threatening circumstances. While we are instinctually programmed to mobilize our defenses in response to acute stress, there is no equivalent relaxation response in the human body; your organism does not necessarily quit protecting itself after a danger has passed. In fact, relaxation is a learned response; muscles do not know when they no longer need to protect. It requires awareness to consciously release tension after the body has been quickened by a threat of imminent danger. Without recovering our awareness of the instinctual fight or flight mechanism and without conscious assessment of the accuracy of our perceptions of danger, the body holds on to unnecessary tension.

Our bodies can cope with high anxiety for short periods; however, as suggested above, when the perception of threat becomes habitual and the survival response is continually activated, we get locked into a state of chronic stress and all the physiological reactions that accompany it: the heart beats faster and pumps more blood to produce the energy needed to fight or flee; the digestive, reproductive, and immune systems switch off or function at a reduced or elevated levels that can only be sustained for short periods of time. When the organs and glands continually function at a suboptimal level and the cervical and lumbar curves become chronically stressed and rigid, the entire organism is subject to premature breakdown. It is critical to your physical health and overall well-being to acknowledge the sources of chronic stress that bear upon you and to create strategies that allow you to respond to stress with awareness, rather than to remain in unconscious, habitual reactions that further reinforce suffering.

In addition to chronic anxiety and unresolved fight or flight muscle patterns, another factor that contributes to fatigue in the cervical and lumbar curves is weak abdominal muscles. When the abdominal muscles forget that it is their duty to support the spine, the muscles of the low back are forced into performing a job that they were not designed for. Another factor that compromises the health of the spinal curves is lifestyle choices. For example, wearing shoes with elevated heels exaggerates the lumbar curve by tilting the pelvis forward, shortening the muscles supporting the lumbar spine. Slouching in poorly designed chairs that don't support the spine forces the muscles of the low back to overstretch and the upper body to stoop. Carrying excess weight in the belly pulls the center of gravity forward and forces the upper trunk to lean backward to counterbalance the weight.

The purpose of the inquiries in this chapter is to support the body to relax and to remind the neuromuscular response centers along the cervical and lumbar spine of their natural functional relationships to one another. Muscles that are either not used at all or are not used properly have likely forgotten their nature and function; many of the movement patterns in these inquiries are habitual and are performed unconsciously. The explorations in this chapter will reveal the connections between the subtle ways that you may be holding on to unconscious tension in your neck, shoulders, and low back and will stimulate awareness of how to move with greater range of motion, flexibility, and freedom in your spine. When provided the opportunity for exploring new options, the body—specifically the neuromuscular system—will always let go of inefficient habitual patterns to reorganize into higher levels of efficiency, effortlessness, and pleasure.

These explorations are organized according to the way your body is designed to move when it is free from the posture of anticipating danger or unconsciously maintaining a defensive or aggressive preparedness. By constantly consuming your energy, maintaining continuous fight or flight posturing in the body actually decreases your ability to respond to perceived threats with maximum strength. When you consciously resolve fight or flight posturing by breathing and relaxing into the muscles and organs, your cells have the opportunity to release accumulated lactic acid and other toxins and receive a fresh supply of oxygen and nutrients that restore balance and even begin to repair the cellular damage brought on by overexertion.

The first set of explorations in this chapter, Opening the Middle and Upper Back, expands the upper body for greater ease in yoga postures such as Downward Dog, Eagle, Yoga Mudra, and Spinal Twist. The second set of explorations, Mobilizing and Synchronizing Movement in the Neck and Pelvis, balances the abdominal and lumbar muscles and opens the bowl of the pelvis for a free flow of prana to rehabilitate chronic imbalances in the digestive, eliminative, and reproductive sytems. Essentially every seated or standing yoga posture requires stable balance in the pelvis. The Cat tilt required in front extensions such as the Cobra, Bow, and Camel poses counterbalances the Dog tilt required in forward-bending postures such as Seated Posterior Stretch,

Standing Forward Bend, and Yoga Mudra. When muscles that stabilize the pelvis and low back are working efficiently, the muscles of the cervical spine are free to do their job of supporting the head. Without this stable foundation in the lower body, the neck and shoulders have to do additional work of pulling upward to support the middle and upper back. The result is greater rigidity and decreased flexibility in the entire spine.

The Pelvic Compass and the Cranio-Sacral Balance explorations here provide a highly supported and therapeutic condition for releasing unnecessary muscular contractions along the spine and for differentiating and toning muscles that are underused. The foundation you establish in reeducating the cervical and lumbar spine to work in relationship to one another is essential before moving into reverse yoga postures—such as Shoulderstand, Plow, and Headstand—which place increased pressure on the fragile structures of the upper back and neck.

Opening the Middle and Upper Back: Folded Empty Coat Sleeves

Inquiry: How do the lumbar and cervical curves work in a balanced relationship to one another?

These explorations take you back to embryonic time, a period in your development when your organism was one long spine with a mouth at one end and a tail at the other. With only the undulations of the spine to propel movement, every segment of the spine moves in sequence and rhythm. Building on this pattern, the movement of the head and shoulders gets differentiated from the rest of the trunk, freeing prana to release restrictions from the shoulders up through the cervical curve. In the last phase, the lumbar spine is freed to move independent of the trunk, completing a full release of restrictions along the spine. This sequence increases flexibility and openness in yoga postures that require a fluid relationship in movement of all segments of the spine.

Exploration 1: Opening the Upper Back by Spreading the Shoulders

1. Begin by lying on your back, legs long on the ground (fig. 6.4). Suggest to your logical mind that this is a time for attuning to the sensations that arise within your body. Are there any adjustments to make that will help you settle into gravity? In this exploration, you will encourage your shoulders to spread wide across your back, freeing the spine from the movements of the shoulders.

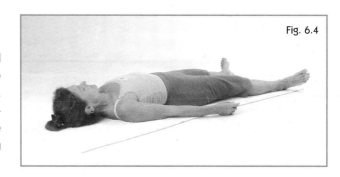

Fig. 6.4

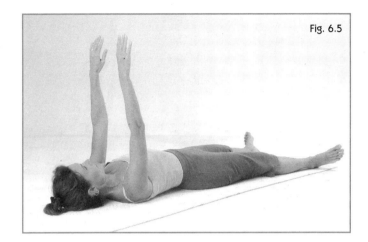

Fig. 6.5

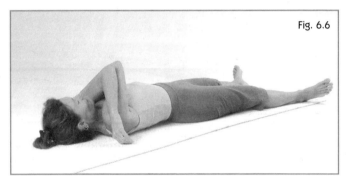

Fig. 6.6

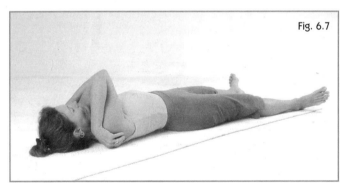

Fig. 6.7

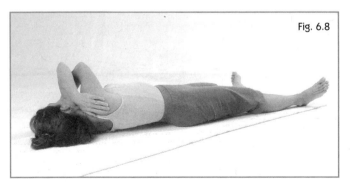

Fig. 6.8

2. Imagine the impression your body makes on the ground. Scan your body to observe any areas that resist the pull of gravity or are holding on in some way. Let any resistance be as it is—there is no need to alter your experience as you begin to enter deeper levels of awareness.

3. Sending your kinesthetic awareness to the curve at the low back, can you sense how much space there is between your low back and the ground? Could you roll a grapefruit through that arch? how about a golf ball? How much space is there between the ground and the spinal curve at your neck? Could you roll a marble through that arch?

4. As you bring awareness to your breathing, notice how your upper and middle back moves with the breath. Can you feel the backside of your rib cage and shoulder blades? How heavy are your shoulders? Take note of how your body feels at this moment.

5. Open your eyes and establish a visual reference point on the ceiling. Reach both arms upward to that point, inhaling as you extend (**fig. 6.5**). Bend at the elbows and fold your arms across your torso as though they were empty coat sleeves. Imagine the way coat sleeves would look if there were no arms inside of them; play around with the placement of your arms to see if there is a way to leave your elbows folded over your chest without having to hold them in place (**fig. 6.6**). You can move the elbows higher, over your collarbones, or even fold them across your chin. When you have your arms in a comfortable folded position, pause and notice your breathing.

6. As you rest your arms in this position, notice how your shoulder blades are spreading apart on the backside of your body. How far down your spine does your breath move in this position? Notice the contact the backside of your rib cage makes with the ground.

7. Now grasp your shoulders with your hands (**fig. 6.7**). Focusing your gaze on your reference point, begin to move your elbows from side to side in a pendulum-like motion (**fig. 6.8**). Make sure you are firmly grasping your shoulders with opposite hands. As the elbows move to one side, notice how the opposite shoulder comes up and off the ground. Exaggerate the movement a bit to see how much of the opposite shoulder you can get up and off the ground.

8. Release the movement, making note of which elbow was on top. Stretch your arms out to your sides and notice any effects from this movement.

9. Fold your elbows again, this time with the opposite elbow on top. Does this feel a little more awkward than the first side? Generally, we choose the familiar side first and the second side feels a bit awkward in the beginning. Pause and let the weight of

your arms ride on your rib cage as your chest rises and falls with the breath. As you allow your arms to get heavier, can you sense the ribs softening and the breath moving into the backside of your ribs?

10. Focus your gaze above you; as you are ready, begin the pendulum movement of your elbows side to side, seeing how much of the opposite shoulder you can get up and off of ground. Notice how your legs

Elbow Compass

Here is a very interesting way to open the shoulder girdle. This movement is particularly effective for releasing tiredness after too many repetitions of Downward Dog by bringing awareness to the reciprocal, or complementary, muscles.

Begin lying in a comfortable position on your back. Reach your right hand overhead, placing your fingertips and palm near or under your shoulder. You can place your fingertips closer to your shoulder by increasing the bend of your elbow. Reach your left hand over to take hold of the knob of your right elbow **(fig. 6.10)**. Hold the elbow securely, right hand under your shoulder. With more flexibility, more of your palm will come closer to the floor.

Experience the stretch in your wrist and shoulder, and anywhere else that you notice any unusual sensations. This may be a position you have never placed your arm and shoulder into before. Slow down and enjoy the novelty of the sensations.

Using your left hand to initiate the movement, notice how you can move your right elbow into different

angles. Move the elbow from side to side, finding east and west on an imaginary compass. Try this a few times and notice your range of movement.

Now move your elbow to the north and south **(fig. 6.11)**. The elbow is a complex joint; in the up-and-down movement the elbow will move only a fraction of an inch. Do not force or push beyond your comfort zone. Notice where the limitations exist. Breathe into the sensations. Scan the rest of your body to see how this movement affects the way your body is positioned on the ground.

Release the elbow to the ground and notice the effects by comparing the difference in the way the two arms and shoulders feel on the ground. Now repeat the shoulder compass with your right hand holding your left elbow.

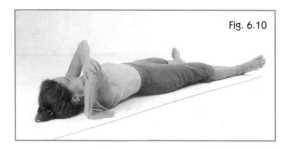

Fig. 6.10

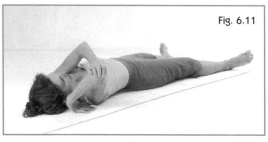

Fig. 6.11

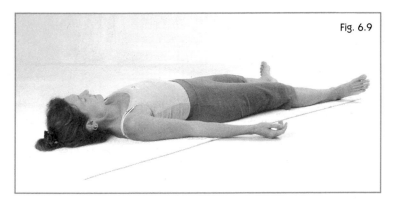

Fig. 6.9

want to get involved in the movement. Do the back of your heels want to exaggerate the movement by pressing into the ground?

11. Right now you are performing a very

contained movement. By allowing the movement to stay contained in this way, you are reminding the spine and nervous system of a time early in its evolutionary development when you had no arms or legs to move through the water. Like a fish, the wavelike motion of the spine propels you through the waters.

12. Release the movement when you feel ready and relax your arms back down to the ground (**fig. 6.9**). What sensations do you notice along your spine? How much space is there now between your low back and the ground? between your cervical curve and the ground? How is the backside of your body moving with your breath?

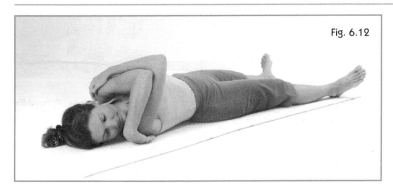

Fig. 6.12

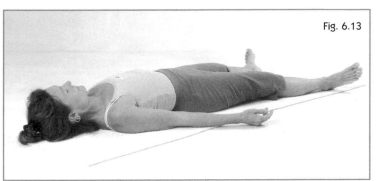

Fig. 6.13

Exploration 2: Balancing the Cervical and Lumbar Curves

1. Lying on your back, fold your arms over your torso and grasp your shoulders. Begin to move your elbows from side to side. Keep this movement going but this time allow your eyes and head to roll in the same direction as your elbows are going (**fig. 6.12**). Look with your eyes to the place on the floor where your ear would touch. Does this allow you to get more of the opposite shoulder up and off of the ground? How does it feel to allow your gaze to go with you, rolling your head in the same direction as the elbows?

2. Release the movement, noticing which elbow was on top. Bring the opposite elbow on top and repeat the movement a few times, allowing the eyes and head to roll with you. Stretch your arms out to your sides and notice any effects from this movement (**fig. 6.13**).

3. Until this point the focus of your movement has been the middle and upper back. Now we'll involve the low back as well. Bend both knees, sliding your feet a comfortable distance toward your buttocks. Notice the contact your low back makes with the floor. Keeping your knees upright, fold your arms as empty coat sleeves over your chest (**fig. 6.14**). This time your eyes are going to look to the opposite direction as your elbows.

4. Begin the pendulum motion of your elbows moving to one side and your eyes looking to the opposite side (**fig. 6.15**). On each side, look to the place on the floor where your ear would touch the ground. How much of the left shoulder can you lift when you are looking to your left? How much of the right shoulder can you lift when you are looking to your right? Let your knees wobble in response to the movement in your upper body. Experience how much of a twisting stretch can happen along your spine when your heels press into the ground and your head is moving in the opposite direction as your elbows.

5. When you feel ready, release the movement and repeat the sequence with the opposite elbow on top. Changing sides helps to create balance between the left and right sides of the body.

6. When you are ready to finish, release your arms to the ground, stretch your legs long, and begin to receive the flurry of sensations traveling throughout your body. What are you noticing about the way the backside of your body is breathing? Has your lumbar curve relaxed toward the ground? What about your cervical curve?

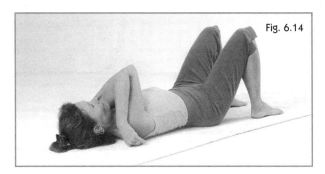

Fig. 6.14

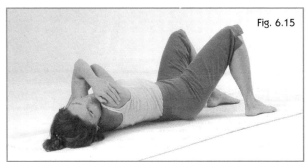

Fig. 6.15

Integration: Reclining Eagle— A Self-Chiropractic Release

1. For this integration movement, fold your arms as in the explorations above, noticing which elbow is on top. Bend your knees; the knee on the opposite side of the body from the top elbow crosses the other knee (**fig. 6.16**). (If the right elbow is on top then your left knee will be crossed over the right knee and vice versa.) Play around with the placement of your legs to find a beginning place that feels grounded. The lower foot remains in contact with the ground as an anchor. If you are familiar with the Eagle pose, experiment with hooking the foot of the upper leg behind the calf of the lower leg (**fig. 6.17**).

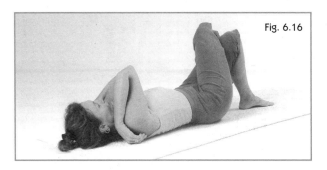

Fig. 6.16

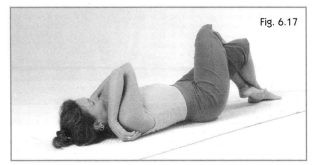

Fig. 6.17

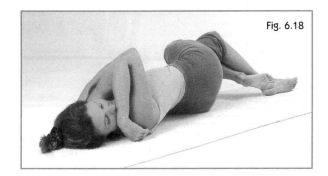

Fig. 6.18

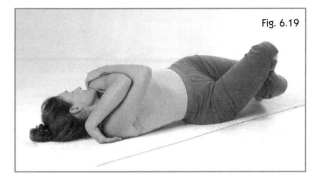

Fig. 6.19

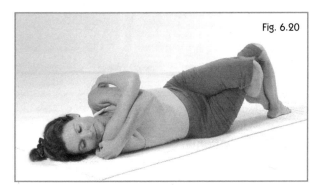

Fig. 6.20

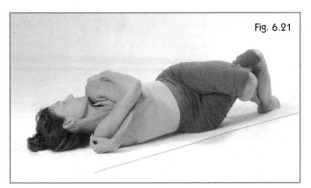

Fig. 6.21

2. Begin the movement by taking the folded elbows to one side and the knees to the opposite side (**fig. 6.18**). Experiment with how far you can relax into the movement without creating discomfort. You do not need to go beyond your comfort zone. When you find the range of motion that feels familiar and effortless, begin to repeat the action side to side, noticing the stretch that happens at the low back. Allow your eyes and head to turn in the same direction as your elbows are moving.

3. After a few repetitions, let the eyes and head roll to the opposite direction as the elbows, looking to the place on the floor where your ear would touch (**fig. 6.19**).

4. After repeating this movement a few times, leave the knees on one side as a heavy anchoring for the lower body while you keep the movement going in the upper body. This phase may give you some spinal adjustments, which you'll likely hear as cracking along the spine. There is no extra charge for your free chiropractic adjustment!

5. Slowly bring the knees over to the other side and repeat the upper-body movement a few times.

6. Bring the elbows and knees to upright and again notice which of your elbows and knees are on top. Reverse the pattern, bringing the other elbow and the opposite knee on top. Begin the movement on this side. Let your body do the movement for you. Find a way to move on this side that feels deeply satisfying all along your spine. Initially let the gaze follow the elbows (**fig. 6.20**), then shift the gaze so that it is looking at the opposite side as the elbows are moving (**fig. 6.21**). Allow any sounds to emerge that want to happen. Slow down and explore any nooks and crannies in your body that get revealed in this interesting movement.

7. When you are ready, return your elbows and knees to neutral, stretch out your arms and legs along the ground, and experience the effects of the movement (**fig. 6.22**). Allow your breath to flow in and out without attempting to control or inhibit the breath in any way. Notice any pulsing, streaming, or tingling sensations.

8. Notice any changes that occur as you lie on the ground; particularly notice the curves beneath your neck and low back. Are they closer to the ground than when you began? How do your shoulders contact the ground? Do you sense more of your spine and rib cage touching the ground?

9. Imagine how it would feel to be standing and entering

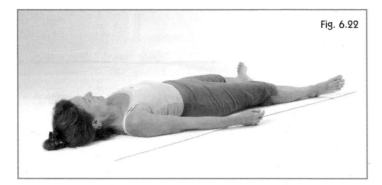

Fig. 6.22

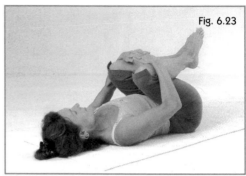

Fig. 6.23

into Eagle pose. How would your arms and legs move to enter the posture with greater ease?

10. Begin your return by rocking your ankles from the inner anklebones to the outer anklebones. Roll your wrists from the inner wrist bones to the outer wrist bones. Roll your head from ear to ear.

11. Deepen your breath and bring up a good stretch. Allow any sounds that happen spontaneously as you stretch. Curl your knees into your chest **(fig. 6.23)**, rock from side to side, and roll up into a sitting position **(fig. 6.24)**. Open your eyes and notice whether your vision has changed in any way.

12. Slowly come up to standing **(fig. 6.25)**. Do you feel any taller? How do your shoulders hang? Does your head feel more centered over your body? Take a few steps and notice the way your feet contact the ground. Notice the way your hips and pelvis move as you walk.

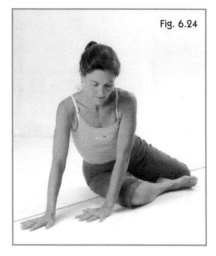

Fig. 6.24

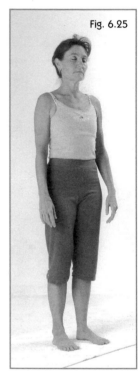

Fig. 6.25

13. Experiment with moving into Eagle pose. Notice the effects of this inquiry on your ability to hold Eagle pose with easy stability.

Mobilizing and Synchronizing Movement in the Neck and Pelvis

Inquiry: What experiences arise when freedom and mobility are restored in the neck and pelvis?

The pelvic bowl houses the most potent concentration of prana in the body. The reproductive organs contain the power to produce new life. In addition to the many structural issues described above, the pelvis is also the place from which we express (or suppress) our natural sexual energies; thus, the pelvis is intimately tied with our feelings of being safe with regard to the appropriate expression of our sexuality and being accepted or desirable in our relationships. By restoring the natural range of motion to the pelvis and becoming comfortable with its pendulum-like motion, the body regains the ability to engage in the Cat tilt and to retract in the Dog tilt.

Exploration 1, the Hip Thump, brings awareness to the hips, creating permission to experience the size, shape, and weight of the hip bones and muscles and providing a way to differentiate their movement from one another. The Pelvic Compass exploration awakens full, circular range of motion in the pelvis. This exploration is the single most effective movement for releasing low-back pain and stabilizing the muscles by bringing up the natural tone of the pelvic floor, and gives the added effect of balancing the abdominal muscles with the muscles of the low back. The Cranio-Sacral Balance sets up a communication link between the low back and the neck, which encourages a deeply relaxing flow of energy throughout the entire spine. Yoga postures that are affected by these movements include all front extensions (for example, Cobra, Bow, Wheel, and Camel) and all forward bends (including Hero, Chin-to-Knee, Posterior Stretch, and Standing Forward Bend). Standing postures, such as Downward Dog, Mountain, and the Warrior series, are benefited due to the increased stability in the pelvic floor.

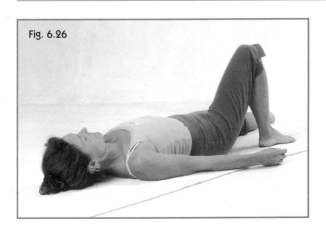

Fig. 6.26

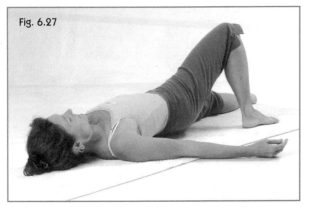

Fig. 6.27

Exploration 1: Hip Thump

1. Lie down on the ground with your legs long. Notice the contact your body makes with the ground as you settle. Sense the shape your body makes on the ground. Observe any areas that seem to resist the pull of gravity or are holding on in some way. Let any resistance be as it is.

2. Engaging your kinesthetic awareness, sense the distance between your low back and the ground. Bend the right knee, sliding your foot along the ground until the foot is standing a comfortable distance from your right buttock (**fig. 6.26**). With your knee upright toward the ceiling and your foot grounded, notice the contact your foot makes with the floor. Imagine that you are standing on this foot.

3. Leaving this foot standing, press into the heel to lift the right hip ¼ inch off the ground (**fig. 6.27**). Inhale as you press and lift; exhale and let the hip thump back down to the ground. Feel for the entire weight of your hip to release downward with the thump. When your hip is as heavy as it can be, press into the heel, lift, and let it thump again.

4. Now put a little speed into the movement, lifting and releasing the hip for a steady "thump, thump, thump."

5. Let go of the movement as you slide the foot along the floor and stretch your right leg long (**fig. 6.28**). Notice the difference in the way your two legs feel on the ground.

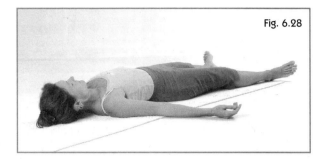

Fig. 6.28

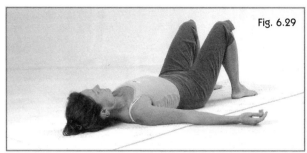

Fig. 6.29

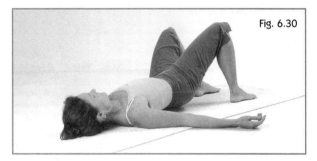

Fig. 6.30

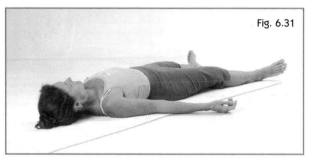

Fig. 6.31

Does one leg feel longer or heavier than the other? Observe any pulsing, streaming, or tingling sensations.

6. Before moving on the other side, tell yourself that this is a new side. Allow the two sides to be as different as they actually are. Now bend the left knee and repeat the Hip Thump on the left side.

7. When you've completed the movement on both sides, bend both knees, bringing your feet a comfortable distance from your hips **(fig. 6.29)**. With both feet standing and your knees pointed toward the ceiling, notice whether the curve in your low back has lengthened down toward the ground.

8. Imagine a ball bearing situated in the hinge of your right hip. As you press into your right heel and lift the right hip slightly off the ground, that ball bearing rolls downhill to the hinge of the left hip **(fig. 6.30)**. Lower the right hip to the ground in a thump. Wait for it to get heavy. Then repeat on the other side: pressing into the left heel to lift the left hip slightly and imagining the ball bearing rolling downhill to the right hip. Alternate back and forth a few times until the image and sensa-

tion of rolling the ball bearing back and forth becomes clearly distinguishable.

10. Continue the movement but let go of the image of rolling the ball bearing. We are going to locate east and west on an imaginary compass. Imagine that the contact your right hip makes with the ground is east; where your left hip contacts the ground is west. Lift and lower your right and left hips back and forth to find east and west on your imaginary compass.

11. Let go of the image of a pelvic compass and put a little speed in the movement. Experience what happens when you let go of the control of the movement, when you let your mind get out of the way and allow the movement to take over. Let anything that wants to happen through your body emerge.

12. Stretch out both legs and come back into stillness **(fig. 6.31)**. Observe any pulsing, streaming, or tingling sensations.

13. Notice any changes or effects that occur as you lie on the ground. Particularly notice the curve beneath your low back. Is it closer to the ground than when you began?

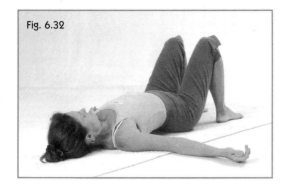

Fig. 6.32

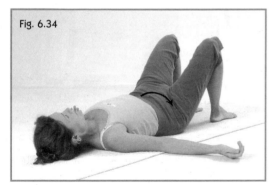

Fig. 6.33

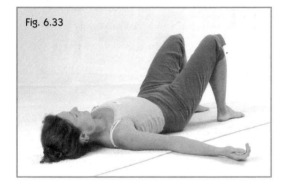

Fig. 6.34

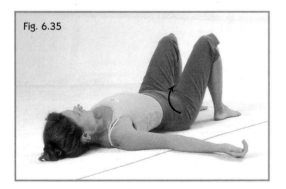

Fig. 6.35

Exploration 2: Pelvic Compass—Finding North and South Pole

1. Bend both knees, standing your feet a comfortable distance from your buttocks. With both knees upright toward the ceiling and your feet grounded, notice the contact your low back makes with the floor.

2. We are now going to establish the poles of an imaginary compass on the ground. The tip of your tailbone is the south pole. Press into your heels and arch your low back off the ground, bringing the tip of your tailbone toward the ground (**fig. 6.32**). The place where your belt cross the back of your spine is the north pole. Lengthen your low back to the ground and press the belt line toward the ground to find the north pole (**fig. 6.33**).

3. Repeat this movement from south to north pole by alternately arching and enlongating your low back. Notice how your breath wants to get involved in the movement. Inhale in one direction and exhale in the other direction. Observe whether any other part of your body is tensing or trying to help. Experiment with localizing the movement to your low back, allowing the rest of your body to remain heavy and relaxed.

4. Now we are going to locate all four directions of the compass. Recall that the right hip contacts the floor to the east; the left hip contacts the floor to the west. Begin the movement by setting the compass at the north pole, pressing the belt line into the floor. Rotate your pelvis from north to east (**fig. 6.34**) and then return to north. Go back and forth several times until you feel connected with the movement in this quadrant of the compass.

5. Set the compass to east by pressing the right hip into the floor and then roll to the south pole, pointing the tailbone to the ground and arching the low back (**fig. 6.35**). Move back and forth in this quadrant from east to south. Repeat enough times that you feel connected with the movement in this quadrant of the compass.

6. Move now from the south pole around to the left hip, or west (**fig. 6.36**). Repeat the movement back and forth until it feels familiar.

7. Complete the last quadrant by moving from west back up to the north pole (**fig. 6.37**). When this movement feels familiar through repetition, rest for a moment. Reflect: which quadrant felt easier? Notice which quadrant was fuzzier in your awareness or felt less mobile. Return to that quadrant and repeat the movement a few times, going very slowly and noticing each point on the floor around the compass.

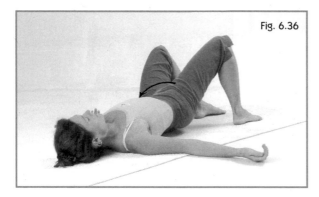

Fig. 6.36

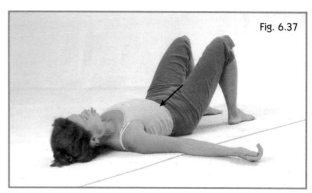

Fig. 6.37

8. Set the compass to the north pole by pressing the belt line toward the floor. Moving very slowly, go all the way around the compass, imagining each point in the circle. Repeat until the circular movement of your pelvis and hips against the ground feels familiar. Then reverse the movement and circle in the opposite direction. Notice any awkward or "fuzzy" points along the compass; go back and forth in that area until it becomes familiar. Keep the breath flowing naturally as you move.

9. Let go of the image of a pelvic compass. Put little speed in the movement, letting go of all conscious control. Experience what happens when you let the movement take over. Allow any expression that wants to emerge through your body.

10. Pause and rest a moment. Notice any pulsing, streaming, or tingling sensations that arise anywhere in your body.

11. Stretch out both legs and come back into stillness. Observe the effects of these movements throughout your whole body. Notice any changes or effects that occur as you lie on the ground. Particularly notice the curve beneath your low back. Is it closer to the ground than when you began?

Integration: Cranio-Sacral Balance

1. Lie on the ground on your back. Bend both knees and slide your feet a comfortable distance from your buttocks. Bring your kinesthetic awareness to the cervical curve, the spinal curve at your neck. Can you sense the tilt of your head by observing the angle of your nose? If you had a paintbrush extending from your nose, would the paintbrush be angled down toward your chest, up toward the wall behind you, or straight up toward the ceiling?

2. As the pelvic compass brings awareness and relaxation to the low back, the cranial compass brings awareness to the cervical curve. To locate the poles of the cranial

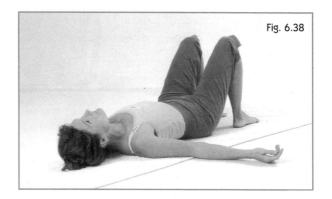

Fig. 6.38

compass, we will be using the nose as a pointer. Arch your neck slightly, pointing your nose toward the wall behind you **(fig. 6.38)**. This is north. Point your nose down toward your

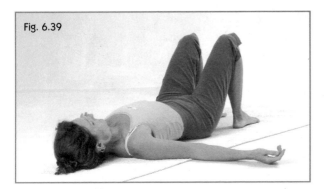

Fig. 6.39

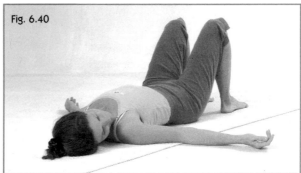

Fig. 6.40

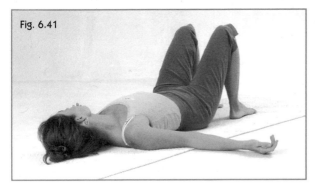

Fig. 6.41

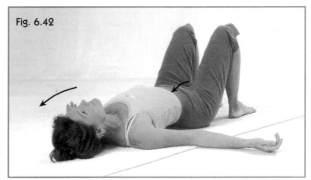

Fig. 6.42

chest (**fig. 6.39**). This is south. Rock the bowl of your head forward and back, alternating between north and south. Can you bring breath into your movement by inhaling in one direction and exhaling in the other? Breathe freely as you continue the movement.

3. Pause and experience the sensations in the back of your neck, or anywhere else you notice an effect in your body.

4. Now point your nose toward your right side, moving your right ear down toward the ground (**fig. 6.40**). This is east. Move your nose along the horizon of your vision, turning to point the nose over toward your left side and bringing your left ear down toward the ground (**fig. 6.41**). This is west. Roll your head back and forth from ear to ear, from east to west. When the movement becomes familiar, pause.

5. Set the compass to north by pointing the nose upward toward the wall behind you. Begin rotating the nose slowly toward the

right ear, moving from north to east, repeating back and forth a few times. Proceed through the quadrants of the compass—east to south, south to west, west to north, and north to east—noticing which movements seem more fluid and which seem fuzzier in your awareness. Repeat through the rotation a few times.

6. Set the compass to north and make full circular rotations, finding every point along the compass. Move slowly enough to visualize each point along the way. After several rotations, reverse the direction.

7. Let go of the movement and notice the effects. Observe any pulsing, streaming, or tingling sensations.

8. Now we are going to synchronize the movement between the pelvic compass and the head compass. Set the pelvic compass at north by pressing the belt line toward the floor, and set the nose compass at north by pointing the nose up toward the wall behind you (**fig. 6.42**). Inhale a

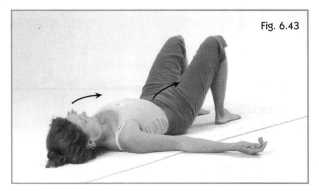

Fig. 6.43

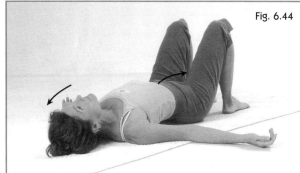

Fig. 6.44

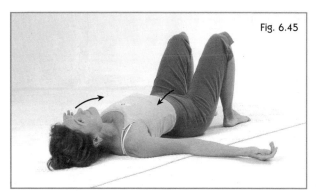

Fig. 6.45

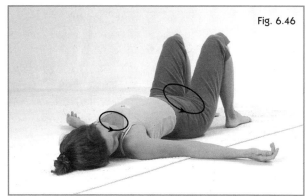

Fig. 6.46

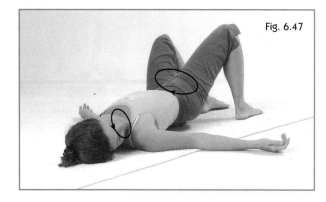

Fig. 6.47

deep breath. As you exhale, move both compasses to their respective south poles: to the tailbone and the chest (**fig. 6.43**). Alternate back and forth a few times until you become familiar with the synchronized movement.

9. Now we are going to differentiate the movement of the head and free it from the movement of the pelvis. Set the nose compass at north and the pelvic compass at south (**fig. 6.44**). Exhale as you reverse, moving the nose to south and the pelvis to north (**fig. 6.45**). This can be confusing. Allow the confusion to simply be; just experiment with the movement until it becomes familiar. Do you notice how this movement flexes and elongates the whole spine?

10. Now let the nose compass and the pelvic compass make full circular rotations in the same direction, all around the points of the compass (**fig. 6.46**). Repeat until the movement becomes familiar. Then reverse, moving both pelvis and nose in the opposite direction.

11. Experiment with letting the nose compass move in one direction and the pelvic compass move in the opposite direction (**fig. 6.47**). Play with this; if it becomes confusing, go back to synchronizing the movements in the same direction. When this pattern of movement becomes familiar, pay attention to your breathing. Allow your breath to flow freely as you move. Keep your jaw, shoulders, and fists relaxed and unclenched while you do the movement.

12. Pause and rest a moment. Notice any pulsing, streaming, or tingling sensations that arise anywhere in your body.

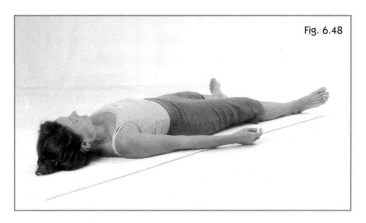

Fig. 6.48

13. Stretch out both legs and come back into stillness. Observe the effects of these movements throughout your whole body (fig. 6.48).

14. Notice any changes that occur as you lie on the ground. Particularly notice the curve beneath your low back. Is it closer to the ground than when you began? Notice the curve behind your neck. Does it feel closer to the ground?

15. How does it feel to synchronize the movements of your head and pelvis? As you give permission for all parts of your experience to be present, notice how quickly and effortlessly your body settles into relaxation. Observe how deeply your mind begins to slow down to attune to the sensations that are arising in your body. Where does your awareness travel as your body relaxes and your mind slows down?

16. As you receive from the wisdom of your organism, do you notice how you might use this experience to release stress in your neck and low back? Suggest to your logical mind that you will be returning with the knowledge and wisdom of your organism. You will be returning with the feeling of having had a healthy, rejuvenating sleep. You'll be returning wide awake, fully alert and ready to move on to the next events of your day.

17. Slowly begin your return, rocking your ankles from the inner anklebones to the outer anklebones. Roll your wrists from the inner wrist bones to the outer wrist bones. Roll your head from ear to ear.

18. Deepening your breath, bring up a good stretch, allowing any sound to emerge as you move. Curl your knees into your chest and rock from side to side. Roll to your side and up into a sitting position.

19. Notice the speed and momentum of your thoughts and thinking. Notice your mood. When you open your eyes notice whether your vision has altered in any way: are colors brighter or duller? shapes clearer or fuzzier? As you transition to your next activity, carry with you an awareness of having restored the natural curves in your spine.

Before Moving On . . ..

The inquiries of this chapter lead you to begin restoring the natural, shock-absorbing balance of your spine. By inquiring as to how the body's long-term response to stress has lodged tension in the cervical and lumbar spine, in the middle and upper back, and in the abdominal and pelvic floor, you gain access to movements that release rigidity and restore greater freedom of motion in your spine, and even in your entire body. Can you notice any differences in the way you now stand and move? Do you feel any taller or more buoyant in your step, or do you feel heavier or more grounded in any way? Do you notice any differences in the way you now carry your head or in how your shoulders and arms hang?

In addition to the physical and kinesthetic openings that result from these inquiries, you have just given yourself the opportunity to notice some of the emotional energies that are present in these areas of your body and perhaps have come upon issues that you will want to give more time and attention to. Many of our deeper feelings, thoughts, and insights that arise during these inquiries have waited a long time to surface into conscious awareness. To receive the fullness of the wisdom that is coming to you, you may want to chronicle your insights in your journal or choose to revisit particular experiences in this chapter.

When the body begins to awaken to its natural, unimpeded state, energy is released to travel into new territories of self-awareness. As your energy flow begins to pick up momentum, you may be faced with questions of what to do with all of this newfound vitality. The next chapter will give you ways to direct your energy toward the "solar battery" in the center of your belly. When you establish a sense of home base in your belly, you will notice a deepening of trust in your ability to venture further in inquiries that open you to an ever-increasing flow of prana.

7 Recharging the Body's "Energy Battery" in the Belly

How does accessing the creative fire of prana open new choices for being?

OUR SUN, THE STAR AT THE CENTER OF OUR SOLAR SYSTEM, has been worshiped as the source of life since the earliest humans developed the intelligence to track phenomenon occurring in the natural world. Buried deep in the epicenter of the human body is a complex network of nerves that generate enough combustion to power the metabolic processes of our entire organism. This vital center is called the solar plexus because the heat generated by the chemical and electrical reactions in this core has the same effect on our physical bodies that the sun has on our vast galaxy. Located at the intersection between the upper and lower extremities, between the right and left sides of the body, and between the front side and the back side, the solar plexus is known in many ancient cultures as the body's center, the "brain" of the cells.

Not only does the fire generated in the belly have the capacity to power the digestive processes of the physical organism; it also has the psychic potency to fuel the process of individuation in our personalities. In Japan this part of the body is known as the *hara*; in Japanese culture a person is not considered an adult until he (or she) has "made his belly." Making your belly means finding a sense of self in the middle of the continuous flow of life experiences that knock you off center—a place to return that feels like home when even the most challenging forces come against you. We in the West refer to people who have courage and conviction as having "guts." And in an absence of psychic strength to face challenges, we say that a person does not have the "stomach" for taking definitive action. We are made "sick to the stomach" when repulsed by behavior or circumstances over which we perceive that we have no control. The agony of indecision ties our belly into knots.

These physical, psychic, emotional, and personality states are summarized by one term in yogic philosophy: *ahankar,* or the sum total of all of our likes and dislikes, the characteristics that make us distinctly recognizable as individual egos. Without a healthy ego, the organism has no possibility for survival; however, when the power of fulfilling likes and dislikes consumes a person's entire identity, life becomes absorbed in accumulating the power to control circumstances and people to maintain a steady flow of getting what we want and avoiding what we fear or dislike, even at the expense of harming others. Developing a strong sense of worthiness to fully receive what we have together with owning our capabilities for getting what we want create self-confidence. But focusing on acquiring what we want can become a trap when we fixate entirely on getting what we want at all costs. By not allowing ourselves to fully enjoy our power to have and to get, we develop unconscious fears that we will never have enough, or that we must get everything we want to prove that we deserve it. The unconscious fears of unworthiness and insecurity actually have the effect of starving the belly's energy center, resulting in impotence to cause either beneficial or harmful effects on the world around us. In extremes, the fixation on personal power eclipses deeper dimensions of our being—our capacities for compassion, love, service, and surrender to mystery.

The purpose for strengthening the fire in the belly center is to generate an abundant supply of energy to fulfill both the survival needs of the body and the personality needs of a balanced ego. As human beings we are endowed with infinite capacity to channel energies to get what we want. Unless we validate our needs and desires, we go through life feeling unworthy to have what we are given, guilty for wanting other than what we have, or going unconscious with greed and jealousy. Unless and until we realize and accept that we are powerful beings who have the capacity to create what we want, we will go on looking for something outside of ourselves to fulfill a deeper longing for awakening to our whole self. When we enjoy what we have and who we are, when we feel that we deserve to have what we want, we can move on to noticing that there is more to life than wanting, getting, and having. We have a surplus of conscious energy that allows us to get curious about what lies beyond the preoccupation of manipulating our world to get more.

What happens when we suspend the reflex to get more? In this pause arises the possibility for what psalmists articulated as "Thy will be done." Surrendering to the greater mystery unfolding is an action that does not arise out of impotency. It arises out of abundance, out of a plentitude of physical, mental, and emotional energy.

Locating the belly center and becoming aware of the qualities of energy present in the solar plexus are the intentions behind the inquiries in this chapter. You will notice that you have choices about nurturing your connection to the infinite source of creative wisdom that flows through your organism. Self-confidence, self-reliance, resourcefulness, emotional availability—these are qualities that describe a person who begins to strengthen his or her belly center. As well, your yoga practice will benefit from the increased physical stamina and endurance. Yoga postures that are especially affected by having belly strength include all of the standing leg lifts, such as Heron, Extended Leg Warrior, and Tree, and reclining leg lifts, such as Upward Boat and Bicycles.

Hara Breathing

Breathing from your hara can recruit strength for entering and holding the most challenging of yoga postures. Even pronouncing the word *hara* engages the belly center. Ordinarily, yogic breathing emphasizes inhaling and exhaling through the nose but when you need an extra jolt of energy directly from the belly try the hara breath: inhale through the nose, then exhale through the mouth with the sound "h-a-a-a-a-a-a-a-a-a-h!"

Remember counting how many sit-ups you could do in gym class? Using the hara breath is going to make that experience a lot easier, perhaps even effortless. Lie on the floor with your knees bent; hook your feet under the edge of a sofa to anchor your legs and to protect your low back. (We didn't have a sofa or chair in the photo studio.) Do a few sit-ups in whatever way you can. Pause and notice how much effort is required. Now close your eyes and bring your arms on the floor overhead (**fig. 7.1**). Relax into your breath as you bring awareness into the center of your belly. Imagine that you are about to pick up a ball and throw it by using the momentum of your arms to lift you up to sitting and then hurling the ball out over your legs and beyond your feet for yards. Take in a deep breath through your nostrils. As you exhale, squeeze your hands into fists and, making the sound "h-a-a-a-a-a-a-a-a-a-h," sit up and hurl the imaginary ball way beyond your feet (**fig. 7.2**). Pause for a moment and experience the energy pulsing in your belly center. Repeat this Hara Sit-up a few times, noticing how making the sound allows you to move from the core of your being.

Reflect on how this experiment demonstrates the power of hara breathing. Consider how many ways you can use this teaching for generating energy and strength in your belly.

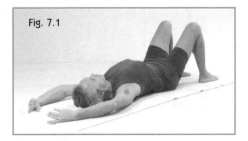
Fig. 7.1

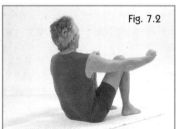
Fig. 7.2

Locating and Energizing the Belly Center

Inquiry: Where is my center of power and strength?

In the first exploration below, we take a step toward kinesthetically locating the belly center. Much of our explorations up to this time have used gravity to align the body from a supine position, with the spine on the ground. To energize the belly center, Spinal Lift reverses the pull of gravity by elevating the hips and pelvis. In Spinal Lift, the abdomen is higher than the neck and shoulders, creating a massaging effect on the fluids in the tissues and organs of the belly. With Hara Pump we allow the body's brain in the belly center to take over our movement by pumping the abdominal cavity using breath, sound, and movement to infuse this vital center with a fresh flow of energy. The power surge of energy generated with this exploration is then directed into the head, neck, and shoulders by holding the pelvis elevated in the Bridge pose.

This inquiry is a powerful tonic for discharging stagnant physical, emotional, and mental energies lodged in the belly and for rejuvenating the entire organism. Using this experience before entering reverse yoga postures, such as Bridge, Plow, Shoulder Stand, and Fish, has the effect of opening the flow of energy in the body for a deeper movement of prana in those postures.

Preparation: Locating Center in Crossing Diagonal Lines of Energy

1. As you lie on the ground, notice how quickly and deeply your body begins to release into contact with the ground (**fig. 7.3**). Scan your body to notice any discomforts or resistance that might be present, letting your experience be precisely as it is. Suggest to your logical mind that this is a time to honor the wisdom of your organism by simply noticing what is.

2. Noticing your breath and your breathing, travel to the place in your being where the impulses to inhale and to exhale arise. Release all control over your breath and simply notice how the body is breathing. Notice the speed and momentum of your thoughts and thinking, allowing any thoughts or concerns to be present, precisely as they arise.

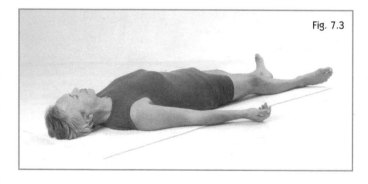

Fig. 7.3

3. Suggest to your logical mind that you are about to cross over a time boundary to experience the slower time in which the body actually lives. Thank your mind for supporting you by focusing awareness on the sensations you'll be noticing. Now, spiraling to the center of your belly, your center of physical and emotional well-being, notice your mood in this moment. What are the colors, textures, or shapes of any

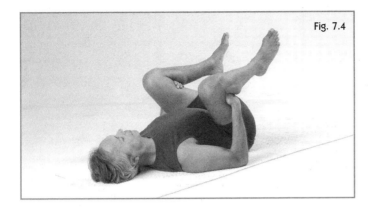

Fig. 7.4

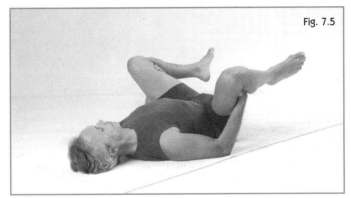

Fig. 7.5

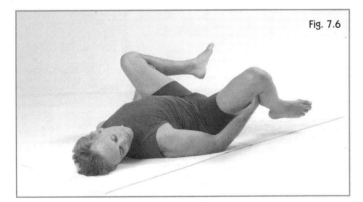

Fig. 7.6

feelings that are present? Suggest to your logical mind that it is safe, desirable, and even pleasurable to expand awareness to include all of your feelings, all dimensions of your being in this moment. Notice how it feels to become interested in the center of your belly. Can you sense the pulse deep in your belly? Notice how your awareness of the pulse enhances the flow of prana into the core of your being. Now we will enter into movements that will reveal a precise sensation of the center of your body.

4. Bend both knees and bring them in over your torso. Keeping your thumb in contact with your index finger, use your hands like a scoop to grasp under the crease of each knee **(fig. 7.4)**. Adjust your grip so that you can continue using your hands in this way while keeping your shoulders relaxed down to the ground.

5. Now open your knees wide apart and see if your elbows can come close to or actually rest on the ground while you continue supporting your knees with your hands **(fig. 7.5)**. Pause here to make any adjustments that will allow you to relax the weight of your legs down into your hands. You'll notice that it's easier for your elbows to settle on the ground the wider you spread your knees apart. Allow your legs to get heavier and heavier in your hands.

6. How are you breathing? Is it easier to support your legs in your hands if you hold your breath? Notice how the effort relaxes as you allow the breath to flow. Using your kinesthetic awareness, can you feel how your low back is elongated on the ground? Make the "yes" movement by rocking on the back of your head, pointing your nose down toward your chest and up toward the wall behind you. Let your head rest now in the neutral, relaxed position.

7. Holding your knees firmly, begin to roll your head from ear to ear, releasing the shoulders down and away from your chin to create more space for the head to roll. Bring your ear as close to the ground on each side as possible. Look with your eyes to the place on the floor on each side where your ear would touch **(fig. 7.6)**. Repeat the head roll from side to side four or five times and then return your head to neutral center. Notice how much of the weight of your legs has released down into the support of your hands.

8. If you notice any strain or discomfort, take a break and release your legs and arms to the ground and notice the sensations arising in your body. When you are ready to resume, bend your knees and scoop your hands under the creases, elbows relaxed to the ground.

9. Continue to hold the crease of your right knee, with your right elbow and shoulder relaxed on the ground. Lower your left foot to the ground, leaving your knee bent and the foot placed on the floor a comfortable distance from your hip. Reach the palm of your left hand behind the back of your head (**fig. 7.7**). Let the weight of your head sink down into the bowl of your palm. Relax and allow all of the weight of your head to slowly let go into your palm. Experiment with letting the left shoulder and elbow stay heavy and relaxed on the ground while your palm receives the weight of your head.

10. Imagine lifting your head, using your left arm and shoulder to do the lifting, while your neck muscles remain relaxed. Now actually lift the head about one inch off the ground (**fig. 7.8**) and then lower it back down. Wait until the entire weight of your head, shoulder, and elbow have dropped back down to the ground and then repeat the lift. Inhale as you lift, pause for a moment, then lower your head and wait for it to get heavy again.

11. Repeat this lift several times, until you have a sense of lifting your head by using your arm rather than your neck muscles.

12. Initiate the lift again. This time begin to angle the left elbow over toward your right knee as you lift, then return your head and elbow to the ground (**fig. 7.9**). Each time you lift your head, bring the elbow across your body toward the knee (but don't touch the knee). The knee remains passive, supported under the crease by your right hand. Repeat this lift a few times; on the last repetition, keep the head lifted as you inscribe a circle around the knee with the left elbow (**fig. 7.10**). Then return back to the floor and let the head and shoulder get heavy again.

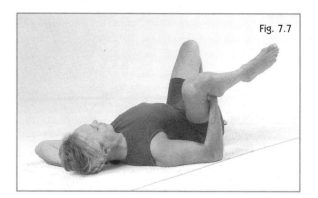

Fig. 7.7

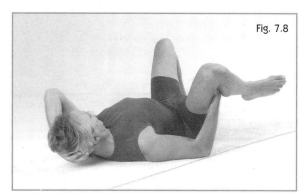

Fig. 7.8

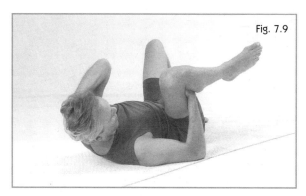

Fig. 7.9

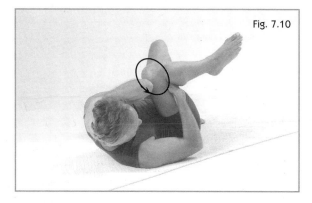

Fig. 7.10

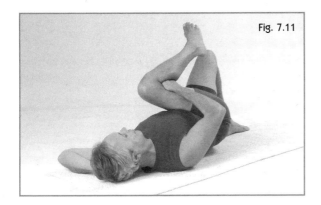

Fig. 7.11

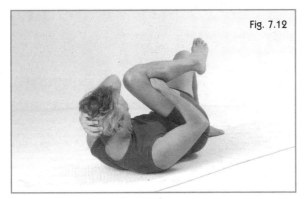

Fig. 7.12

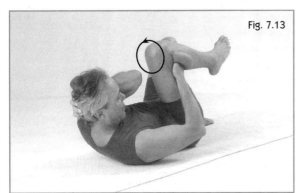

Fig. 7.13

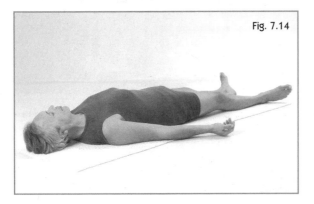

Fig. 7.14

13. Now leave the head resting in the palm of your left hand on the floor and bring your right knee toward your left elbow (**fig. 7.11**). Your range of motion will be limited so only bring the knee as far across the midline as you can without using force or struggle. Repeat this movement a few times, then take a rest.

14. Now lift the right knee toward the left elbow and the elbow toward the knee, (**fig. 7.12**) then lower both of them back down to the ground. Do not allow the elbow and the knee to touch. When you practice this movement, experiment with lifting both elbow and knee at the same time, distributing the effort equally between the upper body and the lower body. Notice the tendency for one segment to dominate or to lead. Continue this movement until you are satisfied that both are lifting at the same time. On the last lift, circle the knee around the elbow (**fig. 7.13**). Reverse direction of the circles, hold, and then release knee and elbow back down to the ground.

15. Stretch both legs long on the ground and bring your arms alongside your body (**fig. 7.14**). Observe any sensations as they arise. Do you notice a diagonal line of energy moving across your body? Where does this diagonal cross your spine—above the navel or below the navel? Take an internal picture of where you notice the diagonal line of energy crossing the midline of your body.

16. When you are ready, bend both knees and repeat this sequence of movements on the other side of your body. Take all the time you need to fully experience each aspect of the exploration. After you feel satisfied with completing this new side, once again stretch out both legs and release your arms down to the ground. Immediately sense the diagonal line of energy moving on the new side. Where do you feel the line of energy crossing the midline of your body? Recall the diagonal energy line from the original side. Using your kinesthetic sense, travel to the place in the center of your being where these two diagonal lines intersect.

17. Allow your full attention to remain focused on the sensations emanating from the epicenter where these counterbalancing lines of energy integrate. Are you aware of any pulsing or streaming sensations?

18. In this state of deep, relaxed awareness, notice how it feels to be at home in the center of your being. Notice how you are open to receive from the wisdom of your organism.

19. When you are ready, initiate your return by rolling to your side and up to sitting or continue with the following exploration.

Exploration 1: Spinal Lift

1. Lying on the ground, bend both knees and bring them a comfortable distance from your buttocks **(fig. 7.15)**. Notice the angle of your nose. If you had a paintbrush extending from your nose, would the paintbrush be angled down toward your chest, up toward the wall behind you, or straight up toward the ceiling? Allow your head to relax into the neutral position.

2. Bring your awareness to both heels. Inhale and press into the heels, lifting the tailbone off the floor slightly. When you lift the tailbone, the low back elongates and presses into the floor; do not lift the tailbone so high that your low back comes off the ground. Play with this movement until you can lift the tailbone by pressing into the heels and still leave the lower back elongated on the ground.

3. When you lift the tailbone, do you notice that your nose points up toward the imaginary north pole? In this movement you will want to keep the nose angled down toward the south pole.

4. Now as you press into the heels, inhale and bring a little more of your spine off the ground, lifting until the belt line is off the ground **(fig. 7.16)**. Maintain awareness of keeping your neck long by angling your chin down toward your chest, toward the south pole. Exhale as you roll back down the spine, individually placing each segment of the spine back down on the ground. Repeat a few times, lifting only the low back and hips and then lowering the spine to the ground.

5. Begin to lift the middle back off the floor **(fig. 7.17)** and roll back down. Stay with the sensation of each vertebra lifting off the floor on an inhaling breath and each vertebra returning to the floor on the exhale.

6. Now lift high enough to feel the bottom edges of your shoulder blades coming off the ground **(fig. 7.18)**. Check to see that your nose is pointed toward your chest. Exhale as you roll back down the spine.

7. Let the movement build until you are lifting as much of your spine off of the ground as is comfortable in one in-breath, holding the breath for a moment at the top of the lift and then exhaling as you roll down the spine. Do you notice any segments along the spine that want to move as a unit instead of individually, vertebra by vertebra? Repeat the movement a few times in these areas until you notice more freedom arising.

8. The next time you lift, keep the pelvis elevated enough to make the pelvic compass while remaining off the ground. (If you need to refresh your memory, see the Pelvic Compass exploration on page 104.) Find the north and south poles by arching

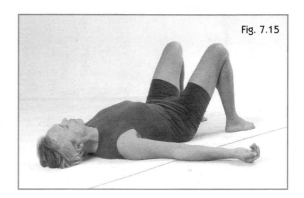

Fig. 7.15

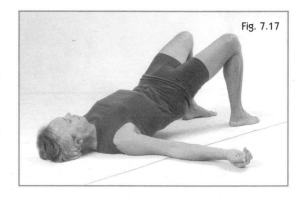

Fig. 7.16

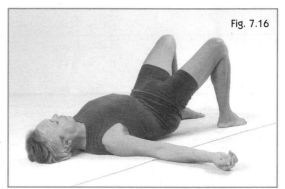

Fig. 7.17

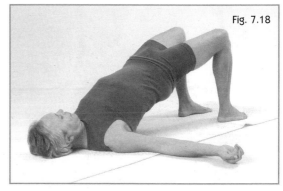

Fig. 7.18

and elongating the low back. Find east and west by alternately lifting one hip slightly higher than the other. Then find all the positions around a circular compass. Move in one direction a few times, then reverse directions.

9. Now lower your spine to the ground. Stretch your legs long and experience the internal effects of your movement. Allow your awareness to ride the waves of sensation that play along your spine. Particularly notice the curve beneath your low back. Is it closer to the ground than when you began? Notice the curve behind your neck. Does it feel closer to the ground?

10. Slowly begin your return, or move on to the next exploration.

Exploration 2: Hara Pump

1. Lying on the ground, bend both knees, standing your feet a comfortable distance from your buttocks. Bring your awareness to both heels. Inhale and press into the heels, lifting the tailbone off the floor slightly. Don't lift the tailbone so high that your low back comes off the ground; when you lift the tailbone the low back elongates and presses into the floor. Play with this movement until you can lift the tailbone by pressing into the heels and yet leave the low back elongated on the ground (fig. 7.19).

2. When you lift the tailbone, do you notice that your nose points up toward your imaginary north pole? As in the Spinal Lift, you want to keep the nose angled down toward your chest, your "south pole."

3. Gradually begin the Spinal Lift described in exploration 1, including more and more of your spine as you roll up (fig. 7.20) and roll down (fig. 7.21). Exaggerate the breath in as you roll up and the breath out as you roll down.

4. When the lift feels familiar, begin to put a little speed into the movement up and down. Emphasizing the flow of your breath in, begin to lift and lower the spine rapidly, as fast as you can go without using force or struggle. Let the breath power the movement.

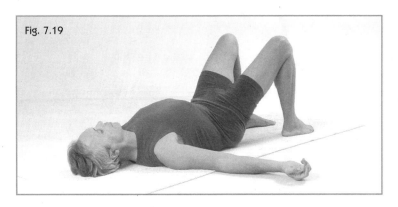
Fig. 7.19

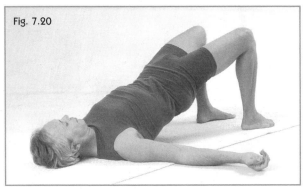
Fig. 7.20

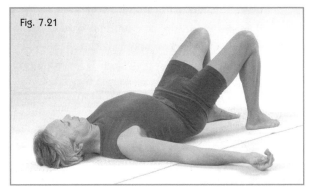
Fig. 7.21

5. Continue the movement, imagining that the movement is pumping the breath. When you feel ready to pause, lower the spine and notice the steady stream of sensations that arise in your body. Relax long enough to allow your breathing to return to normal. Repeat this sequence a few times, gradually extending the length of time you keep it going. This movement will oxygenate your blood and revitalize your lungs by expelling all residual air.

6. Moving now to the next level of energizing your belly, your hara, begin by inhaling as you lift your pelvis and middle back off the floor. Relax as you hold this position while taking in several long, deep breaths. Keep your pelvis and middle back elevated as you begin a pulsing movement in your pelvis, letting your pelvis spring up and down. Imagine that you are using the up-and-down motion of your hip bones to keep a basketball bouncing off your pelvis without letting it fall to the ground. Open your jaw and let out a sound—"hah-ah-ah-ah-ah-ah-ah-ah-ah-ah"—until you exhale all of the breath. Repeat this movement four or five more times, inhaling a big breath in and making the bouncing movement and sound: "hah-ah-ah-ah-ah-ah-ah." Moving up and down like this while you let your pelvis and belly hang is invigorating to all of your abdominal organs. Each time

you repeat the movement and sound, gradually extend the length of time you keep it going.

7. When you have repeated the pumping movement enough to feel energized and comfortable with the mechanics, roll the spine back down into full contact with the ground. Notice how much energy is pulsing through your entire organism. Can you feel how your mood has altered by opening to this much energy?

8. When your breath has returned to normal, stretch your legs long and allow your awareness to ride the waves of sensation that course throughout your body. Notice how it feels to have this much sensation. Imagine that the energy of all of your sensations as well as all thoughts and feelings about this experience are flowing into your center, becoming a welcomed part of all that you are. Every part of your experience has a place in your center in this moment. Suggest to your logical mind that it is safe, desirable, and pleasurable to have this much energy pulsing through your being. Notice how it feels to be at home in the center of your being, full of energy.

9. When you are ready, slowly begin your return by rolling to your side and coming up into a sitting position, or continue on with the following integration.

Integration: Bridge Posture (*Setu Bandhasana*)

1. Lying on the ground, bend both knees and slide your heels a comfortable distance from your buttocks. Place your feet parallel, as though you were standing upright in the Mountain pose. Lengthen your arms alongside your body, close to but not touching your legs (**fig. 7.22**). Suggest to your logical mind that you are now crossing a time boundary to enter a deeper level of communication with the many dimensions of your whole being. Now is the time to receive the effects of the Spinal Lift and the Hara Pump by directing the flow of prana into the base of your

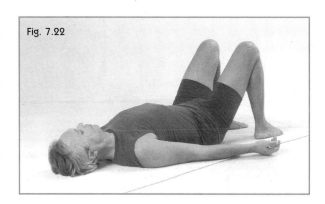

Fig. 7.22

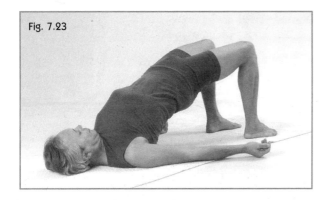

Fig. 7.23

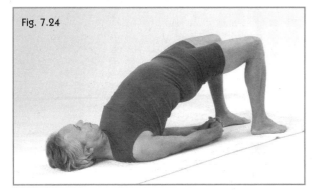

Fig. 7.24

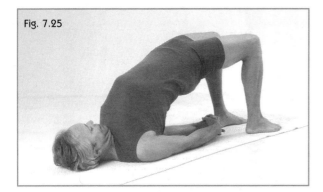

Fig. 7.25

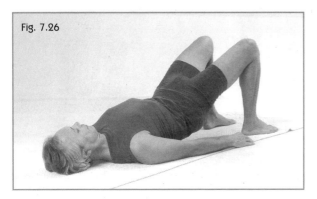

Fig. 7.26

throat. Notice how your organism is communicating its wisdom to you in this moment. Open your awareness to listening for any messages of insight or guidance that may come to you over the next few moments.

2. Exhale all of the breath. On an inhale, press into your feet and begin the Spinal Lift, allowing each vertebra to lift up and off the ground in sequence (**fig. 7.23**). Take as many breaths as you need as you continue lifting the spine a comfortable distance off the ground. Pause and take a few more relaxing breaths. Make the "yes" movement by rocking the back of your head on the ground, releasing any holding in your neck or shoulders.

3. When you are ready to continue, lift the hip bones up toward the sky. Bring your arms together behind your back so that you can interlace your fingers (**fig. 7.24**). Experiment with how you can squeeze your shoulder blades together as you walk your arms and shoulders away from your head and ears. Do not walk your shoulders so far away from your head that the back of your neck is flattened onto the ground.

4. Settle into this phase of Bridge pose for a moment. Relax into your breath. Again make the "yes" movement by rocking the back of your head up and down on the ground to release any holding or tension in the neck or shoulders.

5. In the final few breaths of holding this pose, press your arms into the ground as you lift your sternum toward your chin (**fig. 7.25**). Lift your hip bones toward the sky. Notice how energy of the front side of your body is flowing like a river down from the pubic bone, pooling into the well at the base of your throat. Notice how energy of the back side of your body is flowing like a river downward from the tip of your tailbone to the base of your skull.

6. Before releasing Bridge pose, take in a full, deep breath. Hold the breath in for a few seconds. Take in a little more breath and hold; then, as you release the breath with control, release your hands and arms to your sides and begin to roll the spine back down along the ground (**fig. 7.26**). Keep your chin tucked in just slightly so the back of your neck stays long and relaxed. Take as many breaths as you need while the spine continues its long descent back down to the ground.

7. When the spine is in full contact with the ground once again, pause to receive the effects of this exploration. Do not censor any of the thoughts, feelings, or sensations that cross the screen of your awareness. Allow your experience to be precisely as it is unfolding. Witness the many layers and dimensions of your being as they communicate through the wisdom of your organism.

8. Remain in this position for as long as you wish. Then stretch your legs long on the ground. Make any adjustments in your body that allow you to settle into the ground. Allow your awareness to travel anywhere in your being that calls your attention. Notice how deeply relaxed your body becomes as you journey to the center of your being.

9. Suggest to your logical mind that you can return to this state of deep, relaxed awareness at any time in your life, under any circumstances, simply by recalling the way you feel in this moment; at home in the center of your being.

10. When you are ready, slowly begin your return. As you gradually roll up into a seated position, experience how all of the effects you are noticing have a place in your center—your center expands to include all feelings, thoughts, and insights that are surfacing in this moment. As you move about your day notice how you are engaged with the world around you and grounded in your center at the same time.

Before Moving On . . .

The inquiries of this chapter have helped you to locate your belly center as both a physiological center of gravity and an epicenter where physical, mental, and emotional energies intersect. An infant gains its first healthy sense of self through the steady flow of care for its needs, receiving nutrition, loving contact, and physical stimulation. Without the reliable flow of energy in these forms directed personally to the child, mistrust, shame, and insecurity color the child's life experiences and ability to develop autonomy and self-reliance.

By bringing awareness to your own belly center, you are facilitating greater communication between your mental, emotional, and physical needs. In developing a strong relationship with your energy center, you are establishing a home base that serves as a place of safety in an ever-changing world. Rather than being pulled in one direction in some activities and in another direction by other activities, you have the possibility of initiating all activities from the belly center, remaining in contact with your vital source of energy. The Spinal Lift, Hara Pump, and Bridge are ways to recharge your internal battery, supplying a fresh and abundant supply of energy for sustaining and nurturing your body as well as fueling your need for operating in life with a strong sense of personal power, self-confidence, and determination to accomplish your life's work. Bringing concentrated focus to the energetic center of your body in this way, you are signaling to your mind and ego that awakening to yourself, your power, and your creativity are worthwhile, that you are worthy as a unique individual, and that you have the capability to realize your deepest longings and awaken into your fullest capacities. On the flipside, without a strong belly center you may move through life feeling discontent and out of place, indecisive about where and how best to respond to the world around you.

As your communication with the belly center develops further, you will notice in your yoga practice that by stabilizing the muscles of the abdominal core you simultaneously experience an increase in your physical strength, balance, stamina, and endurance. The inquiries of the next chapter guide you into the next step in which you gain practical experience in initiating movement from your center. The movements you will explore are the same movements that, as an infant, allowed you to roll from one side to another and from being on your back to rolling up to a sitting position.

8 Releasing into Movement from the Center of Being

How is it possible to be in the world without getting uprooted from my center?

THE INTERPLAY BETWEEN BEING AND DOING has been a subject of inquiry since human beings have been stirred by intuitions of an ultimate consciousness. On the side of merging into pure "beingness," some have embodied the yogic ideal as an austere withdrawal from sensorial stimulation in favor of making a solitary journey into the interior of one's own experience. On the side of doing, others have embodied the spirit of yoga as dedication to selfless service in the world. At the heart of both poles in this paradox lies the intention to realize one's capacity to use experience, be it internal or external, as an opportunity to awaken to inherent wholeness as the essence of one's true nature.

In an ancient yoga sutra we catch a glimpse of how yogic practice aims to address this paradox at the heart of human experience. The sutra states: "Although she moves, she is ever still."

Self-Awakening Yoga takes its inspiration from the As Is principle—Awareness of Sensation through Internal Scanning. In becoming aware of our bodily felt experience, our experience at the level of sensation, we begin to ground awareness in the concrete, in the present moment. The body lives in the present, while the mind is free to travel throughout multidimensional time. From this bodily anchor in physical reality, other layers of the self become revealed. Awareness of sensation expands to include awareness of prana, the subtler energy movements in the body. Noticing how the energy of prana can be directed by mind, we become aware that on some level we are participants in the creation of events in our world. Where the mind goes, prana flows. Studying how and why we create what we create reveals a personality at work, an ego that is structured to avoid pain and to seek pleasure. Studying the cause-and-effect relationship of the choices we make begins to open a deeper capacity for fulfillment, a dimension of being beyond wanting, getting, and having. We start to notice that fulfilling our own needs has an impact on others. Taking responsibility for our actions engages the witness, that aspect of our being that operates from discriminative wisdom. In the climate of radical self-acceptance for the survival functions that our egos fulfill, we begin to awaken to deeper levels of choice in our lives.

A sense of bliss emerges when we follow the discriminating wisdom that arises from witnessing our lives, our choices, and our creative possibilities. This bliss is not necessarily a constant euphoric or utopian jubilation but a calm and quiet sense of harmony in the midst of paradoxical circumstances that are constantly and unpredictably changing. Yogis say that it is possible to remain in radical self-acceptance of the many dimensions of our experience amid the unruly events of life. This radical self-acceptance is described as a lotus blossom. The unfolding flower of consciousness is rooted deep in the mud of life.

Swami Kripalu described the intentions of yoga in a slightly different manner. "When a yogi is lying down, the yogi is lying down. When a yogi is sitting, the yogi is sitting. When the yogi is standing, the yogi is standing. When the yogi is walking, the yogi is walking." In other words, when you are lying on the ground in the supine position in the midst of an inquiry into the sensations of heaviness, you are not using the quiet time to think about the shopping you have to do for tonight's dinner. Later, when you are in the grocery store shopping for your family, you are not wishing you were lying on the floor doing your yoga inquiries.

Self-Awakening Yoga provides access to the actual experiences that arise on the screen of consciousness from moment to moment. This includes the moments that we notice ourselves being projected into a hundred other future or past moments. Noticing that our awareness travels throughout many dimensions and accepting that phenomenon is the doorway for returning to the actual experiences in this moment. Being who we are as we are opens a doorway for accessing deeper levels of choice and possibility.

Jesus taught his followers to "be in the world, but not of the world." Yogi Patanjali describes the possibility of witnessing our experience without being identified with it. With our lives already being lived in full progress, how do we begin to return to an internal center from which we can cultivate a witness perspective? How do you recognize your internal center?

Let's begin with some more concrete questions that might lead to an answer to the ultimate inquiry here. As you deepen into your practice of Self-Awakening Yoga, do you notice a developing sense of confidence in your ability to get interested in your actual experiences? With permission to witness and to learn through your experience, have you noticed a lighthearted sense of humor beginning to supplant self-criticism or seriousness? Do you hear yourself beginning to say, "Isn't that interesting?" Is fascination and curiosity about your experiences opening windows to possibility where apathy and indifference or boredom might have won out at other times in your life? Can you sense the presence of novel responses emerging in the place of previously habitual reactions to circumstances? As you begin to acknowledge these qualities in your yoga practice and your life practice, you can recognize that your sense of living at home in your center of being is beginning to crystallize.

You may notice that the inquiries up to now have already begun to open this witnessing capacity. The inquiries in this chapter provide an opportunity to experience how you can move in every direction while staying rooted in your center. As this awareness of your center develops, you are creating the means to return home into this core whenever you feel yourself drifting away from yourself. You will notice that in postures such as Triangle, Rotated Triangle, Half Moon, and Standing Warrior Twist—postures in which the body is extending in several directions at once—your ability to stay grounded will be enhanced with the awareness of remaining in contact with and moving from your center.

Moving from the Center

Inquiry: How does freeing prana in the sacrum encourage free-flowing movement from the center?

Have you ever wondered how the sacrum got its name? First, let's locate the sacral bone. The sacrum is actually five vertebrae that are fused together; the sacrum is located at the base of the spine. When you bring your palm to the base of your spine with your middle finger pointing down toward the tailbone, the heel of your hand will be positioned near the top of the triangular-shaped sacrum, which points downward. At the bottom of the sacrum is the coccyx, the tailbone. Although the tailbone is attached to the sacrum by dense cartilage, it retains some movement possibilities. The sacrum is stabilized on either side by the hip bones, the ilium—bones that fan outward like elephant ears.

The sacrum is designed to move in the hip girdle, although in many adults one or both of the sacroiliac joints, where the sacrum articulates with the hip bones, are fixed in place. The loss of movement in these joints shows up in yoga postures as limitations in forward bending or in "sidedness"—when it is easier to stand, balance, or initiate spinal twists on one side than the other.

Loss of movement at these joints occurs for many different reasons, with injury from a fall being the most common. We don't notice that soreness after a fall will sometimes linger, causing a preference to bear more weight on one side of the body in order to protect the injury. While the injury is in the process of healing the sacrum glides over to fixate on the protected side, leaving the supporting side to do all the work of articulating. Lifestyle habits create other reasons for the sacrum fixating to one side or the other. Have you ever held a baby in one arm with a telephone at your shoulder while you stirred dinner with the other arm? In these kinds of daily movement patterns, the load-bearing side arranges itself to support the body while the other side is left free for movement articulation. What about shifting your weight onto one leg while waiting for the bus? Or sitting at a computer and using one hand to manipulate the mouse while the other hand rests? All such movement habits and preferences create bilateral imbalances that begin to show up in the sacrum.

Now, why is this bone called the sacrum? The name comes from the word *sacred*, or the "sacred bone." In yogic philosophy this bone is considered sacred because it contains the energy of our evolutionary potential. Think for a moment about how humans evolved from locomoting on four legs to standing and walking on two legs. The five fused bones comprising the sacrum are the vestigial remains of a long tail that used to be an essential appendage for hanging in trees, counterbalancing a trot or gallop, or signaling sexual availability. The evolutionary need for the tail has withdrawn to a potent distillation of energy that is housed in the coccygeal nerve plexus. Yogis identify a latent, concentrated form of prana that lies dormant in the sacrum that, when awakened, travels up through the spine and opens the higher centers of human and divine consciousness. Called the *kundalini*, many of the traditional yoga practices are designed to awaken and channel this energy for the conscious evolution of the whole person. In Self-Awakening Yoga we are gently knocking on the doorway of this sacred bone, awakening the concentrated energy of prana so that it may flow more freely throughout the physical body, enhancing the functioning of all systems.

In the Sacrum Release below, you will discover a simple and pleasurable way to restore movement in the sacrum. Reach and Roll allows you to use this freedom of movement as a fulcrum for rolling your body from side to side. The movement builds into a spiral that carries you right up into our first seated postures. Moving in this way allows you to access the seated postures, such as Butterfly, Pinwheel, and Half Lotus, with greater balance between the two sides and greater flexibility in the hip joints.

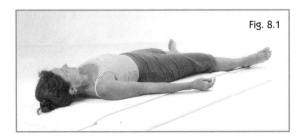

Fig. 8.1

Exploration 1: Sacrum Release

1. You may want a little extra padding for the explorations in this inquiry, as you will be rolling on the ground. Come to a comfortable position lying on the ground (**fig. 8.1**). As you begin to settle, making all the adjustments that support your comfort, begin to scan the many dimensions of your present moment. Notice the contact your body makes with the ground, witnessing any physical sensations that call your attention. Imagine that you are checking in with your body, as you would check in with a good friend, becoming interested in whatever you begin to notice.

2. Become aware of your breath and breathing, noticing how your body moves in response to your breath. Notice how quickly and deeply your body begins to relax as you attune to the sound and the sensation of your breathing. As you sense the speed and momentum of your thoughts and thinking, notice any particular thoughts that may be present for you in this moment. Appreciate your logical mind for participating in this inquiry as witness to your experience.

3. Attuning to the pulse deep in the center of your belly, notice your mood; notice the texture, color, and shape of any feelings or emotions that are present. Suggest to yourself that it is safe, desirable, and pleasurable to expand your awareness to include all of your feelings, all dimensions of your actual experience.

4. Imagine what you might have felt as an infant, lying on your back and exploring the sensations of reaching with your fingers and toes, your arms and legs. What are the sounds and the movements your organism makes as you play?

5. Bend both knees and bring them over your torso. Grasp the knob of your right knee with your right hand, your left knee with your left hand (**fig. 8.2**). Throughout this exploration, your hands will be in continuous contact with the knobs of your knees. The more you use your hands to support your knees, the more your legs will have permission to relax into their own heaviness. As your hold your knees, how much of the weight of your legs can you release into the support of your hands? How are you breathing? Can you feel how your low back is elongated on the ground?

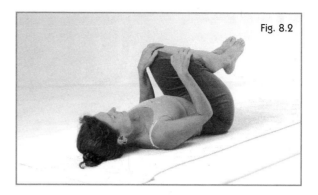

Fig. 8.2

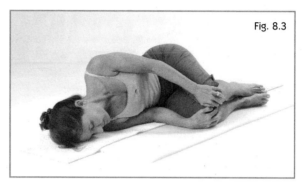

Fig. 8.3

Make the "yes" movement by rocking the back of your head on the ground and release your head in the neutral position.

6. Tie an imaginary string around your ankles, keeping the ankles in close contact. Holding on to your knees firmly and keeping the ankles together, roll over onto your right side. Keep your knees stacked one on top of the other and bent, as though you were sitting on a stool (**fig. 8.3**). Without letting go of your knees with your hands or letting the ankles come apart, explore the sensations of being in this position. What feels comfortable and what feels uncomfortable about the position? Particularly notice the position of your head relative to your right shoulder. Does it rest comfortably or awkwardly on the shoulder?

7. Keeping the ankles stacked one on top of the other and maintaining a firm grip on the knobs of your knees, you are going to begin a subtle movement in which the left leg slides out toward the floor over the right leg

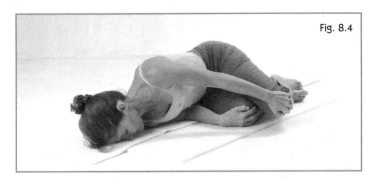

Fig. 8.4

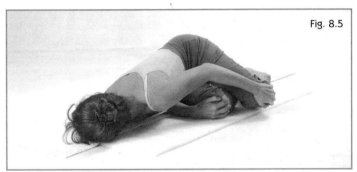

Fig. 8.5

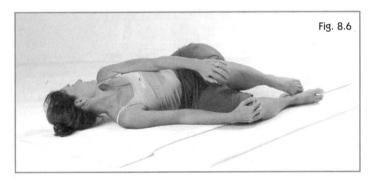

Fig. 8.6

gle-shaped bone at the base of your spine, pivots between the hip bones.

8. When the movement becomes freer, your head will roll forward as the left knee slides out toward the floor. You can tuck your chin slightly and allow your head to roll all the way under to see behind your body (**fig. 8.5**). When you drag the left knee back the head will roll again, this time to see all the way over your left shoulder (**fig. 8.6**). When your head begins to roll from side to side with greater range of motion, you will experience how the left ear can come close to the ground on each side.

9. Keep the movement going long enough to sense how the right shoulder capsule becomes soft and pliable, allowing your head to roll over it without discomfort. Release your jaw and your tongue. Release all expressions on your face and enjoy the freedom of movement that comes in this unique position.

10. Moving now to the other side, allow the left leg to reach up toward the sky, crossing over the body's midline and rolling you to the left side. The right leg stays heavy and only comes over to the left side when it has to. Reestablish the position of your body on this side: see that your knees are bent and stacking one on top of the other; tie an imaginary string that will keep your ankles together. Holding on to your knees, explore the sensations of being on this side. Do you notice any difference in temperature on this side? Is the quality of light any different? Do you sense a difference in mood on this side in relation to the other side? What feels comfortable and what feels uncomfortable about the position? Particularly notice the position of your head relative to your left shoulder. Does it rest comfortably or awkwardly on the shoulder?

11. Keeping the ankles stacked one on top of the other and maintaining a firm grip on the knobs of your knees, begin sliding the

(**fig. 8.4**). The tendency will be to let the ankles come apart or to lift the left (upper) leg, but you want to contain the movement to what you can do with the ankles remaining in contact. Slide the left knee out and drag it back, experiencing the inner thighs moving against each other. Start the movement slow and small; as it begins to feel familiar and comfortable, let the sliding gradually get bigger. If you allow your head to get involved, it will start to roll back and forth over the bump of your right shoulder in response to the pivoting that is occurring in your hips. Notice how the sacrum, the trian-

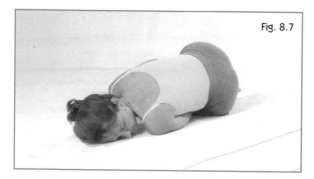

Fig. 8.7

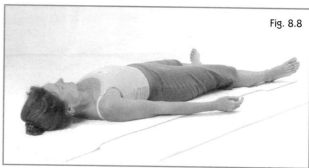

Fig. 8.8

right leg out over the left leg. Don't let the ankles come apart or lift the upper leg; instead, contain the movement to what you can do with the ankles remaining in contact. **12.** Continue the movement exploration on this side, experiencing the growing freedom in your hips and shoulders as the movement becomes more familiar. Keep the movement going long enough to sense how the left shoulder capsule becomes soft and pliable, allowing your head to roll over it without discomfort (**fig. 8.7**). Release your jaw and your tongue. Release all expressions on your face and enjoy the freedom of movement that comes in this unique position. **13.** When you are ready, roll onto your back,

stretch your legs and arms long, and experience the effects of the movement (**fig. 8.8**). Notice any pulsing, streaming, or tingling sensations that occur. Can you picture how the sacrum has released to move in cradle of the hips? **14.** Do you notice the curves of your neck and low back being any closer to the ground than when you began? How do your shoulders contact the ground? Imagine how you have freed the low back and sacrum to move more freely when you are walking. **16.** When you are ready, slowly begin your return, or continue into the following exploration.

Exploration 2: Reach and Roll

1. Lying on your back, bend both knees and bring them over your torso. Begin by moving into the Sacrum Release movement described in the previous exploration. Repeat a few times on each side and notice how much more familiar the movement is becoming as you recall the details of keeping the ankles in contact with each other and allowing your head to roll.

2. Holding your knees, roll over onto your right side. Pause for a moment. Now reach your left knee out over the right knee; continue to reach with the left knee, making a semicircle up toward the ceiling and all the way over to your left side (**fig. 8.9**). Let the right knee stay heavy on the ground until it has to come up in response to the left knee reaching and rolling over to your left side. The same is true for

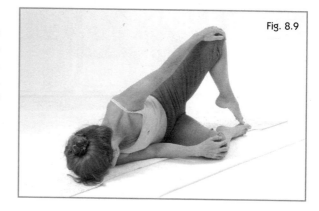

Fig. 8.9

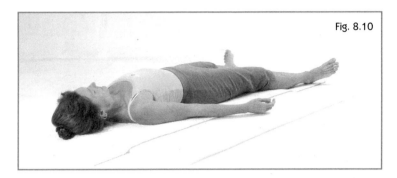

Fig. 8.10

your head—leave your head on the right side until it is moved in response to the reaching and rolling of the left knee.

3. When you land on the left side, stay there a moment. Make sure both hands are firmly holding both knees. Now begin to reach the right knee out over the left knee, in a semicircular stretch up toward the ceiling and all the way back over to the right side. Now you have landed back on your right side.

4. Continue reaching with the knee that is on top and rolling all the way over to the opposite side. Repeat this movement several times, allowing the speed to be determined by the rhythm of your breath and the natural time it takes to discover how to propel the movement. Continue until the movement becomes familiar and effortless and you feel energized.

5. When you are ready, roll onto your back, stretch your legs and arms long, and experience the effects of the movement (**fig. 8.10**). Allow your breath to flow in and out without attempting to control or inhibit the breath in any way. Notice any pulsing, streaming, or tingling sensations that occur.

7. Notice the way you feel when your body is free to reach and roll when you propel the movement from the center of your pelvis. Make a mental reminder to notice how tall you feel and how your shoulders hang to your sides when you come up to standing; imagine the way your head will feel centered over your body.

8. Slowly begin your return, or continue to the integration exploration that follows.

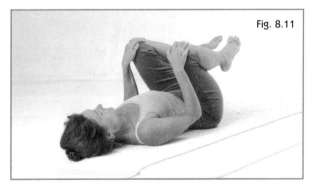

Fig. 8.11

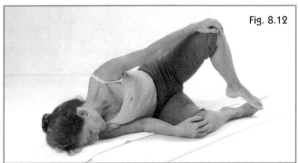

Fig. 8.12

Integration: Spiraling up to Sitting

1. From a position of lying on your back, bend both knees and bring them in over your torso. Grasp the knob of your right knee with your right hand, your left knee with your left hand (**fig. 8.11**).

2. Holding your knees, roll over onto your right side. Pause for a moment. Begin the Reach and Roll movement as in the previous exploration, reaching with your left knee out over the right knee. Continue to reach with the left knee, making a semicircle up toward the ceiling (**fig. 8.12**) and all the way over to your left side. Let the right knee stay heavy on the ground until it has to come up in response to the left knee reaching and rolling over to your left side. Leave your head on the right side until it is moved in response to the reaching and rolling of the left knee.

3. Continue reaching and rolling from side to side, allowing your breath to flow freely. As the momentum builds, begin to notice the precise place on the ground where your elbow touches the ground on each side.

4. Once you have developed an awareness of the contact your elbow makes with the ground, press into the elbow and see how this pressing begins to lift your torso up toward a sitting position (**fig. 8.13**). Continue reaching and rolling from side to side, pressing a little bit in the elbows to lift into sitting and then rolling back down and through to the other side.

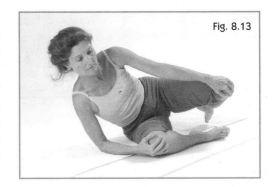
Fig. 8.13

5. After you experience the lift on each side that comes from pressing into the elbow, you are ready to power the movement with the top knee. You will still be using your elbow as a fulcrum to guide the movement, but this time let the momentum come from "throwing" the top leg up and over to bring you all the way into sitting. Once you are sitting, check to see that both knees are still bent at approximately right angles (**fig. 8.14**). Allow the "working" knee to reach further back, beyond the lower knee.

6. To come down, bring the working knee on top of the lower knee and roll back down to the floor, using your elbow as a pivot to guide you back down (**fig. 8.15**).

7. Explore reaching and rolling up to sitting from side to side until the movement becomes familiar and effortless.

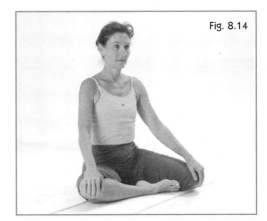
Fig. 8.14

8. This movement is a natural progression from the Sacrum Release and the Reach and Roll. Now your whole body is getting involved as you spiral up to sitting. Allow room for some confusion in the beginning. Go back to earlier stages of the Reach and Roll and allow the natural dynamics of your body to guide you into the movement. This movement can be exhilarating and a lot of fun. Enjoy the discovery process of how to make it a continuous flow from one side to the other. There are hundreds of ways to roll up to sitting from side to side. If this way does not work for you, invent a way to do it that feels natural and comfortable.

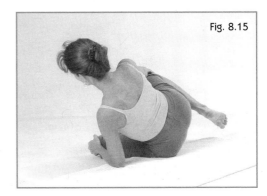
Fig. 8.15

9. When you are ready, roll onto your back, stretch your legs and arms long, and experience the effects of the movement (**fig. 8.16**). Allow your breath to flow in and out without attempting to control or inhibit the breath in any way. Notice any pulsing, streaming, or tingling sensations that occur.

10. Now is the time to receive from the wisdom of your organism. Whatever your experience has been as you explore moving from your center in this interesting way, allow the results to be precisely as you are experiencing them. Suggest to your logical mind that each time you return to this movement, it will continue to integrate at deeper and deeper levels of effortlessness.

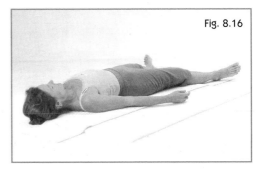
Fig. 8.16

11. Now relax the muscle of your mind and allow all thoughts and thinking to dissolve into the steady stream of sensation that is flowing throughout your body. Allow the wisdom of prana to spiral you into the center of your being.

12. Before beginning your return, notice the way your body looks and feels when you are free to move from the center of your being. Suggest to your logical mind that you can return home to your center at any time and under any circumstances by simply recalling the way you feel in this moment. Suggest that you will be returning with the feeling of having had a deep, relaxing, rejuvenating sleep, and that you'll be returning feeling fully energized, wide awake and ready to move on about your day.

13. Slowly begin your return by rocking your ankles from the inner anklebones to the outer anklebones. Roll your wrists from the inner wrist bones to the outer wrist bones. Roll your head from ear to ear. Bring up a good stretch. Allow your breath to deepen and let any sounds come out that happen spontaneously as you stretch.

14. Curl your knees into your chest, rock from side to side, and roll up into a sitting position. Is it any easier now to roll up to sitting? Open your eyes and notice whether your vision has altered in any way.

15. Slowly come up to standing. Do you feel any taller? How do your shoulders hang? Does your head feel like it is more centered over your body? Take a few steps around and notice the way your feet contact the ground. Notice the way your hips and pelvis move as you walk.

Before Moving On . . .

Locating the center of energy in your belly in the previous chapter prepared the foundation for the inquiries in this chapter that provide awareness for moving in different directions while remaining grounded in your belly. As you experiment with bringing this awareness of being centered in your belly into other aspects of your life, you might observe how often you find yourself returning to your belly center as a way of gathering greater concentration, perspective, and strength in all kinds of different situations. On the days that your yoga practice seems scattered or your priorities confusing, you might take a few minutes to return to Sacrum Release and Reach and Roll to regain your sense of center in the middle of it all.

Building on your capacity to roll up to sitting while remaining in contact with your center, the next chapter begins to explore greater opening and flexibility in the hip joints. Opening the hips for comfortable seated postures creates a flow of energy down into the legs and begins to balance the lower body with the upper body.

9 Opening the Hip Joints for Seated Postures and Simple Spinal Twists

How does releasing my leg muscles open my hip joints for more comfortable sitting?

THE EXPLORATION SPIRALING UP TO SITTING in the preceding chapter uses momentum generated from the center of gravity to propel the torso up into the Seated Pinwheel. This seated yoga posture is inspired by the image of a wheel with its spokes spiraling from the center. The image of the wheel of life appears universally in ancient wisdom cultures from every corner of our world. The name of the posture describes its effect: opening to a synchronized state of being in which all aspects of the person are in harmony with one another. In Sanskrit, this wheel is known as the *swastika*; the Sanskrit name for the yoga posture is *swastikasana*. In yoga, the word *swa* means "total health."

Before going further, we must acknowledge the horrific associations now existing with the word and the image of the swastika, a word ripped from its native context and profoundly distorted by Nazi ideology. The emotional contradiction of considering a state of total well-being alongside the symbol used to provoke utter darkness is intensely challenging. As we begin to explore all dimensions that are inherent in our nature, we are inviting awareness of the shadow that coexists with the light. In pausing to honor the presence of the many paradoxes that exist within our own human nature we must acknowledge that unfathomable suffering exists in our world, as does sublime peace and compassion.

The arrangement of our bent legs in the Seated Pinwheel allows for a deep exploration of the contact the sitz bones make with the ground. By orienting to one side first and then to the other, you give yourself the opportunity to notice how different the two sides of your body are. The particular positioning of your legs in the Seated Pinwheel provides both support and leverage to clearly differentiate the various movements available in the hip joints. Greater freedom of movement in the hips allows the sitz bones to remain grounded, supporting the spine to elongate and to move freely. Noticing the asymetries between the two sides reinforces the physiological phenomenon that we are bilateral beings. The two sides of our body specialize to support our being in different ways. Each side carries different information; when they are in communication, the wisdom of the organism reveals the interdependencies that interact to give us our wholeness.

Having flexibility in the hips means that the ball joint of the long upper thigh bone, the femur, is free to rotate in its socket. This circumduction, or rotational movement, includes all the angles in which the leg can move in the hip socket—adduction and abduction, extension and flexion, and medial and lateral rotation. The movements you will experience from the Seated Pinwheel affect the entire range of motion in the hip joints by releasing the deep, intrinsic muscles that predominantly determine overall flexibility: the gluteus minimus, iliacus, quadratus femoris, gemellus superior and inferior, and obturator externus and internus. The larger, superficial muscles—including the psoas, gluteus maximus, hamstrings, and quadriceps—are strengthened and toned as well.

Locating and Anchoring the Sitz Bones for Grounded Seated Postures

Inquiry: What movements allow me to release my leg muscles and open my hip joints?

In allowing the two sides of the body to be as different as they are, we create a bridge for communication and learning to occur from side to side. As each side learns from the other, both sides are elevated to higher levels of organizational efficiency. Noticing the natural openness and freedoms that arise on one side of the body provides an opportunity for the other side of the body to release holding patterns that are no longer necessary to the organism.

In the first exploration, Knee Thump, you'll be knocking on the door of some of the deepest holding patterns in the adductor and abductor muscles of the legs. When you were first learning to walk, the inner knees were particularly vulnerable to bumps and falls and to injury. This movement says to the knees that you are safe in this position. You are asking the knees: "How do you move when you don't need to continue protecting me from falling?" Releasing the inner knees oftentimes dramatically increases flexibility and range of motion in the entire hip socket. Hip Swing and

Cradles transfer the grounding from the sitz bones up into the various segments of the spine, creating the potential for freer movement between spinal segments. Knee-to-Chest Figure 8s is a coordinated movement that integrates the patterns from both sides of the body by synchronizing movements across the body's midline.

Exploration 1: Releasing the Hamstrings and Quadriceps—Knee Thump

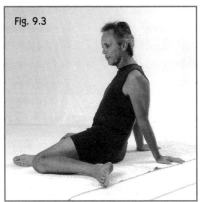

Fig. 9.1

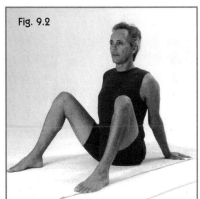

Fig. 9.2

1. Sit in a comfortable position on the ground. Reach your hands behind you and plant them on the floor a comfortable distance from your spine (**fig. 9.1**). Allow your arms to begin supporting the weight of your upright torso.

2. Stand your feet on the ground in front of you with your knees upright toward the ceiling (**fig. 9.2**). Separate your feet so that they are wider apart than your hips. Lower both knees toward the ground on your right side (**fig. 9.3**). If your left knee runs into your right leg or ankle, separate the legs so that both knees can move toward the ground. If you feel any strain in either knee you may place a cushion under the knee for support. If your wrists get tired you may also wish to place a cushion behind you for support.

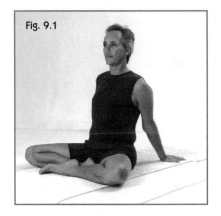

Fig. 9.3

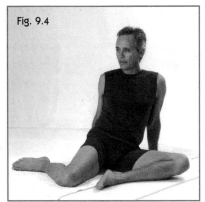

Fig. 9.4

3. With both knees lowered to the ground on your right, observe the shape your legs make—like one side of a pinwheel. Slide your left hand into the space under your left hip. Take an informal measurement of how high that hip is off the ground. Could you roll a lemon under the space? Could an elephant walk under your hip? Make note of this distance, because it is likely to change in the next few minutes.

4. Bring both knees back to upright and lower them over to the left side

toward the ground (**fig. 9.4**). Position your legs wide enough apart that both bent knees are on the floor or the cushion. Slide your right hand under your right hip and measure that space. Notice how different the space under the hip on this side might be in comparison with the left side.

5. Bring both knees back to upright and lower them over to the right side again. Gently lift the left knee and tap the inner knee on the ground, as though you were using that surface to knock on a door (**fig. 9.5**). Keep the

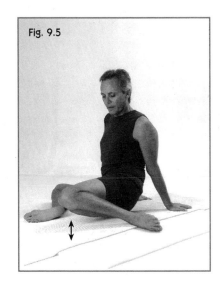

Fig. 9.5

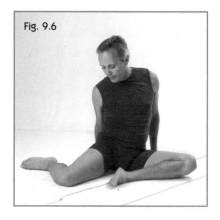

Fig. 9.6

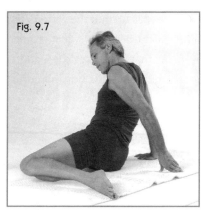

Fig. 9.7

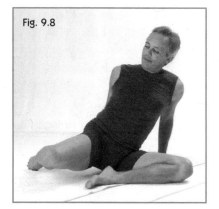

Fig. 9.8

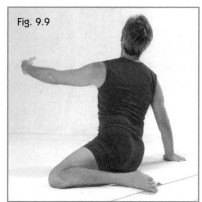

Fig. 9.9

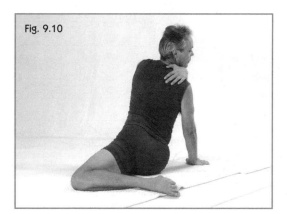

Fig. 9.10

circle on the floor in one direction a few times and in the opposite direction a few more times.

7. Now slide your left hand under your left hip and notice whether that hip has begun to drop toward the floor.

8. Bring both knees back to upright and lower them over to the left side. Gently lift the right knee and tap the inner knee on the ground, repeating the same exploration on this side.

9. When you stop the tapping, slide your right hand under your right hip and notice if it has begun to drop toward the floor.

10. Now, to integrate the two sides of your body, lift both knees to upright and then lower them back and forth from one side to the other (**figs. 9.6 and 9.7**), letting the inner knee tap as you lower it to the ground.

11. Alternating side to side, begin to lengthen the inner knees away from your hips. Imagine the knob of the knee is a tennis ball flying through the air; as the knee/ball comes toward the ground, reach the knee away from the hip a few inches before lowering the knee to the floor (**fig. 9.8**). The action of exaggerating the reaching stretch with each knee will begin to bring your back hand off the ground and your torso forward (**fig. 9.9**). Notice how the hand and arm want to swing around as the hand comes off the ground. Give in to this swinging movement, allowing the hand to come all the way around to the opposite shoulder for a nice pat on the back (**fig. 9.10**). Back and forth, side to side, deliberately

tapping going. The inner knees are the location of many strains and injuries and so are usually held in a protective muscle pattern. Tapping in this manner tells the knee that it is safe to let go in this position.
6. Send the knee out a little further from the hip and tap it back in closer to you. Back and forth, let the knee tap on the floor. Finally, let the knee tap a

swing each arm all the way around to pat the opposite shoulder.

12. Slow the movement until you return to stillness. Are your sitz bones contacting the ground any differently now? Do you feel that your kinesthetic awareness is still moving even though you are seated in stillness?

Do you notice any pulsing or streaming sensations? Has your mood altered in any way?

13. Continue to the next exploration, or take this opportunity to lie on the ground and enter into deep, relaxed awareness, receiving the full effects of these movements.

Exploration 2: Simple Spinal Twists for Releasing the Hip Joints—Hip Swing

1. Sit in a comfortable position on the ground. Close your eyes. Suggest to your mind that this is a time for slowing down and attuning to the sensations that arise within your body.

2. Make any adjustments that help you settle into the experience. Notice the contact your sitz bones make with the ground. Scan your body to observe the areas that require you to effort in some way in order to stay upright.

3. Moving to a deeper level of awareness, begin to press your sitz bones downward into the ground. Does pressing into the sitz bones anchor you to the ground? Do you feel an energetic lift up through the spine when you exaggerate the press in your sitz bones?

4. Imagine that your head is a helium-filled balloon **(fig. 9.11)**. Notice how your head hovers above your spine when you breathe into the "balloon" of your head.

5. Slowly open your eyes. Reach your hands behind you and plant them on the floor a comfortable distance from your spine. Allow your arms to begin supporting the weight of your upright torso **(fig. 9.12)**.

6. Stand your feet on the ground in front of you with your knees upright toward the ceiling. Separate your feet so that they are wider apart than your hips. Lower both knees toward the ground on your right side into the Pinwheel position **(fig. 9.13)**. If your left knee runs into your right leg or ankle, separate the legs so that both knees can move toward the ground. If during this exploration you feel any strain in either knee you may place a cushion under the knee for support; if your wrists get tired you may also wish to place a cushion behind you for support. You will be holding this position for less than a minute; take this time to determine whether you will need the support of a cushion.

7. Moving to the other side, lower both legs to the left and find the Pinwheel position. Again, hold for a minute to determine whether you will need the support of a cushion under either of your knees, or to support the left wrist **(figs. 9.14 and 9.15)**.

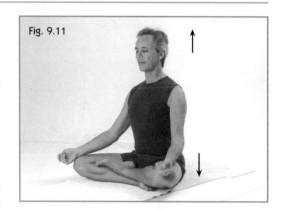

Fig. 9.11

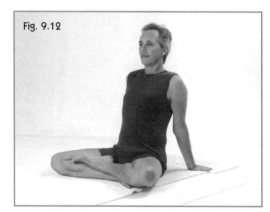

Fig. 9.12

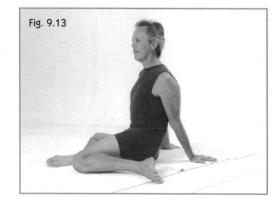

Fig. 9.13

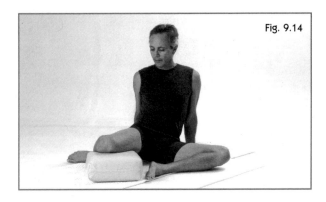

Fig. 9.14

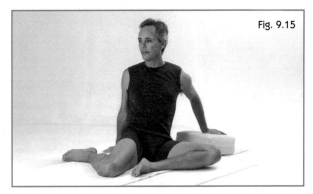

Fig. 9.15

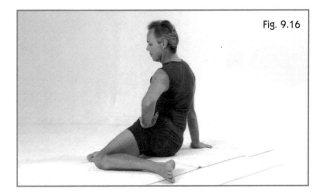

Fig. 9.16

8. Bring both knees back to upright and lower them over to your right side. Place your left hand on your left hip. Inhale and lift your left hip off the ground, allowing your left hand, arm, and shoulder to remain heavy and passive (**fig. 9.16**). You are giving your arm a ride by lifting and lowering the hip.

9. Exhale as you lower the hip. Continue inhaling and lifting the hip, exhaling and lowering the hip. Begin to look in the direction your torso is turning. As you lift the hip, your gaze turns your head to look over your right shoulder (**fig. 9.17**); as you lower the hip, your gaze turns your head back to look over the left shoulder (**fig. 9.18**). Let this movement build, noticing how the breath and looking with your eyes take you progressively deeper into the twisting stretch.

10. Continue this same movement, but this time initiate the turn with your earlobe rather than your eyes. Imagine that you have long Buddha earlobes and that you are being turned by the ear in each direction to hear what is being said. After turning by the ear, add the last little bit of twist by looking with your eyes. Being turned by the ear first and then by the eyes elongates the neck and maximizes the benefits of the movement.

11. Can you let your shoulders and torso move in one direction and your ears, eyes, and head move in the opposite direction? This variation helps to isolate the movement of the various segments of your torso and head.

12. Return to the original movement, torso and head moving in the same direction. Close your eyes and let go of control of the movement. Your shoulder may get very loose, your head can roll (**fig. 9.19**). Relax your jaw and your face. If you put a little attitude into this particular phase of the exploration, you may begin to look like Mae West with her famous hip and shoulder lift. As you let go of the con-

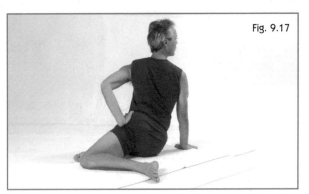

Fig. 9.17

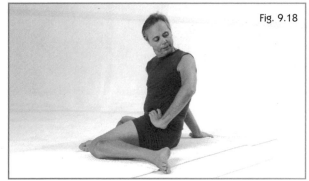

Fig. 9.18

trol over your body, sense how freely and fluidly your body moves. This is movement that comes from the hips and pelvis—you're moving in the way your body is designed to move.

13. Slow the movement down to stillness. Sit with your eyes closed. Feel the effects in your body. Slide your left hand under your left sitz bone and see whether it has released closer to the ground.

14. Bring both knees back to upright and lower them over to your left side. Place your right hand on your right hip. Continue the exploration on this side: lifting and lowering the hip as the arm remains passive; turning to look in the direction of your torso; initiating the movement by turning your earlobe rather than your eyes; and finally letting your shoulders and torso move in one direction and your ears, eyes, and head move in the opposite direction. Then return to the original movement and let go of all control. Sense how fluidly your body can move.

15. Slow the movement down to stillness. Sit with your eyes closed. Feel the effects in your body. Slide your right hand under

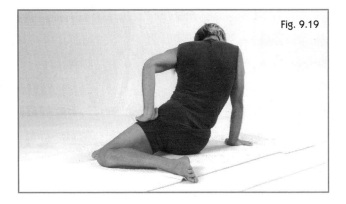

Fig. 9.19

your right hip—has that hip come closer to the ground? Do you notice any other parts of the body that have let go? Can you sense how your sitz bones are contacting the ground any differently? Do you feel that your kinesthetic awareness is still moving even though you are seated in stillness? Do you notice any pulsing or streaming sensations? Has your mood altered in any way?

16. Prepare to continue into the next exploration, or take this opportunity to lie down on the ground and enter into deep relaxed awareness, receiving the effects of these movements.

Exploration 3: Pinwheel to Cradles

1. Sit in a comfortable position on the ground. Close your eyes. Suggest to your mind that this is a time for slowing down and attuning to the sensations that arise within your body. Make any adjustments that help you to settle into your body.

2. Notice the contact your sitz bones make with the ground. Scan your body to observe the areas that require you to use effort in some way to hold yourself upright. Moving to a deeper level of awareness, begin to press your sitz bones downward into the ground. Does pressing into the sitz bones anchor you to the ground? Do you feel an energetic lift up through the spine when you exaggerate

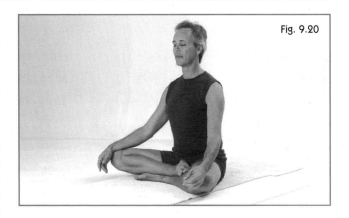

Fig. 9.20

the press in your sitz bones?

3. Imagine that your head is a helium-filled balloon (**fig. 9.20**). Notice how your head hovers above your spine when you breathe into the balloon of your head.

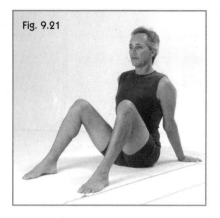

Fig. 9.21

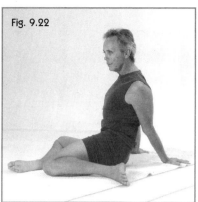

Fig. 9.22

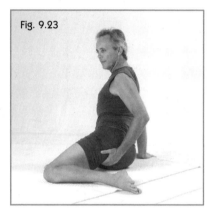

Fig. 9.23

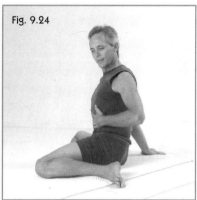

Fig. 9.24

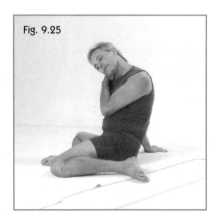

Fig. 9.25

4. Open your eyes slowly. Reach your hands behind you and plant them on the floor a comfortable distance from your spine. Allow your arms to begin supporting the weight of your upright torso.

5. Stand your feet on the ground in front of you with your knees upright toward the ceiling (**fig. 9.21**). Separate your feet so that they are wider apart than your hips. Lower both knees toward the ground on your right side into the Pinwheel position (**fig. 9.22**). If your left knee runs into your right leg or ankle, separate the legs further apart so that both knees can move toward the ground. If you have any strain in either knee, place a cushion under the knee for support; if your wrists get tired you may also wish to place a cushion behind you for support. Moving to the other side, lower both

legs to the left and find the Pinwheel position on that side.

6. Bring both knees back to upright and lower them over to your right side. Place your left hand under your left sitz bone. Inhale as you lift your left hip with your hand (**fig. 9.23**). As you exhale, sit back on the floor into your hand. Repeat a few times and observe how your hand gives feedback to your sitz bone about the lifting and sitting.

7. Bring the palm of your left hand to the right side of your rib cage and take a handful of ribs, turning your rib cage toward the left as you lower the left hip (**fig. 9.24**). The gliding motion of your palm stroking across your rib cage gives your body the idea of rotating through the ribs. Repeat this stroking a few times as you lift and lower the hip.

8. Bring your left hand across the top of the chest to hang on the right shoulder. Let your left elbow become heavy. Lean into your left shoulder, allowing it to lift toward your head while you lower your head to rest on your hand and shoulder (**fig. 9.25**). Give your head a ride by bending the elbow of your right arm, which is supporting your hand and head, and moving the shoulder in a few up-and-down circles. It will feel like you're giving your head a ride. Let your head be as heavy as it can be. Release your jaw and the muscles of your face. Allow any sounds to emerge.

9. Bring your left arm over your head and take hold of your right ear. Allow your hand to cradle the weight of your head. Extend your left elbow up to the sky and begin to make imaginary circles on the ceiling with that elbow (**fig. 9.26**). Notice the tendency for the left hip to engage in an attempt to help perform this movement. Keep the hip relaxed and heavy and allow the work to occur through the upper body. Gradually allow the circles to get larger. Then reverse the direction of the circles and make a whooshing noise with your exhaling breath, putting a little speed and exaggeration into the movement.

10. Bring the movement to stillness. Before releasing your left arm, slide the palm of your left hand down your back. Give yourself a good pat on the back. Reach up with your right palm and grasp the knob of your left elbow. Gently draw the elbow behind your head and toward the midline of your back (**fig. 9.27**). Hold the elbow and take a deep breath in, lifting through the breastbone. Exhale and let the upper body round a little bit (**fig. 9.28**). Inhale again and lift through the breastbone as you firmly cradle the elbow in place (**fig. 9.29**).

11. Release your left arm and let it float back down to your side. Slide your left hand under your left hip and notice whether it has come any closer to the ground. As you sit, pause to notice the openness in your left hip.

12. Bring both knees back to upright and lower them over to your left side. Place your right hand under your right sitz bone. Inhale as you lift your right hip with your hand (**fig. 9.30**). Exhale and sit back on the floor into your hand. Repeat a few times; observe how your hand gives feedback to your sitz bone about the lifting and sitting.

13. Bring the palm of your right

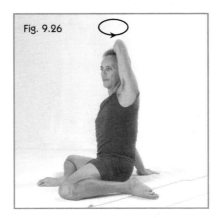

Fig. 9.26

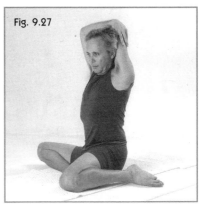

Fig. 9.27

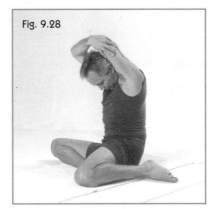

Fig. 9.28

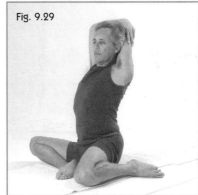

Fig. 9.29

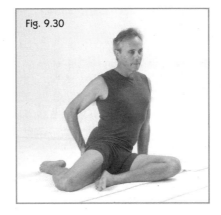

Fig. 9.30

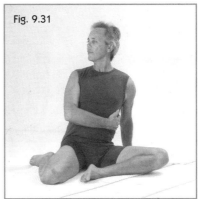

Fig. 9.31

hand to the left side of your rib cage and take a handful of your ribs, turning your rib cage toward the right as you lower the right hip (**fig. 9.31**). Repeat a few times as you lift and lower the hip.

14. Cross your right hand over the upper chest to hang on the left shoulder. Let your right elbow become heavy. Lower your ear and head to rest

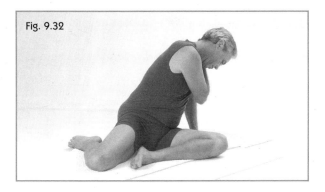

Fig. 9.32

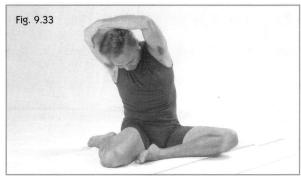

Fig. 9.33

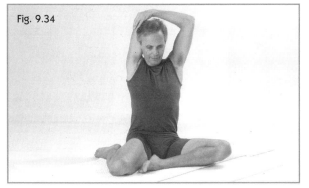

Fig. 9.34

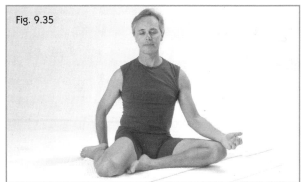

Fig. 9.35

on that hand and shoulder. Bend the left elbow and move the shoulder in up-and-down circles **(fig. 9.32)**. Release your jaw and the muscles of your face. Allow yourself to give voice to any sounds that want to emerge.

15. Bring your right arm overhead and take hold of your left ear. Cradle the weight of your head with that hand. Extend your right elbow up to the sky and begin to make imaginary circles with the elbow **(fig. 9.33)**. Do the muscles of the right hip engage to help execute the movement? Keep the hip relaxed and heavy and let the work happen in the upper body. Allow the circles to get increasingly larger. Reverse the direction of the circles and make a whooshing noise with your exhaling breath, putting a little speed and exaggeration into the movement.

16. Bring the movement to stillness. Slide the palm of your right hand down your back and give yourself a good pat on the back. Reach up with your left palm and grasp the knob of your right elbow. Gently draw the elbow toward the midline of your back **(fig. 9.34)**. Hold the elbow and take a deep breath in, lifting through the breastbone. Exhale and let the upper body round a little bit. Inhale again and lift up through the breastbone as you firmly cradle the elbow in place.

17. Release your left arm and let it float back down to your side. Slide your right hand under your right hip—has it come any closer to the ground? Sit with your eyes closed a moment and experience the sensation of breathing into your open right hip **(fig. 9.35)**.

18. Lie on the floor and stretch your arms and legs long. As you lie on the ground notice any effects in your legs, hip joints, pelvis, or low back. Observe how your upper back and shoulders contact the ground. Notice any pulsing, streaming, or tingling sensations that may begin to arise.

Integration: Knee-to-Chest Figure 8s

1. From a seated position, bend both knees and bring them together. Lower your elbows to the ground behind your back, supporting the weight of your torso with your arms and shoulders (**fig. 9.36**).

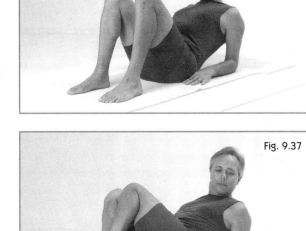

Fig. 9.36

2. Lifting your feet off the ground and keeping your knees together, take your knees to one side of the body and then the other (**figs. 9.37 and 9.38**). Notice how the muscles of your low back are lengthened and how you engage your abdominal muscles to make the movements. The closer your knees stay to your chest, the more intensely your abdominals will be engaged and the more freedom there will be in the movement of the limbs. Continue this side-to-side movement, allowing your head to turn to look in the opposite direction of the knees. Notice your breathing. Allow the movement to synchronize with your breath.

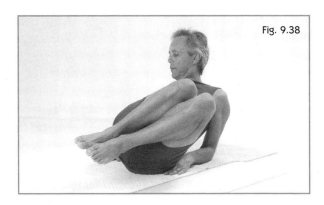

Fig. 9.37

3. Pause for a moment and notice how you are energizing your abdominal center, how you are generating heat in that area. Also notice how this fluid movement goes back and forth across the midline of your body. Crossing the midline in this way stimulates communication between the two sides of the body, integrating both sides into a more efficient whole.

Fig. 9.38

4. Now take the knees in a figure 8 movement. Imagine that a pointer is attached to your nose. Begin to take the head in figure 8s in the same direction as the knees, then in the opposite direction of the knees.

5. Pause and notice how much energy is pulsing in your belly center. The last phase of the inquiry provides a good opportunity for engaging your abdominals to your comfortable limits.

6. Again bend your knees in close to your chest, supporting the weight of your torso with your elbows. Take your knees to one side and then extend your legs, lengthening them to the point that you can hold this position for a moment without undue strain (**fig. 9.39**). Bend your knees and bring them through center to the other side, then once again extend your legs to your comfort zone (**fig. 9.40**). You will notice that it

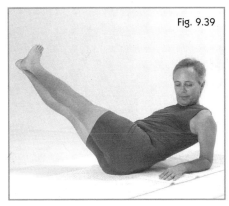

Fig. 9.39

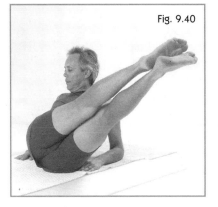

Fig. 9.40

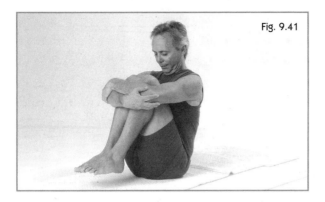

Fig. 9.41

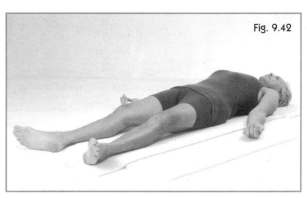

Fig. 9.42

is easier to continue this movement when you allow the eyes and head to look over the opposite shoulder. Repeat this movement until you feel heat accumulating in the abdominal muscles.

7. If you are feeling adventurous, extend your legs and keep them lengthened as you take them from side to side. Use your breath. Allow your head to turn, looking in the opposite direction. Pay attention to keeping your abdominals engaged by bringing the belly button toward the spine, so that your low back does not arch up off of the ground.

8. Bring your knees back in toward your chest and give yourself a good hugging squeeze (**fig. 9.41**). Then stretch your legs long and roll your spine down to the ground for relaxation (**fig. 9.42**).

9. Notice all the sensations streaming though your body at this time. Observe how quickly and how deeply your awareness slows down to ride the waves of sensation. Suggest to your logical mind that this is the time to receive from the wisdom of the organism. Travel in your awareness into the core of your hip joints. Can you sense how the prana is moving in response to the Pinwheel movements? Notice how

your low back, your shoulders, and your neck are releasing into the pull of gravity. Allow all thoughts and thinking to dissolve into the steady stream of sensation.

10. As you begin to prepare for your return, notice the way your body looks and feels when you are at home in the center of your being. Recall the image of a great turning wheel of life, with all the spokes of your experiences connected to your center of being. Suggest to your logical mind that you'll be returning with awakened awareness to the way your hips are designed to support your movements.

11. When you are ready begin your return, gradually roll up into a seated position. Notice the way you are sitting and how your spine elongates as it is supported by the sitz bones. Notice the way your head hovers above your spine.

12. While in this position you may wish to move into one of the seated yoga postures, such as Pigeon, Chin to Knee, or the Seated Forward Bend, to notice the effects of this exploration on your execution of the pose. As you stand and begin to move, continue your inquiry into the way your body articulates as result of these explorations.

Differentiating Spinal Movements by Opening the Hips

Inquiry: How do flexible, open hips support exploring freedom of movement throughout the spine?

This inquiry continues the focus on anchoring the sitz bones to support opening in the hip joints. In addition, the explorations introduce larger, whole-body movements that take the limbs into their full range of motion while the pelvis remains grounded. The physical benefits arise from strengthening and toning the abdominals to support the spine so that the legs can relax into sitting more comfortably. With open hip joints and strong core support in the abdominals, the larger movements of the upper body originate from the body's center.

In Dolphin, the spine enters into a rolling flexion and extension over the thigh, hydrating the vertebral discs and inducing rhythmic, sequenced movement throughout its entire length. In Rocking Horse, the sitz bones begin to spread, creating more space for the hip joints to rotate. Serving Tea activates the hip flexors, powerful muscles responsible for lateral lifting of the thigh. These muscles—particularly the piriformis—are hard muscles to get to; this movement zeroes in with targeted efficiency for strengthening, toning, and increasing flexibility. Fire Truck and Airplane Lifts are simple spinal twisting movements that differentiate the body segments, allowing them to move independent of, yet in harmonious relationship with, the whole body. These particular movements alternately contract and release the oblique abdominal muscles.

All the explorations in this inquiry begin in Seated Pinwheel as guided above. As you progress through these explorations, you will want to periodically review the directives for entering a relaxed Seated Pinwheel. The instructions for entering deep relaxation and for your return are at the end of the final exploration in this chapter. Feel free to pause at any point and enter into deep relaxation.

Exploration 1: Pinwheel to Dolphin

1. Come into Seated Pinwheel with your knees lowered over to the right side. Place both hands on your right knee, one hand on top of the other. Using this hand "sandwich," press your knee into the ground **(fig. 9.43)**. Press it several times and release after each press. Do you notice how your torso moves out over your right thigh to get leverage for a strong press?

2. Let the pressing and releasing begin to move through your torso in a wavelike motion. Exaggerate the wave as it ripples through your body: dive out over your knee with

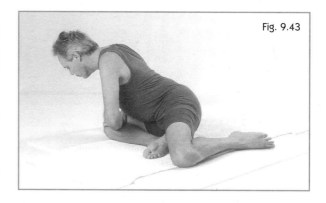
Fig. 9.43

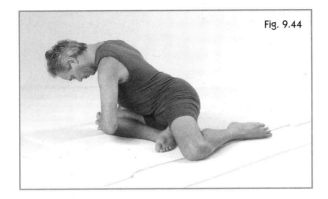

Fig. 9.44

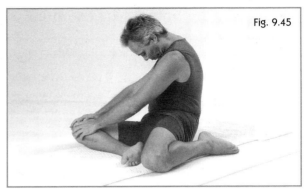

Fig. 9.45

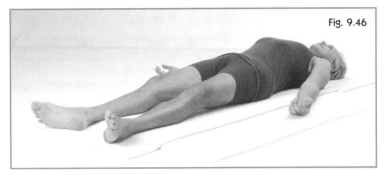

Fig. 9.46

your breastbone lifting away from your thigh (**fig. 9.44**), then curl your spine backward, chin toward your chest, as you release the press (**fig. 9.45**). Imagine a dolphin taking a dive deep into the ocean and then sweeping up and out of the water as you curl back into your sacrum to prepare for the next dolphin dive.

3. Continue this movement, allowing it to get larger and to involve more parts of your body.

This spiraling of the torso can become quite hypnotic, like a perpetual-motion rocking that begins to happen through you rather than by you. Close your eyes, relax your jaw and your face, and enjoy the sensations.

4. When you are ready to bring your body to stillness, sit for a moment and experience how the movement feels as if it continues pulsing through your muscles and nervous system.

5. Bring both knees upright and lower them over to the left side. Repeat Dolphin over your left knee and thigh. When you are ready to come to stillness, experience the sensation of the movement continuing to pulse through your body.

6. Lie down on the floor and stretch your arms and legs long (**fig. 9.46**). Notice any effects that occur as you lie on the ground. Notice any pulsing, streaming, or tingling sensations that may begin to occur.

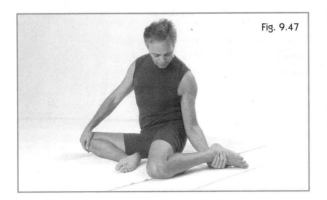

Fig. 9.47

Exploration 2: Pinwheel to Rocking Horse

1. Begin in the Seated Pinwheel with your knees to the right side. Grasp the knob of your right knee with your right hand. Scoop your left hand underneath the heel and inner ankle of the left foot (**fig. 9.47**). Use your thumb as a finger so that your whole palm works as a scoop.

2. With your right hand lift the right knee off the ground a few inches (**fig. 9.48**). Lower it to the ground. Lift the left ankle a couple of inches off the ground, leaving your left knee on the ground (**fig. 9.49**).

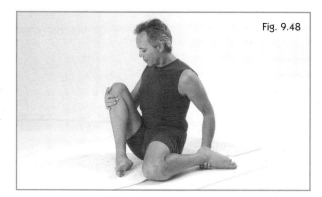

Fig. 9.48

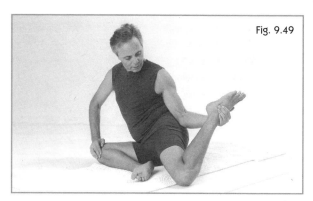

Fig. 9.49

3. Now alternate back and forth, lifting the front knee and then the back ankle. This will take you into a rocking movement called Rocking Horse. When the action takes over, close your eyes and enjoy the sensation of perpetual-motion rocking. Imagine not that you are doing the movement but that the movement is "doing" you. Breathe fully and enjoy the experience.

4. Bring both knees upright and lower them over to the left side, repeating Rocking Horse.

5. When you are ready to bring your body to stillness, sit for a moment and experience how the movement continues pulsing through your muscles and nervous system.

6. Lie down on the floor and stretch your arms and legs long. Notice any effects that occur as you sink your awareness into your sensate body.

Exploration 3: Piriformis Lifts—Serving Tea

1. Begin in the Seated Pinwheel with your knees to the right side. Place both hands on your right knee, one hand on top of the other. Inhale, press into the right knee, and lift the back knee and back ankle a few inches off the ground (**fig. 9.50**). Try to keep the knee and ankle at the same height, as though you were balancing a tray of teacups and a teapot—don't spill the tea! Exhale as you lower the left leg to the ground. This can feel like an intense stretch across the top of the left hip crease. If you experience a cramp, stretch your leg out and say a few swear words, breathe, and wait for the cramp to pass. The cramp is feedback that the muscle is not used to working. It will pass.

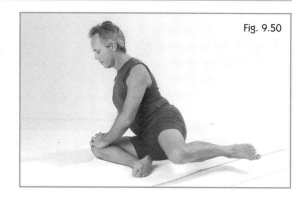

Fig. 9.50

2. Continue for a few rounds, inhaling and lifting the left leg, exhaling and lowering the leg. See how much higher you can lift the leg each time without using force or effort. Repeat until the movement becomes familiar and effortless.

3. Pause and rest a moment. Notice the sensations in the left hip joint.

4. Now inhale and lift the left leg again. Exhaling, stretch your foot as you swing the foot forward (**fig. 9.51**), then flex the heel

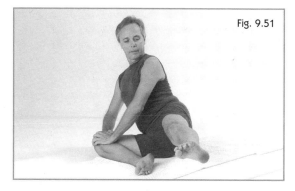

Fig. 9.51

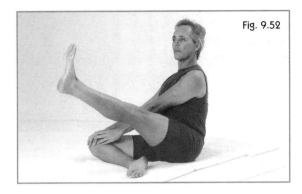

Fig. 9.52

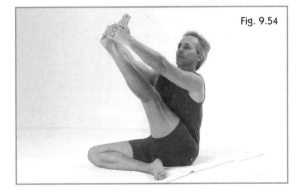

Fig. 9.53

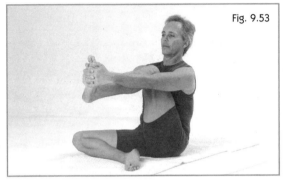

Fig. 9.54

as you extend the leg out in front of you (**fig. 9.52**). Do not let the leg touch the ground. Hold the leg in this position and keep lengthening out through the heel. Use your breath and see if you can make little pulsing lifts to bring the leg a bit higher.

5. Bend the knee and swing the leg back around to the starting Pinwheel position. Now repeat the movement to the front—inhale as you lift the knee; exhale as you swing the leg forward, flexing the heel as you extend the leg out in front of you; then bend the knee and swing it back around to the starting position. Repeat this movement for the next few breaths.

6. The next time you extend the leg out in front of you, reach for the foot and draw your knee toward your torso (**fig. 9.53**). Interlace your fingers around your foot and begin to lengthen your leg from the heel (**fig. 9.54**), then bend the knee back in toward your chest. Repeat this movement a few times and then bring your leg back into the starting Pinwheel position.

7. Before leaving your right knee, do a few Dolphin dives (see exploration 1) over the knee to relieve any tension that may have accumulated in this circular leg lift. When you come into stillness, notice any sensations that arise.

8. Bring both knees back to upright and lower them over to the left side. Repeat this sequence of movements with the right leg forward.

9. Before leaving this side, do a few Dolphin dives over the left knee to relieve any tension that may have accumulated through this leg lift. When you come into stillness, notice any sensations that arise. Does it feel as if the movement continues pulsing through your muscles and nervous system?

10. Lie down on the floor and stretch your arms and legs long. Notice any effects that this exploration might be having on your organism.

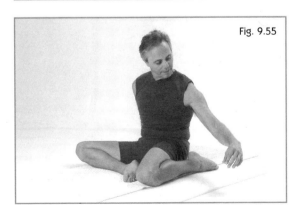

Fig. 9.55

Exploration 4: Simple Spinal Twisting—Fire Truck

1. Begin in the Seated Pinwheel with your knees on the right side. Slide your hand under your left hip to take an informal measure of the space between your hip and the floor.

2. Plant your right hand on the floor behind you for support. Pick up an imaginary toy fire truck with your left hand. Run this fire truck along the floor, making a semicircle to the right and to the left (**fig. 9.55**). Let your eyes stay anchored on the movement of your left hand. Keep the left elbow bent and relaxed; release your jaw and the muscles of your face. Inhale in one direction and exhale in the other.

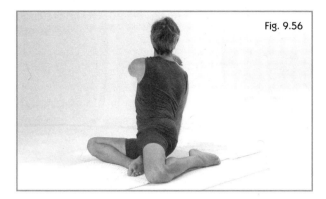

Fig. 9.56

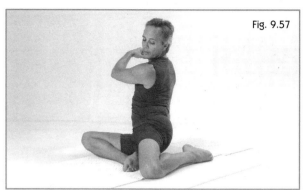

Fig. 9.57

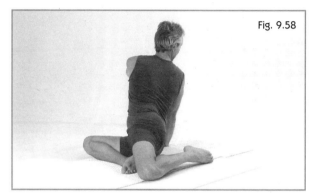

Fig. 9.58

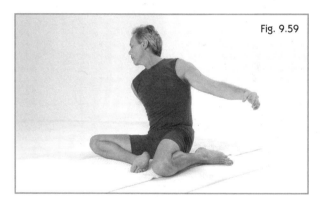

Fig. 9.59

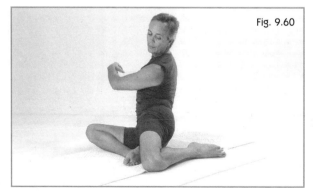

Fig. 9.60

3. Continue this movement, lifting the fire truck off the ground to the level of your elbow. Turn to your right and stay there a moment, looking beyond your hand to find a place on the wall that will help you to mark how far you have turned (**fig. 9.56**). Keeping your left hand and arm in place, look with your eyes up the length of your left arm to your left shoulder and then over your shoulder (**fig. 9.57**). Can you see your foot behind you on the floor? Let your gaze travel back down your left arm to your hand; allow your head to keep turning to your right (**fig. 9.58**). See how much further your head turns this time, now that you have isolated the movement of your head, neck, and eyes.

4. Slowly bring your left arm and head back to neutral and begin the original Fire Truck movement again. After you have the original pattern going, vary it by allowing your eyes and head to look in one direction as the arm and hand with the fire truck move in the opposite direction (**figs. 9.59 and 9.60**). This may be confusing at first; allow the confusion. When you repeat this movement enough to establish a new pattern, the motion will feel effortless and freeing. Breathe and relax into the movement. Notice how much deeper your breath goes when you let the eyes and head turn in the opposite direction as your arm and hand.

5. Release the movement and slide your left hand under your left buttock to see if the hip has released down toward the ground at all. Close your eyes and breathe into the sensations in this hip.

6. Lie down on your back; stretch your arms and legs long. Notice any differences in the way the two sides of your body contact the ground. Does one leg feel longer than the other? Is one hip more released into the ground than the other? Observe any pulsing, streaming, or tingling sensations.

7. Slowly open your eyes. Roll up into the Seated Pinwheel with your knees over to the left side.

8. Leave your left hand on the floor behind you for support as you measure the space between your right hip and the ground. In your right hand, pick up an imaginary toy fire truck. Run this fire truck along the floor, making a semicircle to the right and to the left. Continue through the sequence of movements on this side.

8. Release the movement and slide your right hand under your right buttock to see if the hip has released toward the ground. Close your eyes and breathe into the sensations in this hip.

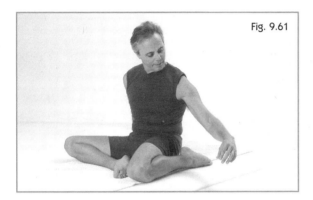

Fig. 9.61

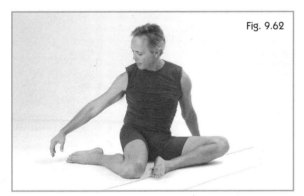

Fig. 9.62

Integration: Side-to-Side Simple Spinal Twisting

1. Come into Seated Pinwheel with your knees to the right side. Plant your right hand on the floor behind you for support. In your left hand, pick up an imaginary toy fire truck. Run this fire truck along the floor, making a semicircle to the right and to the left. Let your eyes stay anchored on the movement of your left hand **(fig. 9.61)**. Keep the left elbow bent and relaxed; release your jaw and the muscles of your face. Inhale in one direction and exhale in the other.

2. Bring both knees back to upright and lower them over to the left side. Put your left hand on the floor behind you for support. Pick up an imaginary toy fire truck in your right hand and run it along the floor, making a semicircle to the left and to the right. Focus your gaze on the movement of your left hand; keep your right elbow bent and relaxed. Inhale in one direction and exhale in the other.

3. Bring both knees upright and lower them over to the right side again. Repeat the fire truck movement to the left one time, then bring the knees upright, lower your legs to the left, and repeat the fire truck movement to your right one time. Alternate the movement back and forth from one side to another **(figs. 9.62, 9.63, 9.64, 9.65, 9.66, and 9.67)** until

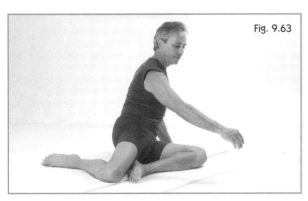

Fig. 9.63

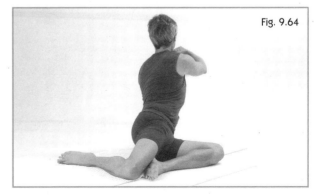

Fig. 9.64

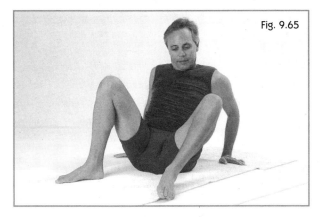

Fig. 9.65

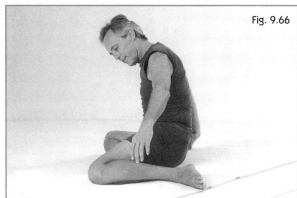

Fig. 9.66

you get the feeling of swinging from one side to another. Let the breath flow in and out with each movement: inhale in one direction, exhale back to center, and inhale to the new direction.

4. Allow the momentum to build until you feel the sensation of perpetual-motion rocking, a movement that is happening through you, not by you.

5. Slow the movement and come into stillness. Lie down on your back and stretch your arms and legs long. Allow your breath to flow in and out without attempting to control or inhibit it in any way. Observe the sensations pulsing through your body.

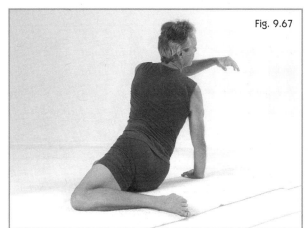

Fig. 9.67

Integration: Lifting into Side Stretching— Airplane Lifts

1. Begin in the Seated Pinwheel with your knees to the right side. Plant your right hand on the floor behind you for support. In your left hand, pick up an imaginary toy airplane, similar to the fire truck in the previous explorations. This airplane, though, is going to lift off the ground and take your torso with you. Run this airplane along the runway to your right, then allow it to lift off, lifting your buttocks off the floor but leaving your right knee in contact with the ground (fig. 9.68). In this semicircular lift to the right let your eyes stay anchored on the movement of your left hand. Hold the lift long enough to feel the stretch, then return back down to the ground and prepare for another lift. Inhale as you lift and exhale as you lower back down to the ground.

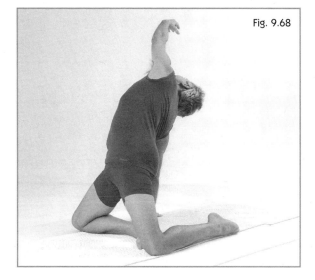

Fig. 9.68

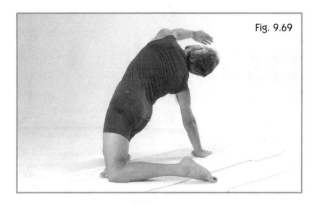

Fig. 9.69

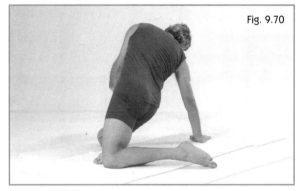

Fig. 9.70

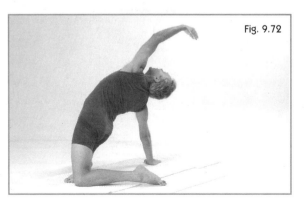

Fig. 9.71

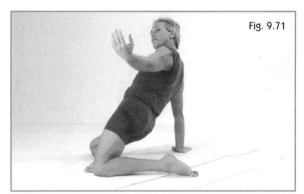

Fig. 9.72

2. Repeat this airplane lift several times to your right. On the last repetition, hold the lift as you make wide, sweeping circles with your arm, keeping your eyes anchored on the motion of your left hand **(figs. 9.69, 9.70, 9.71, and 9.72).** Go in one direction first, then scribe a circle in the opposite direction. Breathe deeply and fully into this magnanimous stretching movement.

3. Come back to the ground and sit with your eyes closed. Experience the sensations that result from this stretch.

4. Bring both knees to upright and then lower them to the left side. Leave your left hand on the floor behind you for support. In your right hand, pick up an imaginary airplane that will lift off the ground and take your torso with it. Run this airplane along the runway to your left, then allow it to lift off, lifting your buttocks off the floor but leaving your left knee in contact with the ground **(fig. 9.73).** In this semicircular lift let your eyes stay anchored on the movement of your right hand. Hold the lift long enough to feel the stretch, then return back down to the ground and prepare for another.

5. Repeat this airplane lift several times to your left, inhaling as you lift and exhaling as you lower. On your last lift, make wide sweeping circles with your arms, keeping your eyes anchored on the circular motion of your right hand. Go in one direction first, then scribe a circle in the opposite direction. Breathe deeply and fully.

6. Return back down to the ground and sit with your eyes closed **(fig. 9.74).** Experience the sensations that result from this whole-body movement.

7. Bring both knees upright and lower them to the right side; repeat the airplane lift once to this side. Change to the left side and repeat the airplane lift. Continue from side to side until you get the feeling of swinging from one side to

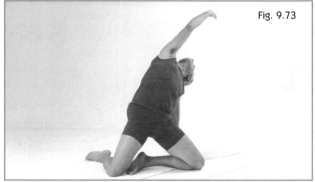

Fig. 9.73

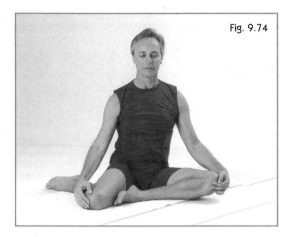

Fig. 9.74

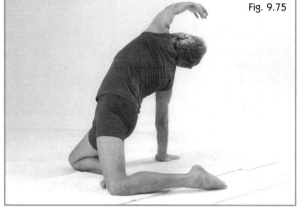

Fig. 9.75

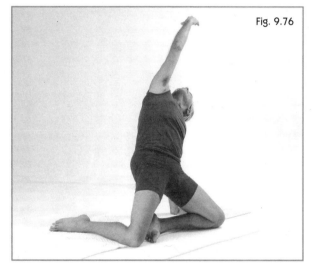

Fig. 9.76

another (**figs. 9.75 and 9.76**). Let the breath flow in and out with each movement. Inhale in one direction, exhale back to center, and inhale to the new direction. Allow the momentum to build until you feel the sensation that the movement is a perpetual-motion rocking that is happening through you.

8. Slow the movement and come into stillness. Lie down on the ground and stretch your arms and legs long (**fig. 9.77**). Allow your breath to flow in and out without attempting to control or inhibit it in any way. Observe the sensations pulsing through you.

9. Notice all the sensations streaming though your body at this time. Observe how quickly and deeply your awareness slows down to ride the waves of sensation. Suggest to your logical mind that this is a time to receive from the wisdom of your organism. Travel in your awareness into the core of your hip joints. Can you sense how the prana is moving in response to the whole-body movements originating from the Pinwheel? Notice how your low back, your shoulders, and your neck are releasing into the pull of gravity.

10. Allow all thoughts and thinking to dissolve into the steady stream of sensation.

11. As you begin to prepare for your return, notice the way your body looks and feels when you are grounded in your center. Recall the sensations of turning and lifting from side to side and returning to your center. Beginning your return to wakeful, alert consciousness, slowly curl your knees in toward your chest and roll up into a sitting posi-

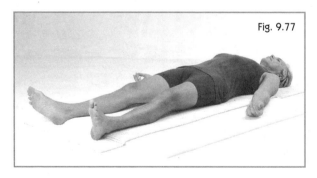

Fig. 9.77

tion. Notice the way you are sitting: can you sense how the hip joints are open, allowing you to feel the contact between your sitz bones and the ground? Do you notice a greater degree of relaxation in your legs, allowing your spine to find its natural length?

Before Moving On . . .

In the preceding chapters you have learned to focus your attention toward energizing your central core in the belly and how to initiate movement from the center while remaining in contact with your abdominal strength. In this chapter your focus has been directed more specifically to movements that open your hip joints to greater flexibility and make it possible to relax the muscles of your legs, gain further strength in the abdominal muscles, and enter seated postures with greater ease and comfort. The movements of this chapter have introduced the spine to simple twisting and side-stretching explorations that prepare the body for entering larger movements with greater awareness.

In the next chapter you will experience the dynamics of lengthening the front side of your body as a way of both protecting and strengthening the muscles of the low back. As you will discover, awareness of lengthening the low back during back bending will give you even more contact with the power and strength in your abdominals.

Having just completed the explorations of this chapter, you may choose to experiment with any of the standing balancing postures, such as Tree, Queen of Dancers, Extended Leg Stretch, or Eagle, to notice the movements of the hip joints that are required to enter these postures with balance and ease. By maintaining awareness of the grounding and stability in your belly, you will notice that many postures you practice will benefit from the openings now occurring for you. When you are ready to move on throughout your day, continue your inquiry into the way your body moves as result of these explorations.

10 Hugging the Planet Earth: Opening from the Belly into Front-Extension Postures

How can core creativity be channeled for birthing new possibilities in life?

WE BEGIN THIS GROUP OF INQUIRIES by making a primary distinction between lengthening the front side of the body through front extension versus compressing the lumbar spine in back bending. What is the difference between a backbend and a front extension? Someone watching you enter into the Cobra, Bow, or Camel pose might not notice that you are entering these postures from the perspective of extending the front side of your body, as opposed to doing what looks like a backbend.

Traditional yoga often emphasizes movements that arch the low back rather than lengthen the line from the pubic bone to the sternum on the front side of the body. The shift in orientation to lengthening the front side of the body can make an important difference in the health of your spine. Chronic low-back pain is a primary contender for on-the-job disability in the American workplace; the inquiries in this chapter can provide relief, support, and education for strengthening this potential "hot spot" in your body.

A backbend encourages the spine to overarch in the low back and the neck, the spine's most flexible (and therefore most vulnerable) areas. The vertebrae of the middle back support the ribs, which wrap around each side of the spine and connect to the sternum on the front side of the body; the rib structure prevents the middle back from bending as much as the low back and the neck.

Picture the discs between the vertebrae, whose job it is to cushion the pressure between bones and to provide lubrication for fluid movement. The discs are round and red, plump and juicy—like water balloons. When you arch backward the fluids in the discs are squeezed flatter on the backside, causing the front side of the discs to bulge. Some squeezing and bulging can be favorable to spinal health—compression and release tones the elastic walls of the discs and stimulates the replenishing of fluids and nutrients to the discs. But repeated, long-term compression can cause the discs to lose their tone and fluidity or to rupture when the spine is overarched. The good news is that low-back conditions, including those that involve the discs, are highly responsive to movements that stimulate physical reeducation.

The energetic differences between these two orientations under discussion are highlighted when you think about the times in your life when you "bent over backward" to please someone. There is a loss of self when you lose connection with your center; the emphasis becomes about what is happening behind your back. When awareness is grounded in your center and you lengthen into an opening from the front side of the body, you sense that you are engaging in life from the inside out, investing your life force and creativity into projects that embody your passion and talent. Rather than haphazardly backing into life, expanding your awareness through your pelvis, belly, and heart encourages you to consciously connect with your interests and take responsibility for your creations. Extending from the womb of the self deep in your belly gives room for the possibility of connecting with an energetic umbilical cord to a continuous and reciprocal flow of nurturance from the universe.

We begin the inquiries in this chapter by humbling ourselves down onto our bellies to hug the planet Earth. The second group of inquiries open the belly and extend the front side from a kneeling position, the posture often associated with prayer.

Lengthening the Front Side to Hug the Planet

Inquiry: How does it feel different to open the front side from the belly versus bending over backward?

In this first exploration you will notice that releasing into gravity in a belly-down position already begins to passively lengthen the front side of the body. As in the gravity scan on your back, Hug the Planet explores the use of gravity and deep relaxation to begin naturally realigning the body. Sphinx brings awareness to the details of lengthening the line from your pubic bone to your sternum, awareness applicable to yoga poses such as Camel, Bow, Cobra, and Wheel. Frog opens the hips and pelvis, allowing for more freedom to lengthen in front extensions. Iguana coordinates upper-body strength with front extensions, preparing the way for yoga postures that require pushing into the hands and arms, poses such as King Cobra and Downward Dog. In these explorations you may be reminded of the movement an infant makes when first learning to push up off of her belly. Spiraling Up to Sitting provides a joyous transition from the belly into the Seated Pinwheel, further establishing your ability to remain in contact with your abdominal strength while rolling up to Pinwheel from another orientation to gravity than you have heretofore experienced in the inquiries.

Exploration 1: Hugging the Planet Earth

1. Lie on your belly on the ground (**fig. 10.1**). Make any adjustments that encourage your body to settle in this position. Observe the contact your belly makes with the ground. Can you sense your abdominal pulse? Can you feel the pulse of the Earth Mother? Suggest to your mind that this is a time for slowing down and attuning to the sensations that arise within your body. When you have settled into the belly-down position, give yourself the message that for the next few minutes you will be scanning your body to observe the way you have organized your body to be on the ground.

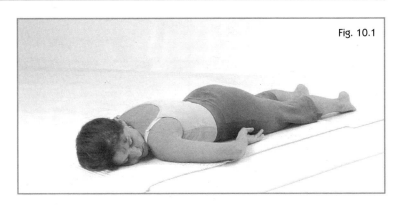

Fig. 10.1

2. Bring your awareness to your feet and notice what surfaces of your feet are touching the ground. Observe the differences between the ways the two feet contact the ground. Sense how far apart your legs are.

3. Moving up to your knees and kneecaps, notice what surface of your knees are in contact with the ground. Notice the difference between how comfortable or uncomfortable each knee feels.

4. Can you sense whether one hip bone is closer to the ground than the other? Do you feel holding in the joint at one or both hips?

5. Observe the way you have organized your arms and hands to be on the ground, particularly noting the difference in the way the arms and hands are each placed on the ground.

6. Now bring your awareness to your head. Notice how your head is placed and what surfaces of your chin, cheekbones, or head are touching the ground.

7. Letting your consciousness travel to your low back, can you sense the rising and falling of the lumbar area as you inhale and exhale? Notice the expansion in the middle back and back of the rib cage as they move in response to the breath.

8. Moving to a deeper level of awareness, scan your entire body and experience the impression your body makes into the ground. Allow your bones to become very heavy; sense your bones gliding down through layers of muscle and tissue in response to the pull of gravity. Observe any pulsing, tingling, or streaming sensations that arise.

9. Slowly reposition your arms, stretching them out to your sides in a T position. Lift

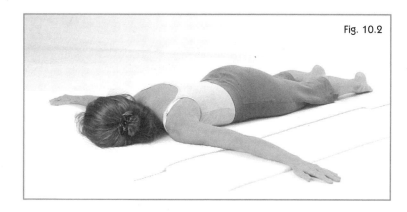

Fig. 10.2

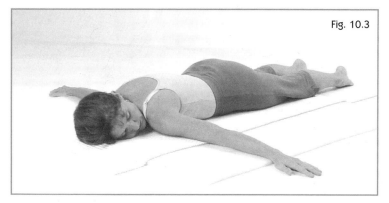

Fig. 10.3

you can let your shoulders become over the next few breaths (fig. 10.3).

12. Lift and turn your head once more, placing the left side of your head on the ground. Relax your jaw and the muscles of your face. Do you notice any difference in the ease of turning and in the quality of the stretch in your neck and shoulders than when you first placed your head in this position?

13. Now bring your awareness down to your feet and legs. Slowly draw your inner ankles together. Squeeze the inner ankle-bones together as you inhale and hold for a moment, then release the heels to roll out to the sides. When you let the heels roll out to the sides, position your big toes so that they are in contact with one another.

14. Lift and turn your head, placing the left side of your head on the ground. Squeeze the inner ankles together as you take in a deep breath. Squeeze the inner knees and the inner thighs together—keep holding the breath. Now exhale and let your heels roll out to the sides. Allow the entire weight of your legs and feet to release down into the ground. Pause here and observe the rising and falling in your low back as you inhale and exhale. Do you notice any difference in the movement from when you first began?

15. Lift and turn your head, placing the right side of your head on the ground. Bring up a strong squeeze at the inner ankles, the inner knees, and the inner thighs and squeeze the lower buttocks together. Hold the squeeze along the entire inner surface of your legs and lower buttocks as you breathe in and out. Exaggerate the squeeze as you imagine pointing your tailbone down toward your heels. Do you notice how the pubic bone gets pressed into the ground? Take a final deep breath in as you squeeze a little more. Then exhale and allow the entire

your head and turn it to place the left side of your face on the ground (**fig. 10.2**). Experience the sensation of being in this position. Observe how your breath is altered by positioning your arms and shoulders in this way. Notice that you are now in a position to feel the gentle curve of the planet earth beneath your embrace.

10. Imagine someone placing sandbags on your shoulders. Experience how much of the weight of your world you can release down toward the ground. Over the course of the next few breaths, allow the shoulders to melt down into the ground.

11. Lift and turn your head, now placing the right side of your head on the ground. Walk your fingertips and palms away from you, lengthening your arms from the shoulders. Imagine stretching your arms from your heart. Place imaginary sandbags on your shoulders again and experience how heavy weight of your legs to release into the ground as your heels roll out to the sides.

16. Notice how much relaxation you feel after you release the squeeze. Can you sense the pulse in your belly getting stronger? Observe the quality of relaxation in your lower buttock muscles. Imagine the lower buttocks opening, like opening a book.

17. Lift and turn your head, placing the left side of your head on the ground. Allow your shoulders to get heavy. Take a deep inhaling breath and bring up the squeeze in your inner ankles, knees, thighs, and lower buttocks. Point your tailbone down toward your heels and press the pubic bone into the ground. Observe the sensation of contracting the lower buttocks and anchoring the pubic bone to the ground. Notice how the low back is lengthened in this exaggerated position. As you exhale, release the legs, rolling the heels to the outside. Release completely.

18. Scan your body and observe any pulsing, streaming, or tingling sensations. Observe the rising and falling of your low back in response to the breath. Experience the way your whole body is opening and lengthening to hug the Earth. Envision the curve of the Earth's surface gently tractioning your spine as you let go into deeper and deeper levels of relaxation.

Exploration 2: Sphinx

1. Lie down on your belly and bring your arms into a T position **(fig. 10.4)**. Slowly slide your arms toward you, lifting the crown of your head toward the ceiling so that you can place your elbows on the ground directly under your shoulders. Adjust your position so that your arms are in contact with your ribs and your forearms and palms are stretched out and parallel on the ground in front of you **(fig. 10.5)**. Notice whether you have contracted the lower buttocks; relax the buttock muscles and settle into this position.

2. Lift your head out of the basket of your shoulders. Press your shoulders down away from your ears and press your elbows down into the ground without allowing your wrists to arch up off of the ground. Take a deep breath in and then relax in this position for a moment.

3. The elbow push-up happens when you press your elbows into the ground and lift your head out of the basket of your shoulders, lengthening the crown toward the ceiling. Experiment with this subtle push-up

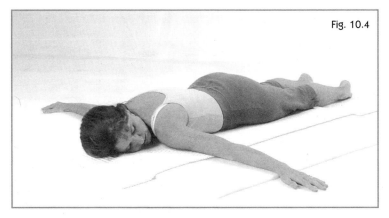

Fig. 10.4

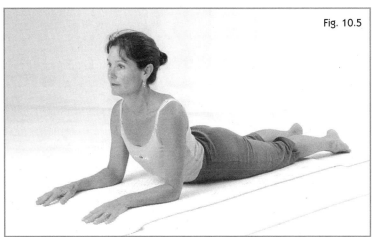

Fig. 10.5

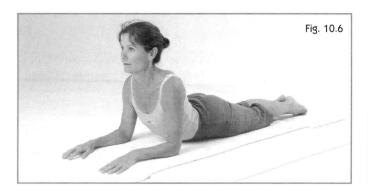

Fig. 10.6

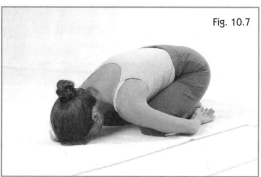

Fig. 10.7

a few times. First press into the elbows, elongating the crown, and then sink your head back into the sling of your shoulders. In this exploration you want to develop the awareness of keeping the head moving up out of the shoulders as you simultaneously press the elbows down into the ground.

4. Continue holding the Sphinx with the elbow push-up engaged. As you hold the pose, roll the inner ankles together and bring up a squeeze to the inner knees, thighs, and lower buttocks. Aim the tailbone down toward the heels and press the pubic bone into the ground **(fig. 10.6)**. Exaggerate the squeeze as you continue to take long deep breaths in and out.

5. Continue holding the Sphinx as you release the squeeze in the lower body, allowing the heels to roll out and the big toes to remain in contact with each other. Pay attention that the elbows are still pressing into the ground and the crown is lifting toward the

ceiling. Your chin is parallel to the ground; softly focus your gaze on the horizon. As you hold this position notice any pulsing, streaming, or tingling sensations, particularly in the kidneys or low back.

6. Take a deep breath in and then press into your elbows and lift your sitz bones back to sit on your heels in Child pose. Draw your arms alongside your body and completely let go of the weight of your torso onto your thighs **(fig. 10.7)**.

7. Can you sense the pulsation in your lower belly? Scan your body, noticing any sensations of heat and cold. Has any part of your body become warm and glowing? Observe your mood and internal feelings. As you release into deeper levels of relaxation in Child pose, consider how you have opened the front side of your body with your belly in close contact with the earth. How does it feel to curl into the fetal position to rest?

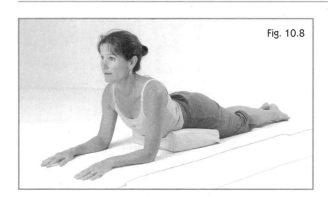

Fig. 10.8

Exploration 3: Opening the Inner Thighs—Frog

1. Come into the Sphinx position. Allow the time it takes to lengthen the front side of your body while angling the tailbone down between your heels. Notice how pressing your pubic bone into the ground and sending the tailbone toward the heels lengthens the low back. For this exploration, you may want to place a cushion under your belly to elevate your hips and decrease the amount of stretch in the inner thighs until you find your comfort zone in this pose **(fig. 10.8)**.

2. Position your legs wider than your hips and bend your knees to bring the soles of your feet together behind you **(fig. 10.9)**. Pivot the lower legs like windshield wipers **(fig. 10.10)**. Experiment with letting them go in the same direction for a while, then allow them to come in and out together. How much of the weight of your feet and ankles can you release into this movement? Do you notice how the inner groin and inner thigh muscles begin to release as you allow the movement to become more playful?

3. Now give yourself some applause for a job well done by clapping the soles of your feet together behind you. Are you ready to open your knees wider apart? The wider your knees, the easier it is to clap.

4. With the soles of your feet touching, press your feet together. Place an imaginary paintbrush between your feet and paint a circle on the wall behind you **(fig. 10.11)**. Can you sense how this movement opens your ankles, knees, and hip sockets? Reverse the direction of the circles. Now make figure 8s. All of these movements awaken different working relationships between the muscles of the lower body and release unconscious holding patterns in your hips.

5. Keeping the soles of your feet together, lower your inner ankles toward the ground, coming to touch the ground if you can **(fig. 10.12)**. This is Frog pose. Breathe all the way down into the lower belly while you hold this position for as long as it is comfortable to do so.

6. When you are ready to release, come back into Child pose by pressing into your hands and sitting back on your heels. Release your torso to hang over your thighs **(fig. 10.13)**.

7. Can you sense the pulsation in your lower belly? Scan your body, noticing any sensations of heat and cold. Has any part of your body become warm and glowing? Observe your mood and internal feelings. As you release into deeper levels of relaxation in Child pose, consider how you have opened the front side of your body by encouraging the hips and inner thighs to come into closer contact with the earth. How does it feel to curl into the fetal position to rest?

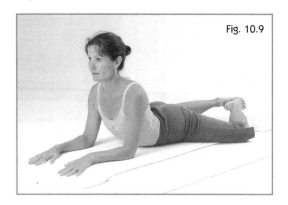

Fig. 10.9

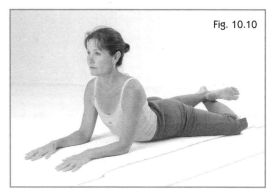

Fig. 10.10

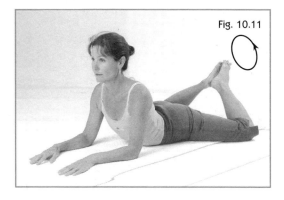

Fig. 10.11

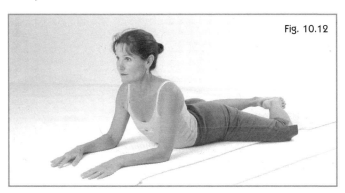

Fig. 10.12

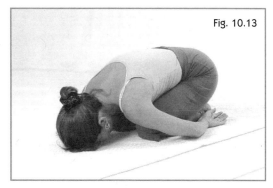

Fig. 10.13

Head Lifting into Baby Cobra

Here is an experiment that will bring awareness to lengthening your head away from your spine in such a way that you won't have to arch or crunch your neck when you go into front-extension postures. These steps are similar to the manner in which an infant learns to lift his head off the ground and push through the hands to come up into the baby's expression of Cobra.

Lie down on the ground and slide your palms under your shoulders, fingertips facing the wall in front of you and your elbows tucked in close to your ribs. Extend the back of your neck by bringing your forehead and scalp line to the floor (**fig. 10.14**). Take a few long and deep breaths and notice how it feels to be lengthening the back of your neck in this position.

Looking with your eyes, begin to focus your gaze on the floor and slowly follow an imaginary line forward on the floor. Notice how your nose and chin brush the floor as the head follows the movement of your eyes (**fig. 10.15**). Look only as far forward on the imaginary line on the floor as you can see with your chin on the ground. Keep your shoulders relaxed and your arms and palms passive on the floor. Take a deep breath in and hold for a moment. Then, exhaling, look with your eyes back toward your chest and curl the chin and nose back in toward your collarbones (**fig. 10.16**).

Imagine a movement you made as a tiny baby when you were learning to lift your head. An imaginary ladybug begins to inch along the floor away from you. See it moving away from you toward the bend where the floor meets the wall. Pause to take in a deep breath, and then exhale and slowly let your gaze travel back in toward your chest.

Repeat the same movement, this time following the movement of the ladybug with your gaze as the ladybug travels up the wall to the place where the wall joins the ceiling (**fig. 10.17**).

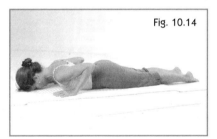

Fig. 10.14

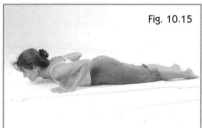

Fig. 10.15

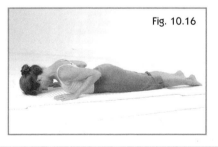

Fig. 10.16

As your chin scoots along the ground and your head begins to lift slightly off the ground, notice how the back of your head lengthens away from your shoulders. Pause to take in a deep breath; as you exhale, return all the way back to the starting position in one breath **(fig. 10.18)**.

Now allow the movement to take your head all the way off the ground, lengthening the crown away from your shoulders as you watch the ladybug move up the wall and onto the ceiling above you **(fig. 10.19)**. Keep your shoulders relaxed and your arms and palms passive on the floor. Take a deep breath in, hold that breath, and then in a single exhaling breath lower your head, following the movement of your eyes back in to look toward your chest. **(fig. 10.20)**. Over the next few breaths repeat this movement, allowing the repetition and rhythm of the movement to take over. Keep your eyes engaged as the initiator of the movement. Stay relaxed in your shoulders and allow your forearms and palms to remain passive on the floor.

Now lower your elbows back down to the ground, stretching out your arms in T position **(fig. 10.21)**. Remaining in this relaxation position, notice the effects of this movement in your low back and belly. Do you sense your abdominal pulse beating any stronger? How is the back side of your body moving as you breathe?

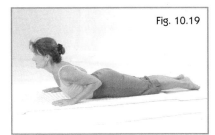
Fig. 10.17

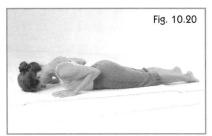
Fig. 10.18

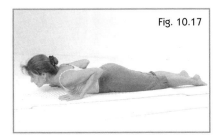
Fig. 10.19

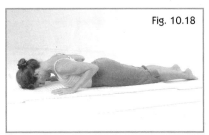
Fig. 10.20

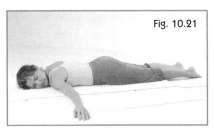
Fig. 10.21

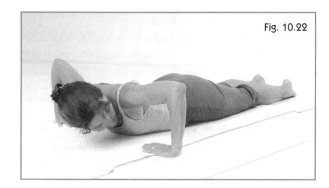

Fig. 10.22

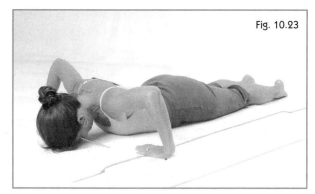

Fig. 10.23

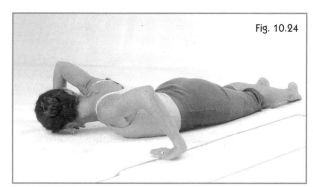

Fig. 10.24

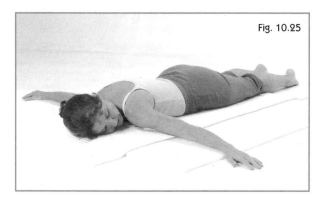

Fig. 10.25

Exploration 4: Iguana

1. Lie on your belly and bring your body into the T position. Extend your arms out to your sides and walk your hands apart. Bend your elbows and plant your palms on the floor in line with your shoulders. Turn your hands so that your middle fingers are pointing at each other (**fig. 10.22**). Play with this unusual position. Notice how your elbows angle out toward the walls on both sides.

2. Slide your hands further and further apart until your elbows form right angles with the floor. Your fingertips remain facing each other and your palms are relatively flat, although you do not want to force or strain the stretch in your wrists or shoulders in any way.

3. Leaving your elbows angled out and your palms on the floor, lower your head, placing the scalp-line of your forehead on or toward the ground. Your chin curls in toward your collarbones (**fig. 10.23**). Leaving your head in this position, alternately press one elbow and then the other forward and back in a winglike motion.

4. Lift and turn your head, placing your left ear on or toward the ground. Look under the window of your right elbow (**fig. 10.24**). Leaving your head in this position, again play with the winging motion in your elbows. Do you notice how one shoulder rolls down toward the ground and the other rolls up toward the sky? Exaggerate that rolling motion in the shoulders.

5. Now lift and turn your head, brushing your nose along the floor and placing the right ear on or near to the ground. Look under the window of your left elbow. Play with the winging motion in the elbows and the rolling motion in your shoulders.

6. Release your arms and return to the T position for a stretch (**fig. 10.25**). Notice any pulsing, streaming, or tingling sensations in your shoulders or neck. Lift and turn your head to bring the left ear toward the ground. Notice the way your spine moves as you breathe.

7. Bend your elbows at right angles, fingertips facing each other and your palms on the ground. Lift and turn your head, placing your left ear on or near the ground. Slide your head under the window of your right elbow and see your right leg and foot along the floor (**fig. 10.26**).

8. Lift and turn your head, placing your right ear on or near the ground. Slide your head under the window of your left elbow and see your left leg and foot along the floor. Bend your left knee and drag your left knee along the floor toward your gaze (**fig. 10.27**). Press into your palms for leverage. Only drag the knee as far forward as is comfortable.

9. Pause for a moment and experience the interesting sensations in your shoulders, hips, and legs.

10. In a rhythmic motion, push the left knee away from you again, turn your head brushing your nose along the ground, and look under the window of your right elbow as you simultaneously begin to drag the right knee along the ground toward your gaze.

11. Pause and experience the sensations generated from being in this position.

12. Alternating from side to side, moving like a giant lizard or iguana, begin to experience the rhythmic motion of looking under one elbow at the oncoming knee, then switching to the other. When the movement becomes familiar to you, begin to use your breath to power the action so you do not strain and can experience an effortless, iguana-like motion.

13. Release the movement and return to the T position for a rest. Turn your head to one side and then the other to experience the sensations that are arising throughout your body.

14. For the final phase of the exploration, return to the movement that you have been making—looking under the window of each elbow and dragging your knee toward you. When this motion is well established, begin pressing your hands into the floor and looking up and over the shoulder toward the oncoming knee (**figs. 10.28 and 10.29**). Start slowly from side to side; let the movement build. As you return through the middle each time, let your chest and head come back down to the ground and brush along the floor before springing up to the other side. Use your breath to power the movement.

15. The next time you come up to look over your left shoulder, stay there for a moment. Roll slightly further so you can balance your weight on your right hip and the outside of your right thigh (**fig. 10.30**). Bend your left knee in as close to your left shoulder as possible. Play with any movement that wants to happen in your right leg as you remain in the position for a few more breaths.

16. Finally, sweep back through the middle and over to look past your right shoulder. Roll slightly further so you can balance your weight on your left hip and the outside

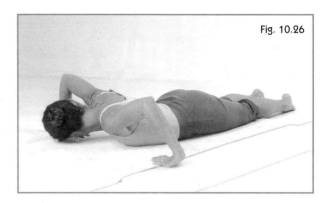

Fig. 10.26

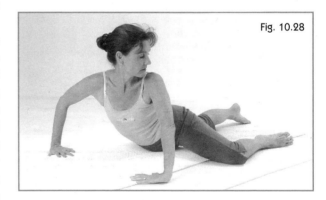

Fig. 10.27

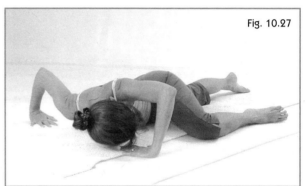

Fig. 10.28

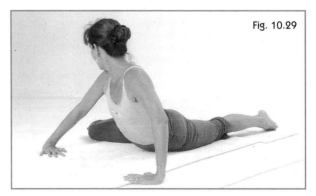

Fig. 10.29

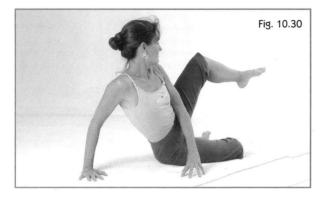
Fig. 10.30

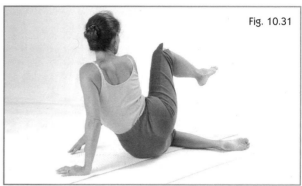
Fig. 10.31

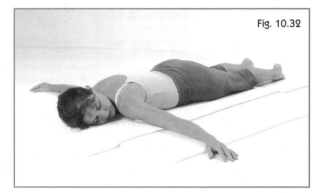
Fig. 10.32

of your left thigh. Bend your right knee in as close to your right shoulder as possible (**fig. 10.31**). Play with any movement that wants to happen in your left leg as you remain in the position for a few more breaths.

17. Now lower your legs back down to the ground and stretch out your arms to a T position. Lift and turn your head, placing your right ear on or toward the ground (**fig. 10.32**). Experience the pulsing, tingling, or streaming sensations through your body. Notice how your lower back lifts and lowers in response to your breathing.

18. Lift and turn your head, placing the left ear on or toward the ground. Do you observe any difference on the two sides of your body? Allow yourself to sink into deeper and deeper layers of relaxation.

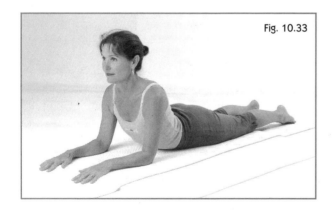
Fig. 10.33

Integration: Spiraling Up to Sitting

1. Begin in Sphinx position, with your arms in contact with your ribs and your forearms and palms stretched out and parallel on the ground in front of you (**fig. 10.33**). Notice whether your lower buttocks are contracted. Relax the buttock muscles and settle into this position.

2. Balancing on your elbows, bring your hands together and interlace your fingers. Notice the thumb and index finger that are on top; this is probably your habitual way of interlacing your fingers. Unlace your fingers and interlace them with the other thumb and index finger on top,

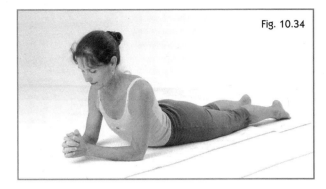

Fig. 10.34

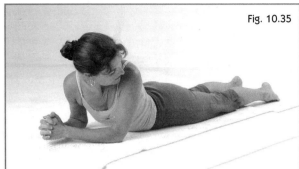

Fig. 10.35

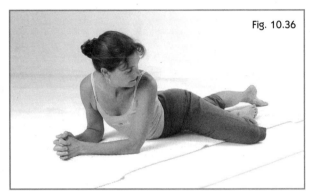

Fig. 10.36

and all of the other fingers falling into the new pattern (fig. 10.34).

3. Close your eyes for a moment and experience the sensation of having your fingers interlaced in the nonhabitual pattern. Does it feel as if you are holding someone else's hand? Does one hand feel thicker than the other? Suggest to yourself that adapting to this new pattern will stimulate a new awareness of the body-mind interactions in your upper body.

4. Holding your hands in this new pattern, turn and look over your right shoulder to see your legs stretched out behind you, then turn and look over the left shoulder to see your legs (fig. 10.35).

5. For the next few breaths, turn and look over each shoulder alternately and begin to bend the knee that is the object of your gaze. As you look to the right, bend the right knee and drag it a few inches toward your right shoulder. As you look to the left, bend the left knee and drag it a few inches toward your left shoulder (fig. 10.36).

6. Return to the Sphinx position. Bend your legs at the knees and bring your inner ankles together. Imagine that you have a string around your ankles keeping your ankles in close contact with one another. Another string is tied around your knees, keeping your knees together. Without letting your ankles or knees come apart, begin to lower your feet to the floor on your right side (fig. 10.37). Experience how close your feet come toward the ground without straining. Notice how lowering your legs together to the right side lifts your left hip up and off the ground. Exaggerate the lift in your hip (fig. 10.38). Feel the stretch along the sides of your rib cage. Leading with your eyes, turn your head to look over your left shoulder

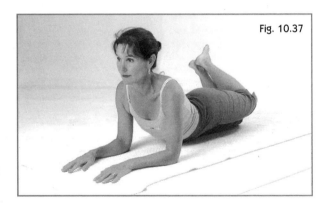

Fig. 10.37

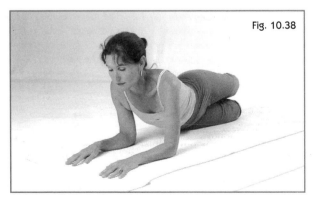

Fig. 10.38

Back Twist

Here is an interesting way to enter a spinal twist from a belly-down position. Lie on the ground and extend your arms from the trunk in a T position. Walk your hands apart (fig. 10.39).

Lift and turn your head, placing your right ear on or near the ground. Bend the left knee and reach your left foot across your body to touch the floor on your right side (fig.10.40). See how close you can come to touching your right hand; feel the intense stretch and twist occurring in your spine. Lower your left leg back to the ground. Pause and notice the sensations. Observe the difference in the two sides of your body.

Now lift and turn your head, placing your left ear on or near the ground. Repeat the twist on this side, bending the right knee and reaching your right foot across your body. When you bring your leg back to the ground, pause and notice your sensations. Now repeat the movement on each side of your body, alternating back and forth between one side and the other. Notice how much easier the movement becomes after you repeat it a few times.

Take a rest. Notice any pulsing, streaming, or tingling sensations that arise in your body. Slow down and let your breath travel all the way down your spine. Can you sense a change in temperature of your muscles and your skin?

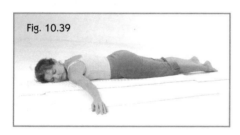

Fig. 10.39

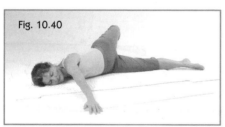

Fig. 10.40

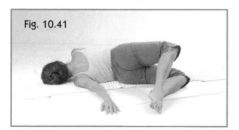

Fig. 10.41

When you feel a return to relaxed and effortless breath, prepare for the final experiment in movement from this position. Bend both knees and, keeping knees and ankles together, reach over to one side of your body with your feet touching or coming close to the ground (fig. 10.41). Return to the center and reach both legs to the opposite side. Go back and forth from side to side until the movement feels familiar and comfortable.

Now lower your legs to the ground and stretch your arms out in a T. Lift and turn your head, placing your right ear on the ground. Experience any pulsing, tingling, or streaming sensations in your body. Notice how your lower back lifts and lowers in response to your breathing.

Lift and turn your head, placing the left ear on the ground. Do you observe any difference on the two sides of your body? Allow yourself to sink into deeper and deeper layers of relaxation.

(fig. 10.42). Notice how this rotation in the upper back and neck completes the twist in your upper spine.

7. Inhale and lift your lower legs back up to the midline, paying attention to keep the ankles together and knees together.

8. Now lower both legs to the left side and notice how the right hip comes off the ground when you keep your ankles and knees together. Again, notice the stretch along the sides of your rib cage. Leading with your eyes, turn your head to look over your right shoulder. Can you see your feet on the ground behind you?

9. Lift your legs back up to the midline and begin to rock your legs from side to side in a pendulum-like motion; when your legs go down in one direction, your eyes and head turn to look over the opposite shoulder (**fig. 10.43**). Go slowly enough to experience the sensation of lifting the opposite hip up and off the ground.

10. Allow the movement to build in momentum until it feels natural and comfortable to be swinging your legs from side to side. Continue the movement until you feel as if you've let go of the control over your body and that your body and its momentum are moving you.

11. Leaving your feet over to the right side, lift the left leg and, in a scissorlike movement, reach back to Pinwheel, touching the floor with your left foot (**fig. 10.44**). This movement is going to be useful later in the exploration in helping to propel you up to sitting without using your hands and arms. To familiarize yourself with the way your leg moves from the stacked knees and ankles position to Pinwheel, move the leg back and forth a few times, stacking the left ankle on top of the right ankle and the left knee on top of the right knee and then reaching back to touch the toes of the left foot to the floor.

12. Return to the "stacked" position, lifting the left leg and placing it onto the right leg, stacking the left ankle on top of the right ankle and the left knee on top of the right knee. Keeping your knees and ankles together and bent at the knees, return to the Sphinx (**fig. 10.45**).

13. Imagine that a string tied around your ankles keeps your ankles in close contact with one another. Another string is tied around your knees, keeping your knees together. This image will help you to learn to use your legs like a pendulum. Without letting your ankles or knees come apart, begin lowering your feet to the floor on the left side (**fig. 10.46**).

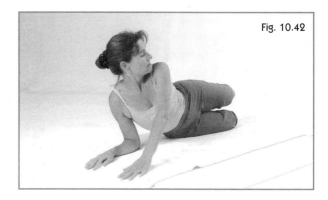

Fig. 10.42

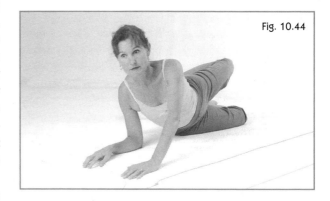

Fig. 10.43

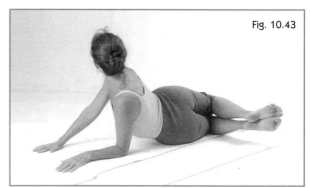

Fig. 10.44

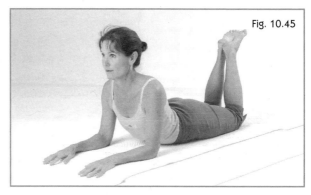

Fig. 10.45

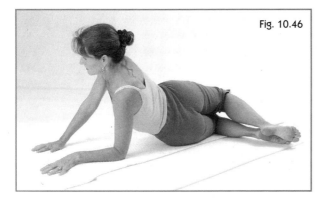

Fig. 10.46

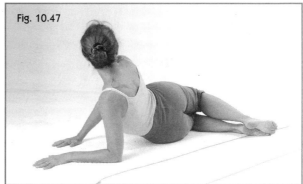

Fig. 10.47

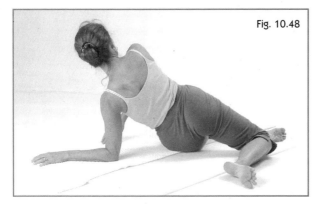

Fig. 10.48

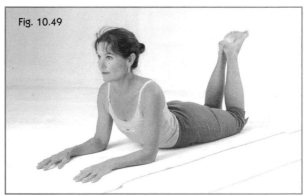

Fig. 10.49

14. Experience how close your feet can come toward the ground without straining. Notice how lowering your legs together to the left side lifts your right hip up and off the ground. Leading with your eyes, turn your head to look over your right shoulder (**fig. 10.47**). Notice how this rotation completes the twist in your upper spine.

15. Leaving your legs over to the left side, lift the right leg in a scissorlike movement, reaching back to touch the floor with your right toes (**fig. 10.48**). To familiarize yourself with the way your leg moves from the stacked knees and ankles position to the Pinwheel, move the leg back and forth this way a few times, stacking the right ankle on top of the left ankle and the right knee on top of the left knee and then scissoring back into Pinwheel. Then bring both legs back to the neutral "stacked" alignment.

16. Keeping knees and ankles together, come back to the Sphinx position. Now, in a pendulum-like motion, swing your legs to the right side; the moment they touch the ground, continue reaching with the left toes toward the floor behind you into Pinwheel. This reaching motion will spiral you back so that your elbows and hands will want to come up and off of the ground.

17. To finish, bring the left knee back on top of the right knee and roll down to the floor onto your belly (**fig. 10.49**). Then immediately swing your legs over to the left side, reaching with the right foot toward the floor behind you (**fig. 10.50**). See if you can reach your right foot far enough to comfortably begin to lift your hands off of the floor.

18. Continue this same movement, spiraling up to sitting on one side, rolling back down onto your belly in the center, and then spiraling up to the opposite side. Your

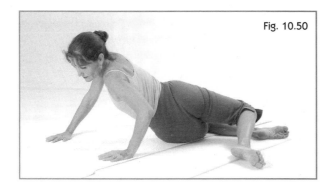

Fig. 10.50

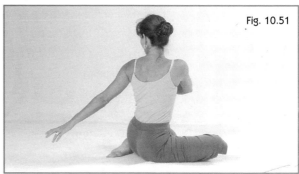

Fig. 10.51

eyes and head look in the opposite direction as your legs (fig. 10.51).

19. Let the movement build until it becomes playful and fun. Each time you come back through the center, lower your belly further toward the ground, then use your hands like a push-up to spring back up to spiral on the opposite side.

20. Slowly let the movement subside. Lower your legs to the ground and stretch

out your arms in a T. Lift and turn your head, placing your right ear toward the ground. Experience the pulsing, tingling, or streaming sensations throughout your body. Notice how your low back lifts and lowers in response to your breathing.

21. Lift and turn your head, placing the left ear on the ground. Do you observe any differences between two sides of your body?

Opening to Life by Engaging the Belly Core

Inquiry: How do I stay grounded in my center while opening into whole-body, front-extension movements?

In this inquiry we transition from front extensions in the belly-down position to front extensions from a kneeling position. Where lying on the ground supplies a surface to press against, there is no such contact with the front side of your body in a kneeling position. This inquiry provides further explorations into ways to enter the traditional backbending postures from the alternative perspective of lengthening the front side, and will help you gain awareness of how to protect yourself from overarching in the low back by extending from the pubic bone to the sternum. Staying anchored in your center allows for deeper relaxation in the midst of any yoga postures or movements that lengthen the front side of the body.

In the first exploration, Kneeling, we explore the details of supporting the low back and neck by focusing awareness on the long, continuous line of the spine as it opens. Sliding Hip Pockets and Windmill prepare the body for gradually entering Camel pose, identifying the limits that are within your safe zone. Forward Lunge combines front extensions with strengthening the legs in preparation for the Standing Runner's Stretch and all of the Warrior postures. This exploration is particularly effective in gaining famil-iarity with aligning the feet for maximum safety for the knees when you move into standing postures that combine hip flexibility with front extensions and standing bal-ance. From a Seed to a Tree integrates the full range of motion from being curled into the fetal spiral of Child pose all the way into opening the belly in the Camel. All of these movements provide checkpoints along the way to assure that you remain connected to your center and do not get tempted to overarch the lumbar or spinal curves.

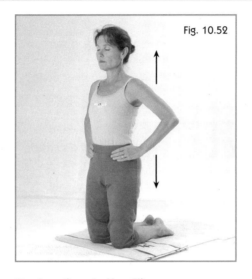

Fig. 10.52

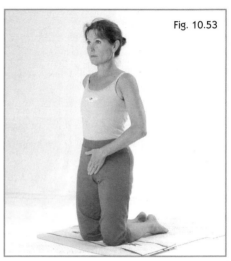

Fig. 10.53

Exploration 1: Kneeling

1. Come up into a kneeling stance. If your kneecaps are sensitive to pressure, use a pad, a cushion, or a folded blanket under your knees.
2. Place your knees directly beneath your hips; make sure your lower legs are parallel to one another. Hook your hands on the outside edges of your hips. Squeeze your hands inward and down toward the ground at the same time. Hold this grip for a few breaths as you close your eyes and "ground" your legs; as you send your legs downward feel the energy in your spine and torso rising upward through the crown of your head. Adjust your chin so that it is parallel to the ground and allows a free flow of sensation through the neck and collarbones (**fig. 10.52**).
3. Open your eyes and softly focus your gaze at a point along the horizon. Leave your hands hooked on your hips as you become aware of the placement of your lower legs

and feet. Notice whether your feet feel stable with the tops stretched out on the floor, or if instead you are more stable with the toes curled under. Experiment back and forth and choose the position that gives you the feeling of balance and stability while kneeling.
4. Bring your right hand to the sacrum, placing the heel of your hand on the upper edge of the sacrum and pointing the mid-dle finger down toward the tailbone. Position your left hand on your lower belly below the navel (**fig. 10.53**). Slide the back hand down the sacrum as though a down-ward-moving elevator is descending from the beltline to the tip of your tailbone. At the same time, slide your front hand upward, as though an upward-moving ele-vator is traveling from the pubic bone to the navel. Repeat this sliding motion a few times to sense how energy moves up the

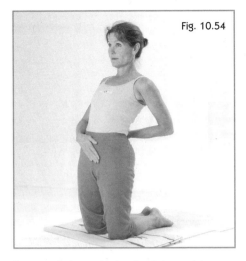

Fig. 10.54

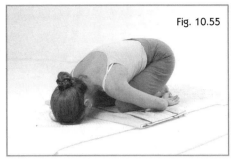

Fig. 10.55

front and down the back of the pelvis, creating stability and groundedness.

5. Tuck your chin in toward the shelf of your chest. This slight tuck will keep the back of your neck long as you begin to lengthen the front side of your body. Bring up a smile in the crease of the lower buttocks and begin to shift your center of gravity forward by pressing the hip bones forward (**fig. 10.54**). The head is very heavy; the further forward you send your center of gravity forward, the greater the tendency is to let the weight of your head hang back. Rather than releasing the head to arch backward, the emphasis here is to keep the head growing out of your spine.

6. Inhale as you shift your center forward; hold the breath in for a moment. As you exhale,

slowly release the hips and chin to neutral.

7. Experiment to see how far forward you can move the hips without losing stability. As the hip bones move forward the sacrum and tailbone lengthen downward, elongating the lower back. Hold this position for several deep breaths. Imagine a wheel of energy turning in the pelvis, moving up the front from the pubic bone to the navel and circling down the back from the belt line to the tip of your tailbone. Experience the sensation in your center and along the front of your thighs.

8. Before you release this position, take a deep breath in and hold the breath. Keep holding and take in a little more breath, tucking the chin a little more. Then exhale and lower down into Child pose (**fig. 10.55**).

9. Slide your arms alongside your body and release the weight of your torso onto your thighs. Observe any pulsing, tingling, or streaming sensations. Notice whether your body heat has increased with this movement.

Exploration 2: Sliding Hip Pockets

1. Come up into a kneeling stance. If your kneecaps are sensitive to pressure use a pad, a cushion, or a folded blanket under your knees. Experiment with the position of your feet and place them in a way that makes you feel stable and grounded, either tops stretched out or toes curled under.

2. Place your knees directly beneath your hips and position your lower legs so that they are parallel to one another. Place your

hands, fingers pointing downward, on your kidneys, as though your hip pockets were very high (**fig. 10.56**).

3. Take a deep breath in as you tuck your chin in toward the shelf of your chest. Press both hip bones forward and squeeze the elbows in toward each other behind your back (**fig. 10.57**). Exhale as you release the press and return to the neutral position. Do you notice how squeezing your elbows

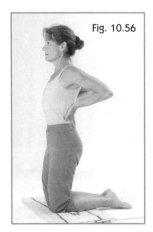

Fig. 10.56

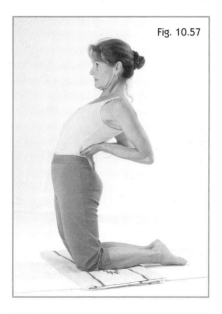

Fig. 10.57

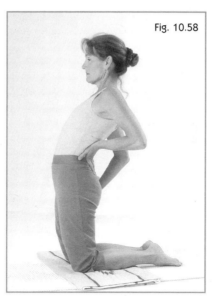

Fig. 10.58

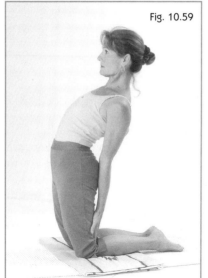

Fig. 10.59

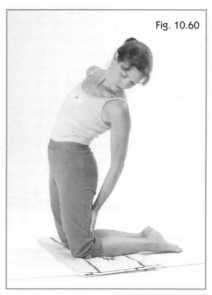

Fig. 10.60

pockets, become aware of the contact your right hand makes with your back. Imagine that your hand is tucked in a pocket; as you exhale, slowly begin to glide this pocket down the backside of your right thigh (**fig. 10.58**). Only go as far as is comfortable without straining. Keep your eyes focused on a point along the horizon in front of you and tuck the chin slightly to protect your low back from arching. Release and glide the pocket back up to the kidney position.

6. For a few breaths, glide the pocket down the backside of your right leg, reaching lower each time until you reach all the way down or close to the crease of your right knee. Glide your hand back up to the kidney position.

7. Now become aware of the contact your left hand makes with your left kidney. Imagine that your hand is tucked in a pocket; as you exhale, slowly begin to glide this pocket down the backside of your left thigh (**fig. 10.59**). Only go as far as is comfortable without straining. Keep your eyes focused on a point along the horizon in front of you and tuck the chin slightly to protect your lower back from arching. Release and glide the pocket back up to the kidney position.

8. For the next few breaths alternate back and forth, sliding the right pocket down the backside of your right leg toward the knee crease, then the left pocket down the left leg. Coordinate your movement so that when one hand is gliding down, the other is gliding upward. Allow as much of the sur-

together behind your back opens up your heart and chest?

4. Repeat this elbow squeeze and forward hip press several times. Hold the inhale longer each time, releasing the breath on the exhale. The more you press your hips forward, the more you squeeze your chin in toward your chest and your elbows toward each other behind your back.

5. With your hands still positioned on your kidney

face of your palms to touch as much of the surface of your legs as possible.

9. When this movement becomes comfortable and familiar, begin to turn and look over your shoulder to watch your hand gliding downward (**fig. 10.60**). Then look over the other shoulder and watch that hand glide down.

10. Release the movement, bringing the hands and arms to hang along your sides. Close your eyes and experience the sensations moving though your body. Notice what is happening in your feet, knees, and the muscles on the front sides of your thighs.

11. Slowly lower down into Child pose.

Exploration 3: Sliding Hip Pockets to Windmill

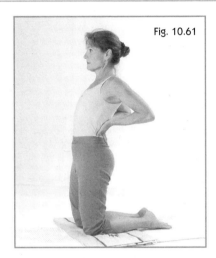
Fig. 10.61

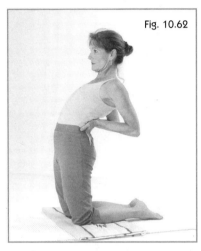
Fig. 10.62

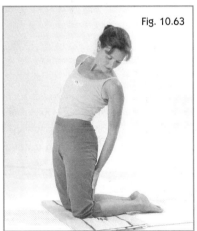
Fig. 10.63

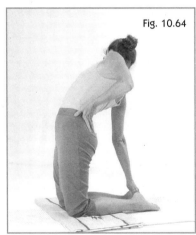
Fig. 10.64

1. Do not progress to this variation if the Sliding Hip Pockets exploration above is not comfortable. Repeat that exploration until you are ready to go to the next level with this one.

2. Come up into a kneeling stance. Place your knees directly beneath your hips and position your lower legs so that they are parallel to one another. Place your hands, fingers pointing downward, on your kidneys (**fig. 10.61**). Take a deep breath in as you tuck your chin in toward the shelf of your chest, press both hip bones forward, and squeeze the elbows in toward each other behind your back, opening your heart and chest (**fig. 10.62**). Exhale as you release the press and return to the neutral position.

3. Repeat this elbow squeeze and hip press forward several times. Hold the breath in longer each time, releasing the breath on the exhale. As you deepen the forward press of the hips, also deepen the squeeze of your chin toward your chest and your elbows toward each other behind your back.

4. Position your hands on your kidney pockets, fingers pointing downward. Begin the hip pocket gliding movement down one thigh, then the other, alternating back and forth and looking over your shoulders (**fig. 10.63**).

5. If this movement is comfortable, the next time you glide down the right leg to the knee crease, keep sliding your right hand all the way to the heel (**fig. 10.64**). Then return to the upright neutral position. Repeat the same movement down

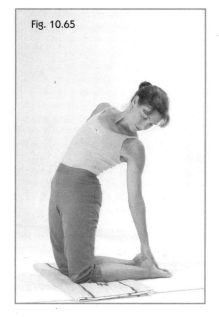

Fig. 10.65

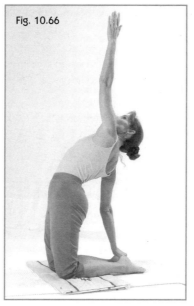

Fig. 10.66

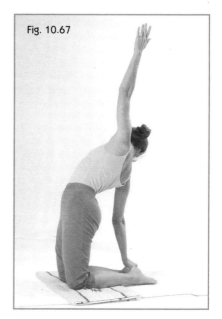

Fig. 10.67

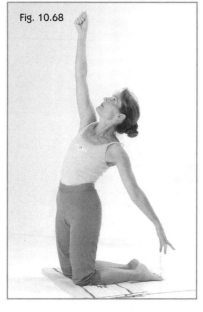

Fig. 10.68

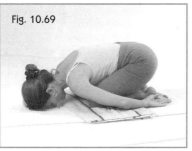

Fig. 10.69

the left thigh toward the left heel (**fig. 10.65**).

6. Alternate back and forth several times until the movement becomes familiar and comfortable. Remind yourself to look over the shoulder and actually see your hands touching your heels on each side.

7. The next time you glide down to the right heel, anchor your hand on your foot and stretch through your left arm up toward the ceiling. Stretch like a windmill upward from the little finger side of your arm. Inhale and allow your eyes to look upward at the airborne thumb (**fig. 10.66**). Exhale and look down at your right hand and heel (**fig. 10.67**). Keep pressing the hipbones forward. The next time you look up at the left thumb, catch hold of an imaginary skyhook and let the skyhook lift you back up into the upright kneeling position.

8. Close your eyes and experience the sensations moving through your body. Notice any difference in sensation between your two legs.

9. Open your eyes and glide your left hand down to your left heel, anchor your hand on your foot, and stretch the right arm upward toward the ceiling. Stretch upward like a windmill from the little finger side of your arm. Inhale and allow your eyes to look upward at the airborne thumb. Exhale and look down at your left hand and heel. Keep pressing the hip bones forward. The next time you look up at the right thumb, catch hold of an imaginary skyhook and let the skyhook lift you back up into the upright kneeling position (**fig. 10.68**).

10. Bring your arms to your side. Close your eyes and notice the effects of these movements.

11. Slowly lower down into Child pose (**fig. 10.69**). Sit for a moment and observe the internal effects of this sequence of movements.

Exploration 4: Kneeling Forward Lunge

1. Come up into a kneeling stance. If your kneecaps are sensitive to pressure, use a pad, a cushion, or a folded blanket under your knees.

2. Place your knees directly beneath your hips and position your lower legs so that they are parallel to one another. Hook your hands on the outside edges of your hips. Squeeze your hands inward like a vice grip and downward toward the ground at the same time (**fig. 10.70**). Hold this grip for a few breaths as you close your eyes and imagine grounding your legs. As you send your legs down, imagine the energy in your spine and torso rising upward, through the crown of your head. Adjust your chin so that it is parallel to the ground and allows a free flow of sensation up through the neck and collarbones.

3. Lift your right knee and stand your right foot solidly on the ground in front of you. Keep your hands planted firmly on your hips for stability (**fig. 10.71**). Moving from your sacrum, imagine a hand behind you gently pressing you forward (**fig. 10.72**). As your center of gravity moves forward, your spine remains erect and elongated, chin slightly tucked. Notice that your knee glides directly over your right foot, rather than to the inside or outside of your foot. Exhale and return to neutral.

4. For the next several breaths, inhale as you glide forward directly out over the foot and exhale as you glide back to the upright kneeling position. As you come back, you may want to bow

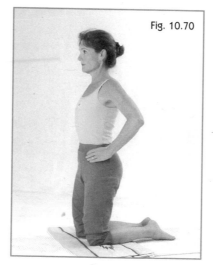

Fig. 10.70

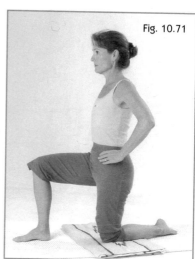

Fig. 10.71

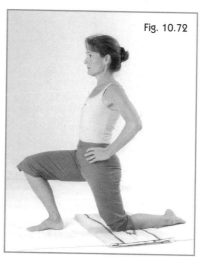

Fig. 10.72

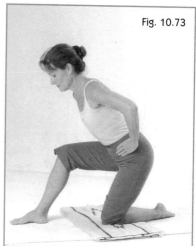

Fig. 10.73

forward slightly and reach your sitz bones back toward your left heel (**fig. 10.73**). Remind yourself to move from your center of gravity or your sacrum and to keep the spine upright as you lunge forward.

5. The next time you return to neutral, reposition your hands, placing one on top of the other on top of your right knee (**fig. 10.74**). Again begin the forward gliding motion, but this time imagine that a string is attached to your sternum and that

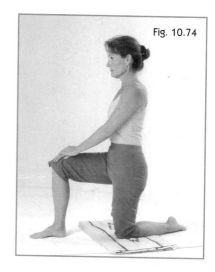

Fig. 10.74

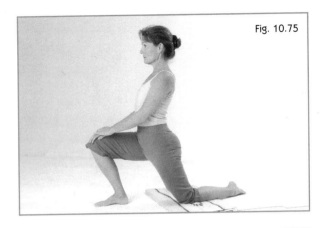

Fig. 10.75

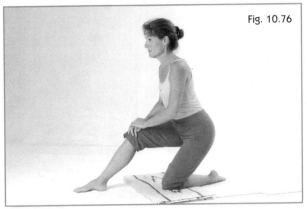

Fig. 10.76

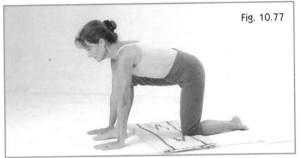

Fig. 10.77

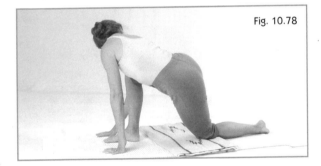

Fig. 10.78

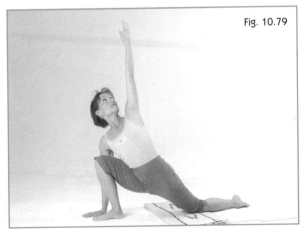

Fig. 10.79

you are being pulled forward by the breastbone (**fig. 10.75**).

6. Exhale and sit back toward the heel, allowing the torso to bow forward slightly (**fig. 10.76**). Repeat this forward-and-backward movement until it becomes familiar and effortless. Experiment with how far forward and back you can go without straining or allowing your front knee to wobble from one side to the other.

7. Now take a dive forward and plant your hands on the floor on either side of your right foot (**fig. 10.77**). Turn and look over your left shoulder and see your left ankle on the floor behind you. Turn and look over the right shoulder (**fig. 10.78**). Deliberately allow the back ankle to roll from the inner anklebone to the outer anklebone as you turn to look from side to side. This rolling of the ankle will release the long upper bone of the leg to rotate more freely in the hip socket.

8. Leave your left hand planted on the floor and extend your right hand toward the sky. Look toward the airborne thumb. Then reverse, planting the right hand on the floor and extending the left arm upward, gazing at the thumb (**fig. 10.79**).

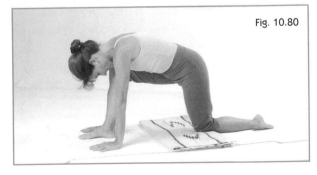

Fig. 10.80

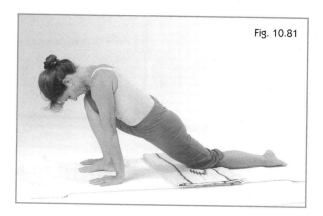

Fig. 10.81

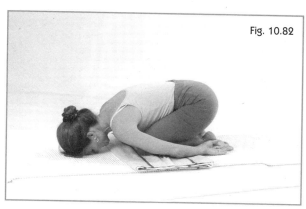

Fig. 10.82

9. Keeping your hands on the floor, lower the weight of your torso onto your right thigh. Wait until your torso becomes heavy. Release the weight of your head to hang (**fig. 10.80**). Relax your jaw and the muscles of your face. Keeping your torso very heavy and resting on your thigh, let your thigh take your torso for a ride forward and back (**fig. 10.81**). Stay heavy and relaxed in the movement.

10. Slowly return to the upright kneeling position, then lower down into the Child pose for a rest (**fig. 10.82**). Notice the effects of the movement. Observe the difference in the two sides of the body. Do you sense any pulsing, streaming, or tingling sensations?

11. Roll your spine to an upright position and then come up into a kneeling position. Repeat the exploration starting with the left knee and foot forward. Finish in Child pose, sitting for a moment and observing the internal effects of this sequence of movements.

Exploration 5: Kneeling Hitchhiker

1. Come up into a kneeling stance. Place your knees directly beneath your hips with your lower legs parallel to one another. Extend both arms perpendicular to your shoulders in a T position. Curl your fingers into your palms and extend your thumbs as though you were hitchhiking (**fig. 10.83**).

2. With a soft gaze, watch your right thumb rolling upward in the hitchhiker's gesture; at the same time roll the left thumb down in the "thumbs down" gesture. Hold this position and exaggerate the rolling in your shoulders

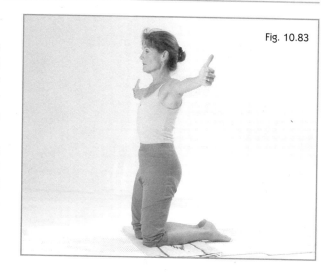

Fig. 10.83

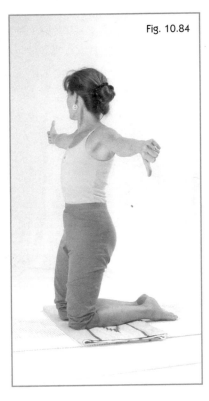

Fig. 10.84

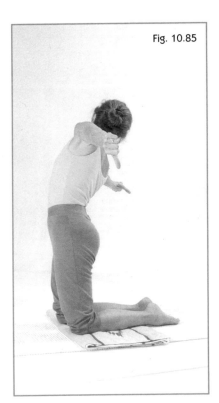

Fig. 10.85

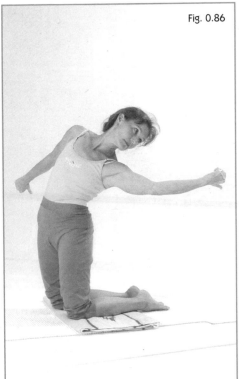

Fig. 0.86

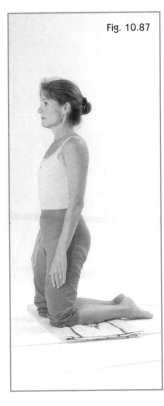

Fig. 10.87

(fig. 10.84). The right shoulder is rolling up and back, the left shoulder is rolling forward and downward.

3. Now simultaneously reverse the position of your hands as your gaze shifts to look at your left thumb rolling upward into the hitchhiking gesture. Hold this position as you breathe into the stretch and exaggerate the rolling in your shoulders.

4. Now begin to change gestures from side to side, exaggerating the rolling motion in the shoulders. Look to each thumb as it is rolling upward.

5. Continue the movement but stretch the arms wider and wider apart, as if you were stretching a towel behind your back **(fig. 10.85).** Feel the shoulder blades widening out from the spine.

6. Now begin to put a little speed into the movement. Allow the elbows to bend and the hips to sway from side to side **(fig. 10.86).** Imagine the wind is blowing you; let your whole body begin to respond to this wringing, winding, fluid movement. Play with the movement until the movement takes over. Let your body flow freely into whatever form of rolling and twisting emerges.

7. Slow the movement down and return to the neutral kneeling position **(fig. 10.87).** Close your eyes and experience the effects in your body.

8. Lower down into Child pose. Reach your palms around to your low back and give the muscles a good massage, releasing any residual tension they may be holding. When you are ready, slowly roll up into a sitting position.

9. Sit for a moment and observe the effects of this sequence of movements.

Integration: From a Seed to a Tree

1. Come up into a kneeling stance. Place your knees directly beneath your hips and position your lower legs so that they are parallel to one another. Extend both arms out from your trunk in a T position. Curl your fingers into your palms and extend your thumbs as though you were hitchhiking (**fig. 10.88**).

2. Roll both thumbs upward in the hitchhiker's gesture and then roll both thumbs down into the "thumbs down" gesture (**fig. 10.89**). Repeat this movement a few times, inhaling as you roll up and exhale, squeezing all of the breath out as you roll the thumbs down. Exaggerate the rolling movement in your shoulders.

3. Now let your head and eyes begin to move with your shoulders. As your thumbs roll up let your eyes look up, stretching your chin toward the ceiling and pressing your hip bones forward (**fig. 10.90**). Squeeze the lower buttocks slightly and elongate the low back rather than arching or contracting. When the thumbs roll down, your chin tucks into the shelf of your chest and your upper back rounds forward slightly (**fig. 10.91**).

4. Gradually allow more of your body to stretch backward in the thumbs up gesture and more of your spine and torso to curl forward in the thumbs down gesture. As you let the movement build, you will curl all the way down into the Child pose, or the "seed" position, on the exhaling

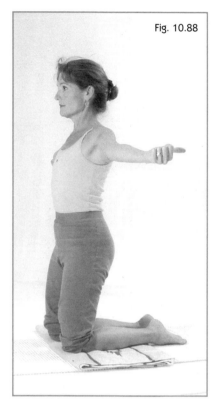

Fig. 10.88

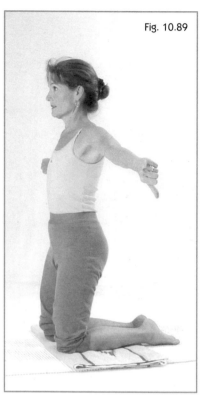

Fig. 10.89

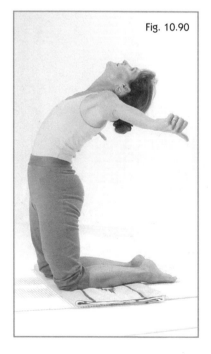

Fig. 10.90

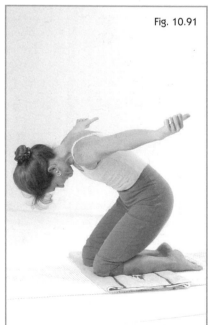

Fig. 10.91

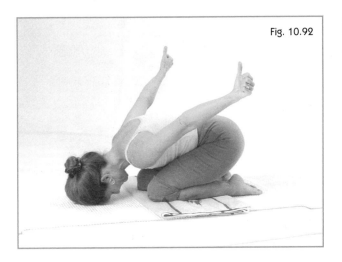

Fig. 10.92

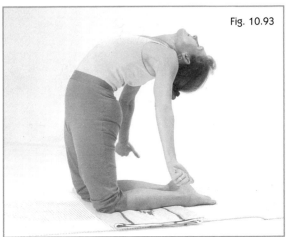

Fig. 10.93

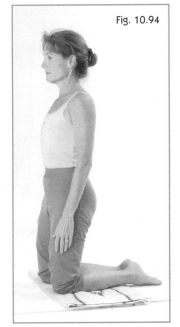

Fig. 10.94

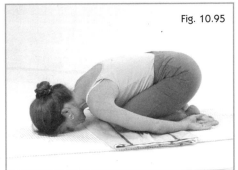

Fig. 10.95

breath (**fig. 10.92**). On the inhaling breath, sprout from the seed all the way back up into the full-grown tree, opening your chest, rolling your shoulders and thumbs up, squeezing your lower buttocks slightly, and pressing the hip bones forward (**fig. 10.93**).

5. Continue the movement until the breath and momentum carry you along. Imagine the energy and vibrancy of moving from a tiny seed to the full-blown expression of a whole tree in one burst of movement and in one breath.

6. Allow the movement to slow down until you return to stillness in the neutral kneeling position (**fig. 10.94**). Close your eyes. Allow your breath to flow in and flow out without any inhibition. Experience the effects of this movement on your whole being. Particularly notice your mood. Do you feel more playful or more energized?

7. Lower back down into Child pose (**fig. 10.95**). Notice how quickly and deeply you are able to relax in this position. Draw your breath down the entire backside of your body, noticing how you lengthen on the inhalations and relax even more deeply into gravity on the exhalations. In your own time, slowly roll back up into a sitting position, observing from within how each part of your spine moves in sequence.

8. Sit for a moment and observe the effects of this sequence of movements.

Before Moving On . . .

In bringing awareness to the difference it makes for the health of your spine to extend the front side of your body as compared to arching backward into backbending postures, you have established a way to experience the belly- and heart-opening effects of backbends without compromising or straining your low back or neck. The movements you learned in Hug the Planet not only bring relief for overworked and overdeveloped low-back muscles, but provide a balanced way to relax and elongate your low back while also hydrating and toning intervertebral discs. By reeducating your spine in this way you may begin to notice an increase in the efficiency and overall range of movement in your whole spine.

As you have now experienced, the same body mechanics that you apply in the prone position are relevant to the front extensions from a kneeling position as well. Rather than avoid backbends in order to protect your low back and neck, you now have some practical ways to approach all backbends and to receive their rejuvenating and energizing effects.

Do you recall a moment during one of these explorations when you felt a noticeable difference in the flow of energy in the way of increased heart rate or a pulsing in your belly or chest? The counterbalance of moving from front extensions down into the Child pose have the massaging effect of stretching and then compressing all the vital organs in your belly and chest. As you open to increased levels of circulation and stimulation in the belly and chest in this way, you are not only releasing some unnecessary protection; you are also inviting a fresh infusion of energy to be directed toward fulfilling your important priorities with greater ease and confidence.

So far in the progression of these Self-Awakening Yoga inquiries you have now located the belly center and learned ways to energize and move from your belly center while lying on your back, lying on your belly, sitting in Pinwheel, and kneeling. The next chapter explores movements that channel the vital strength from your belly into your arms and legs in Table position. As a child pushes and pulls his way up off of his belly and onto all fours, a new set of possibilities for exploring the world begins to open that require developing strength in the arms and legs.

11 Lifting onto All Fours: Balancing Stability with Mobility in Cross-Lateral Movement

How does cross-lateral movement stimulate whole-body balance?

A SIGNIFICANT MILESTONE IN THE JOURNEY OF SELF-AWAKENING occurs when an infant makes the transition from being "ground bound" on her belly to mobilizing through the environment by pushing through her limbs. Lifting the torso off the ground stimulates an explosion of sensory excitation and fuels developmental leaps in gross- and fine-motor skills and brain development. With this rapid increase in nervous-system, muscular, and cellular activity comes a voracious demand for fuel, causing the heart, the lungs, and all the metabolic processes to fire up great volumes of energy.

Pushing into the arms scoots the baby backward. How frustrating this must be when the motivation is to move *forward*, toward attention-grabbing, fuzzy, furry things. Discovering knee and leg actions that break the backward scoot becomes a means for counterbalancing the action of the arms. Digging the knees into the ground to resist the backward locomotion of arm-pushing lands us in sitting, as in the Pinwheel.

With sitting comes the capacity to take in a panoramic view without having to exert continuous arm strength. Sitting stimulates further strengthening of the postural muscles for natural alignment. Attention and concentration give rise to ideational sequencing and expanded awareness of the overall environment—important capacities in and of themselves, but those abilities do not satisfy that nagging urge to reach out and touch that puppy on the floor just out of reach. Waiting for Mommy or a sibling to deliver the puppy does not provide the baby with the immediate satisfaction that the sensorial rouse is demanding. Reaching involves a resolute dive forward into the arms and hands, hurling the baby back to the ground for undertaking more activities geared toward getting him where he wants to go. There's going to be a significant amount of pushing and pulling of arms and legs in inventing a way to move forward toward that puppy. The pushing and pulling develops strength and agility. By the time a coordinated effort to crawl forward emerges, the brain has increased its intelligence by trillions.

In the struggle to move toward a goal—toward this puppy—the problem-solving capacities of the left cerebral hemisphere synchronize with the kinesthetic patterning, image recognition, and interpretive capacities of the right cerebral hemisphere. But the crowning achievement at this age of discovery is the birth of autonomy stemming from increasing mobility: "I see it. I want it. I can get it. I can hold on to it. I can let it go. It is mine." That autonomy holds true for the opposite range of experiences as well: "I see it. I don't want it. I can get away from it." From these primal engagements in the world of a developing self the foundations for an individuated personality are formed. The moment when negotiating a crawl across the floor gets me to the puppy is cause for squealing celebration. This orchestration of body awareness, ideational intelligence, and sense of self is a milestone in awakening into autonomy.

All struggles that we undertake toward developing multidimensional consciousness provide the ground for activating our potentials. Think of a butterfly emerging from its cocoon. Pushing and pressing against the wall of the chrysalis forces fluids into the spiny tubules that will form and harden into wings. If you clip the cocoon in an effort to reduce the pupa's struggle, the wings will not develop the strength to carry the developing butterfly into flight. On a human level, research into brain-mind maturation reveals that the crawling stage in human development is essential for harmonizing the functions of the right and left hemispheres of the cerebral cortex. Children who are prevented from crawling, children who are overly encouraged to walk before their hip joints and sacroiliac joint have developed, and children who are left in walkers for prolonged periods of time are prone to develop a variety of learning disabilities, including dyslexia, attention deficit disorder, and delayed development of physical coordination. Manufacturers of baby walkers are now required by law to place a warning about limiting the amount of time a child spends in a walker, at the risk of creating adverse dependency.

Our intention in this chapter is to return to the wisdom of the organism for clues that will fill in missing links and open the doorway for pleasurable rediscoveries in the simple ecstasy of learning new patterns of movement directly from the body. The cross-crawl pattern of movement involves a sequenced transfer of balance between the upper and lower limbs and a lateral balance across the midline of the body between opposite arms and legs. Some of the adverse effects of walking before one is ready (which unfortunately is the developmental history of far too many people) are reversible by returning to the original learning process and stimulating neuromuscular activity with these basic body-mind bridges.

Several of the explorations in this chapter investigate ways to develop and maintain stability and balance as the center of gravity shifts, to allow for the differentiation and coordinated movement of body segments. Developing upper body strength in the shoulders and arms in the Table position frees the legs to explore the muscular action required for lifting and lowering and for flexing and extending. Pigeon Kicks take each leg into its full range of flexion and extension while the arms and shoulders maintain strength and balance in the upper body. The focus on cross-lateral patterning that is required for coordinated and synchronized movement is provided by Thread the Needle and Pigeon Walk; these explorations establish neural pathways for balancing the right and left hemispheres of the brain, preparing the way for the challenges of many yoga postures that require cross-lateral patterning involving the upper and lower limbs, postures such as Cow Head, Eagle, Full Pigeon, and Bound Lotus. As a group, the inquiries in this chapter provide transitions that allow for an unbroken flow of movement from belly down to sitting, twisting, standing, and even going upside down, as in Head Roll.

The organismic genius awakened through uninhibited learning during the crawling stage in our development is echoed in the assertions of yogis who claim with authority that there are more than 180,000 yoga postures. Perhaps in this exaggeration lies the realization that it would be impossible to be in any movement without it being a yoga posture. What elevates any particular movement to the designation of yoga is the quality of awareness in the experience. I once witnessed Swami Kripalu reaching for a pen. He slowed his movement down to a pace that became so absorbing it sent an audience of five hundred people into deep, meditative awareness. By slowing down to notice what is happening through the body in any given moment, regardless of how seemingly mundane the activity might appear, consciousness of the inherent genius of prana awakens spontaneously. Awakening to yogic awareness is your birthright by virtue of living in your body. Notice what happens in you as you enter the following inquiries.

Stabilizing the Upper Body

Inquiry: How does crawling prepare us for whole-brain thinking?

This inquiry sequence begins in a different way from previous explorations. With the preparation inquiry you will have a few moments to recreate some of the early movement investigations you likely made as an infant. Then, moving like a caterpillar does, arm and shoulder strength will bring you from Child pose to Table pose. Although the explorations here are guided to mobilize various body segments, such as flexing and extending the pelvis in Cat and Dog and rotating the rib cage in Peanut Butter Jar, these movements provide the foundation for a greater range of coordinated actions that synchronize to move the whole body, such as in dancing or in just about any sports activity. In the inverted position of Thread the Needle you are guided into gently leveraging your body weight onto one shoulder as a way to explore how the movements of your head, neck, and shoulders are integrated into your personal, unique patterns of movement.

Enjoy your plunge back into discovery!

Preparation: Pushing and Crawling into Child Pose

1. Lie on your belly on the ground. A hardwood floor works best for the scooting aspect of this inquiry. Wear long sleeves and thick pants to minimize friction. In the next few moments you will have the opportunity to revisit some experiences that you likely had early in your development. Suggest to your logical mind that it is pleasurable and desirable to enter the mentality of an infant, immersed in the safety of exploring the world through your senses. Before beginning, slow down and follow your breath. Notice the contact your body makes with the ground as you lie on your belly. Make the following explorations that feel interesting to you.

2. How does it feel to open your mouth, releasing your tongue and jaw to make sounds? How would it feel to have permission to drool? What sounds want to come out in this moment? What do your fingers taste like? Using your tongue, explore all of the interior surfaces of your mouth.

3. How warm or cold is the ground? Is there a way to use your toes and feet to explore the texture of the ground? How heavy is your foot when you flop it on the floor? What does your hair feel like? Would you

like to find the texture of your face?

4. Tuck your arms close to your sides and invent a way to roll like a pencil. How fast can you go? What are the sounds your body would like to make as you go rolling?

5. How would pounding, flopping, or hopping happen?

6. Finding your elbows and forearms, is there a way to push that allows you to scoot backward? How much effort is required to actually push your body backward? Can you use your knees as brakes? If you dig your knees in to stop the backward scoot and you keep pressing into your hands, do you come up to sitting in an interesting way?

7. Come from your belly into sitting in a way that you have never done before. Invent that movement. Then invent a way to come back down to your belly.

8. Invent a way to push and crawl from your belly into Child pose. Go back and forth a few times until you find a rhythm and pattern that is interesting to you.

9. Remain in Child pose for a few breaths. Travel inside your impulses in this moment and allow your body to move into any posture or position that arises from your own inner urges. There is no one watching you. See what wants to happen when no one is watching.

10. When you are ready, come onto your back for relaxation. This is the time to notice the sensations that are passing though your body. Notice your mood in this moment. Can you sense how much permission your body has to explore movement as a child? Before returning, thank your logical mind for allowing this opportunity to explore without criticism and without inhibiting your play. Suggest that you'll be returning with fresh insight into how your body wants to move. Whenever you are ready, begin your return.

Exploration 1: From Child onto All Fours—Table Pose

1. Come into Child pose—on your knees with your torso resting on your thighs. Bring your arms alongside your body (**fig. 11.1**). Allow the weight of your torso to rest as comfortably on your thighs as possible.

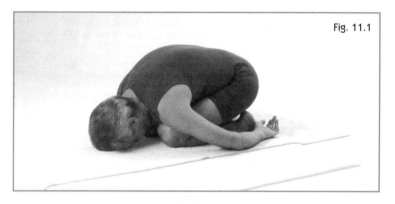

Fig. 11.1

Notice any pressure at your knees or ankles. If you experience strong discomfort in this position, place a rolled towel under your ankles. A cushion between your hips and calves will relieve pressure in the knees. Another option is to place a cushion between the belly and thighs in order to rest the torso more comfortably.

2. After you have made any adjustments that allow you to comfortably be in Child pose, begin to notice your breathing. Suggest to your logical mind that this is a time for slowing down and attuning to the sensations that arise within your body.

3. Begin to notice the contact your belly makes with your thighs. Notice that your head is lower than your hips and belly. Observe any pulsing, streaming, or tingling sensations as gravity moves the fluids in your body down into the bowl of your head. Notice any effort or resistance in your body. Let any resistance be as it is.

4. Moving to a deeper level of awareness, begin to slide your palms along the ground and shift your weight forward onto your knees and hands. Adjust your hands so that your palms are directly beneath your shoulders and not further apart or closer in than the width of your shoulders. Adjust your knees so that they are directly beneath your hips and your lower legs are parallel behind you. Look at your knees and legs and visually scan your posture to see that you are balanced for stability.

5. Bring your attention back to your hands. Spread your fingers apart, stretching your palms open on the floor as if the fingers were stars. The middle fingers are the lead fingers. Look to see that the middle fingers are pointed straight forward and are parallel to each other. Now you are in a stable Table pose.

6. Look at the crook of your elbows. Rotate the crook of your elbows forward toward the wall in front of you (**fig. 11.2**) and notice how this affects the positioning of your shoulders, wrists, palms, and fingers. If the knuckles at the base of your index fingers or thumbs come off the ground to help you get more stretch, press them back down into the star position. We are isolating the rotation in the arms and shoulders by rotating the crook of the elbows forward and leaving the hands in a stable position. In order to keep the hands grounded as you rotate the elbows forward, it is helpful to press the webbing between the thumb and the index finger down into the ground. Are you breathing?

7. Now roll the crooks of the elbows so that they are facing each other. Roll the crooks of the elbows forward toward the wall in front of you and back to face each other for a few repetitions. Exaggerate the rotation that is occurring in the shoulders. Keep the shoulder blades spread wide across your back.

8. Take a deep breath in and hold the breath. Then, keeping the hands in this position, reach your sitz bones back to your heels, returning momentarily to Child pose (**fig. 11.3**). Stretch the entire spine and let out any sounds that want to emerge.

9. Moving like a caterpillar, slide your nose forward along the floor, taking the weight of your torso forward into your hands **fig. 11.4**). Dive your breastbone forward, staying low along the ground (**fig. 11.5**), and then scoop back up into Table pose (**fig. 11.6**). Hold for a moment and then reach the sitz bones back toward the heels (**fig. 11.7**).

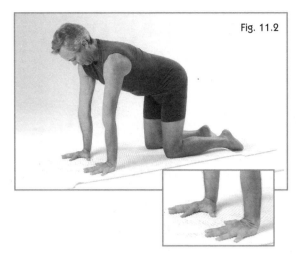

Fig. 11.2

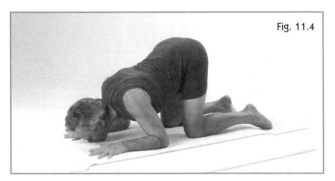

Fig. 11.3

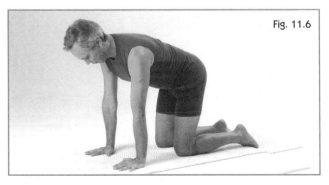

Fig. 11.4

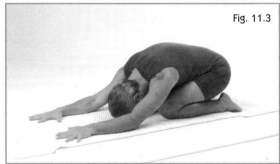

Fig. 11.5

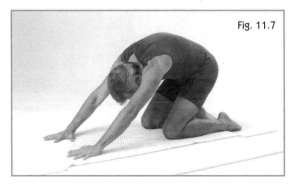

Fig. 11.6

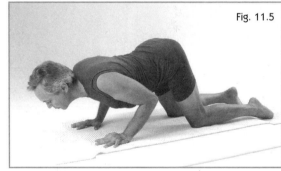

Fig. 11.7

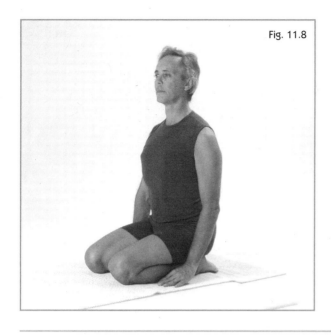

Fig. 11.8

10. Moving like a caterpillar, repeat this circular movement, using your breath to energize your whole torso. Continue until the movement becomes familiar and effortless.

11. The next time you return to Child pose, remain there. Slide your arms alongside your body and release the weight of your torso onto your thighs. Observe any pulsing, tingling, or streaming sensations.

12. Create an image of the way your body looks and feels when you are stable in the Table position and your elbows are rotated forward. Recall the sensation of moving from Child pose to Table pose and returning in a circular rhythm.

13. Begin your return by lengthening your head forward and elongating your spine back up into a sitting position (**fig. 11.8**). Sit for a moment and observe the effects of this sequence of movements.

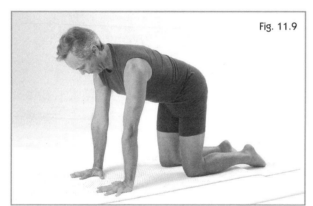

Fig. 11.9

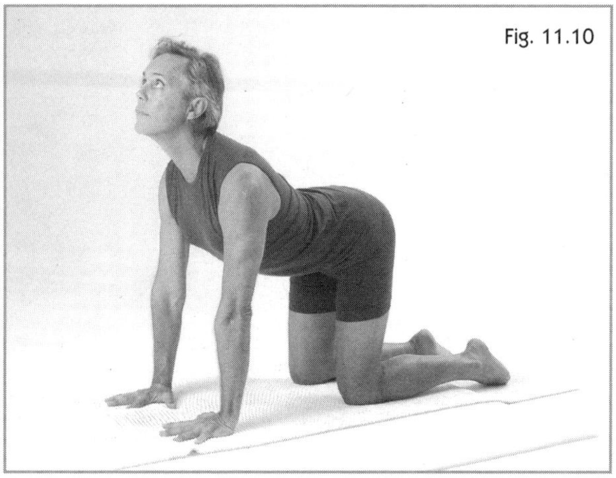

Exploration 2: Cat and Dog

1. Adjust your hands and knees into a stable Table pose (**fig. 11.9**).

2. Inhale and lengthen the front side of your body by bringing the back of your head toward your sacrum as you lift your tailbone toward the ceiling and look with your eyes toward the ceiling (**fig. 11.10**). Imagine that you have a tail that arches upward and that you can see your tail with your eyes. Notice how this image elongates your spine. This is called the Dog tilt of the pelvis.

3. Exhale and round your spine, tucking your hips under. Squeeze your lower buttocks together slightly. Look with your eyes toward your navel and notice how this completes the forward flexion of the spine (**fig. 11.11**).

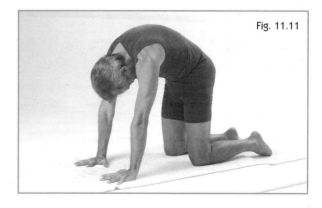

Fig. 11.11

Fig. 11.10

Imagine making the fur on your back stand up as a cat would do. This is called the Cat tilt of the pelvis.

4. Repeat the movement from Dog tilt to Cat tilt several times, looking with your eyes each time to complete the stretch. Inhale fully into Dog tilt and exhale into Cat tilt. Squeeze the breath out and suck the lower abdominal organs in just slightly at the end of the exhaling breath.

5. Continue the movement until it becomes familiar and effortless and you have the sense of arching and flexing your entire spine.

6. Slowly reach your sitz bones back to sit on your heels, returning to Child pose (**fig. 11.12**). Slide your arms alongside your body and release the weight of your torso onto your thighs. Observe any pulsing, tingling, or streaming sensations.

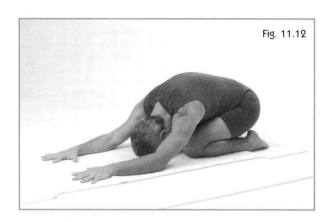

Fig. 11.12

Exploration 3: Windshield Wiper Shinbones

1. Adjust your hands and knees into a stable Table pose (**fig. 11.13**).

2. Transferring your weight forward onto your hands, lift the ankles and shinbones. In a windshield-wiper motion, cross the right ankle over the left, open the ankles apart, and then cross the left ankle over the right (**fig. 11.14**). Repeat this movement several times, until it feels effortless.

3. Lower the ankles and shinbones to the ground and bring your knees together, inner thighs and ankles touching (**fig. 11.15**). Transfer your weight forward onto your hands as you lift the ankles and lower legs. Keeping your ankles together, make a windshield wiper motion from side to side: when your feet move to the left, look around your left shoulder to see your feet (**fig. 11.16**). When your feet go to the right, look around your right shoulder. This lateral stretch is like an accordian that opens the ribs on one side while compressing the ribs on the other side.

4. Repeat this movement several times until it becomes

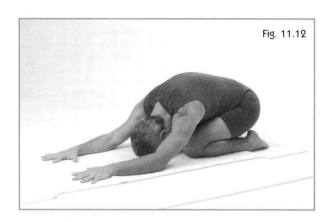

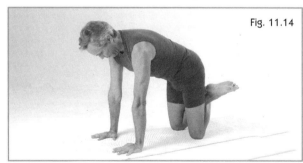

Fig. 11.13

Fig. 11.14

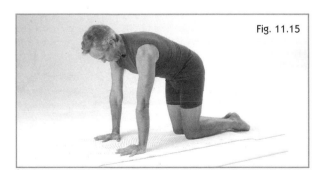

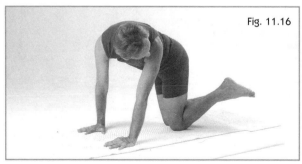

Fig. 11.15

Fig. 11.16

effortless and familiar. Use your breath.

5. Lower the ankles to the ground and reach your sitz bones back to sit on your heels in Child pose. Slide your arms along-side your body and release the weight of your torso onto your thighs. Observe any pulsing, tingling, or streaming sensations.

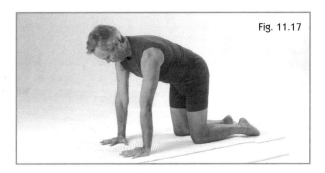

Fig. 11.17

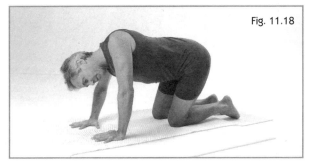

Fig. 11.18

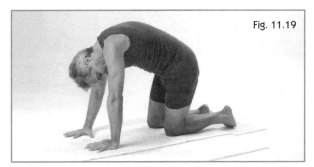

Fig. 11.19

Exploration 4: Peanut Butter Jar

1. Adjust your hands and knees into a stable Table pose (**fig. 11.17**).

2. Allowing your elbows to bend and your head to move freely, begin to take your ribs and torso in a circular motion (**figs. 11.18, 11.19, 11.20, and 11.21**). Imagine that you are inside a peanut butter jar and you are using your rib cage to clean the walls of the jar.

3. Slow down the movement and experience every bit of the stretch. Allow any sounds to come out and breathe into all parts of your torso as you move. Let the circles gradually become larger. Let go of the control of your movement and allow your body to be moved by the breath.

4. Reverse the direction of the circles. Again allow the rhythm to build until you let go of control over the movement. Experience how your body wants to move in this stretch. What parts of the body want to open?

5. Slow the movement and gradually come to stillness in Table pose. Experience the sensations in your body.

6. Slowly reach your sitz bones back to sit on your heels, returning to Child pose (**fig. 11.22**). Release the weight of your torso onto your thighs. Notice the way your shoulders and ribs feel. Observe any pulsing, tingling, or streaming sensations.

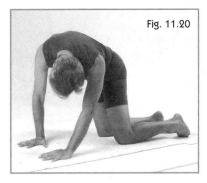

Fig. 11.20

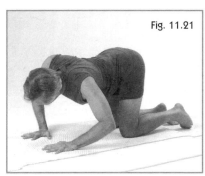

Fig. 11.21

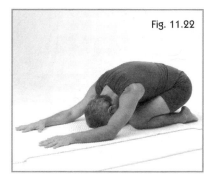

Fig. 11.22

Integration: Thread the Needle

1. Adjust your hands and knees into a stable Table pose.

2. Shift your weight to the left to be supported by the left arm and hand; extend the right arm out to your right side. Let your gaze turn your head to see your arm extended from the right shoulder (**fig. 11.23**). Balance your body as though you were still in the Table pose, with both arms supporting you.

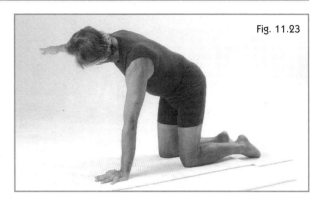

Fig. 11.23

3. Bend the right elbow and slowly begin to lower the backside of your right hand to the floor, sliding it under the window of your left arm and elbow (**fig. 11.24**). Thread the right arm all the way through until your right shoulder is on the ground and you can relax the weight of your head on the shoulder or floor (**fig. 11.25**).

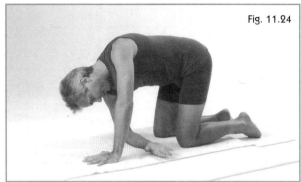

Fig. 11.24

4. Explore the sensation of being in this interesting position. Shift your hips from side to side and roll your head into different positions to notice how much more weight you can let go of when you fully relax into your breathing. How does it feel to release the weight of the world, allowing all holding to melt off the right shoulder and into the ground? Open your jaw; relax your eyes, your face, and even your scalp. Give yourself permission to reposition your knees to find the precise way to provide pleasure and release to this side of your body.

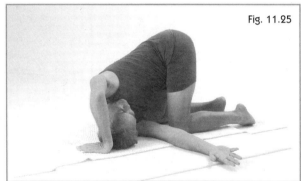

Fig. 11.25

5. Remaining in this position, lift the upper (left) arm to your side and follow the sweeping motion with your eyes (**fig. 11.26**). Do not lose sight of your hand; that way your neck will remain protected in this position. Fold your left arm across your low back and reach to contact the inner thigh of the opposite leg (**fig. 11.27**).

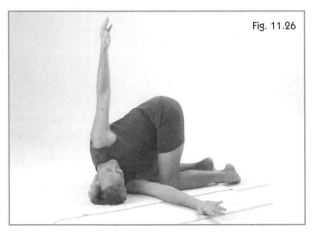

Fig. 11.26

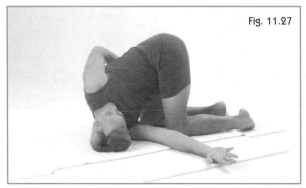

Fig. 11.27

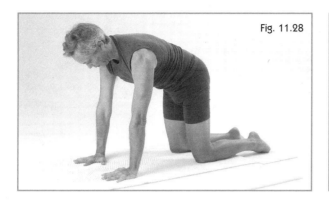

Fig. 11.28

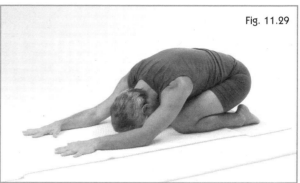

Fig. 11.29

6. Make the "yes" movement with your head. Experiment with ways your body is prompting you to release further.

7. Press back up into Table pose and experience the difference between the two sides of your body **(fig. 11.28)**.

8. Shift your weight to be supported by the right arm and hand; extend the left arm out to your left side. Follow the Thread the Needle movements on this side of the body, experimenting through each position with ways that your body is prompting you toward deeper release. When you have completed the series of movements on this side, press up into Table pose.

9. Slowly reach your sitz bones back toward your heels and rest for a moment in Child pose **(fig. 11.29)**. Move to a deeper level of awareness and experience the effects of these deep stretches. Release the weight of your torso onto your thighs. Notice the way your shoulders and ribs feel. Do you notice any difference in the expansion of your torso as you breathe? Observe any pulsing, tingling, or streaming sensations.

Balancing Upper Body Strength with Flexibility

Inquiry: What movements both strengthen and stabilize the upper body while creating greater flexibility?

Finding the power in our legs occurs long before we learn how to stand. In this set of explorations, all performed on your knees, you will be discovering movements that lift and lower and flex and extend your legs, one leg at a time. When one leg is moving, the other leg is providing stability by drawing upon the strength that has been developing in the core abdominal muscles. As you explore the various movements of one leg at a time, the shoulder and arm muscles are also engaged, balancing upper and lower body strength while stabilizing the upper body.

In and of themselves, Donkey Kicks and Pigeon Kicks are excellent ways to further develop the abdominal strength required in all standing and balancing postures. As the names imply, Puppy Sternum and Hip Stretch and Puppy Push-ups are playful ways to open the chest and provide concentrated stimulation to circulatory and respiratory systems. The Puppy postures help to develop upper body strength balanced by flexibility in the legs, crucial to Downward Dog, by providing a way to differentiate all the movements and dynamics of balance that eventually come into play in this pose.

Pigeon Walk integrates the activity of the right and left hemispheres of the brain by harvesting the energetic effects from the preceding explorations, blending the range-of-motion actions into a sequence of forward and backward walking that crosses the midline of the body. Downward Dog focuses on balancing upper and lower body strength in the apex of the pelvis. When determination is met with sufficient strength in the legs and the arms and sufficient patterning allows for coordinated movement, the child learns to push from a squat into Downward Dog. Pigeon Kicks alternate from sitting to standing, using the arms for balance and counterbalance. The body is open and ready to enter the Pigeon as an integration for all of the movements in this sequence.

Exploration 1: Puppy Sternum and Hip Stretch

1. Adjust your hands and knees into a stable Table pose.

2. Bend your elbows and place your forearms on the ground **(fig. 11.30)**. Walk your arms away from you until you can begin lowering your sternum toward the ground. You will want your hips to stay directly above your knees so that you experience the stretch in your low back and your sternum. Bring your forehead to the ground, lengthening the back of your neck (be careful not to mash your nose) **(fig. 11.31)**.

3. Now deepen your breath and experience the stretch occurring in your torso. As you breathe deeply into your upper and middle chest your torso will move up and down in response to the breath. If you want more stretch, balance on your elbows and place your palms together behind your back in the prayer position **(fig. 11.32)**.

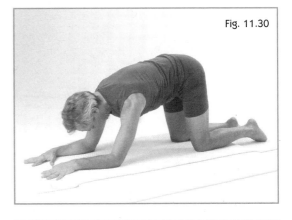

Fig. 11.30

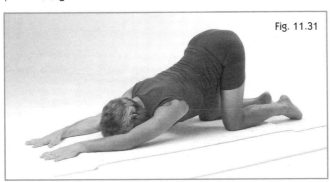

Fig. 11.31

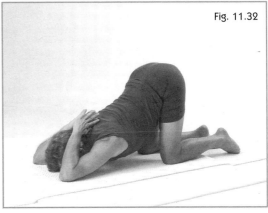

Fig. 11.32

Using Sound Vibration to Relax the Bones of Your Skull

This deeply relaxing position brings a flow of blood to the brain and massages the scalp by combining the use of applied pressure on the cranium with making pleasurable sound.

Begin by coming into Child pose, your torso resting on your thighs. Bring your arms alongside your body (fig. 11.33). Allow the weight of your torso to rest as comfortably on your thighs as possible. Make any adjustments that allow you to be in Child pose as comfortably as possible. Begin to notice your breathing.

Roll onto the crown of your head by lifting your buttocks off your heels (fig. 11.34). Slide your elbows forward to bring your hands under your shoulders (fig. 11.35). Imagine the sensation of beginning a somersault as you roll onto the surface of your skull.

Allow as much weight as possible to press through the head and into the ground. The plates of the skull enjoy pressure. Roll your head from side to side, enough to experiment with bringing sensation and awareness to various surfaces of your skull.

With your lips closed, take a deep breath in and exhale through your nose, humming the sound "h-m-m-m-m-m-m-m-m." Draw the sound out as long as possible and feel the vibration through the bones of your skull. Repeat this humming sound several times, until you feel a sense of pulsing and vibrating in your crown.

Slowly reach your sitz bones back to sit on your heels (fig. 11.36). Move to a deeper level of awareness and experience the effects of directing sound vibrations into the bones of your skull. Release the weight of your torso onto your thighs. Notice the way your head and face feel. Observe any pulsing, tingling, or streaming sensations.

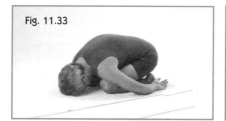
Fig. 11.33

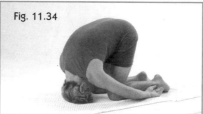
Fig. 11.34

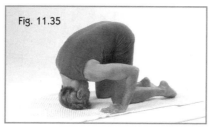
Fig. 11.35

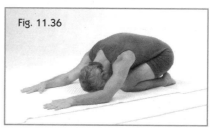
Fig. 11.36

4. Stay in this position long enough to feel the surge of sensation that begins to flood into the upper chest, neck, and head. Keep the breath flowing and experiment with deep, rapid breaths to facilitate a spring action in your chest.

5. Slowly bring your sitz bones back to your heels and release the weight of your torso onto your thighs (**fig. 11.37**). Notice the way your shoulders and ribs feel. Do you notice any difference in the expansion of your torso as you breathe? Observe any pulsing, tingling, or streaming sensations.

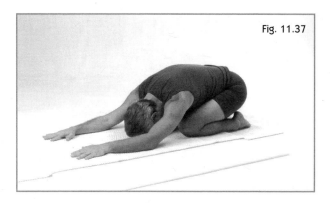

Fig. 11.37

6. Moving now into the Puppy Hip Stretch, bend your elbows and place your forearms on the ground out to your sides so that you can place your palms one on top of the other (**fig. 11.38**). Adjust your position so that your hips are directly above your knees and your sternum can drop down toward the ground. Lower your forehead to rest on top of your hands (**fig. 11.39**). Begin to take long, deep breaths.

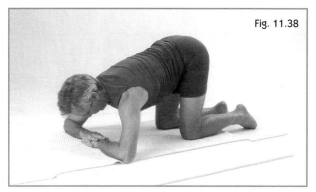

Fig. 11.38

7. Inhale as you press into both elbows; exhale to lower your hips toward the floor on your right side (**fig. 11.40**). Experience the profound stretch along the left side of your rib cage and hip. On the next exhaling breath, press into both elbows and lift your hips back upright over your knees (**fig. 11.41**). Pause and notice the difference between the two sides of your body.

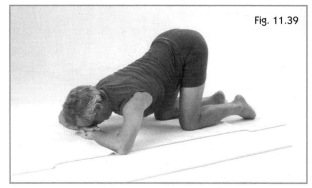

Fig. 11.39

8. Inhale as you press into both elbows; now exhale to lower your hips toward the floor on your left side. Experience the opening stretch along the right side of your rib cage and hip. On the next exhaling breath, press into both elbows and lift your hips upright over your knees.

9. Using the exhaling breath to do the lifting and the

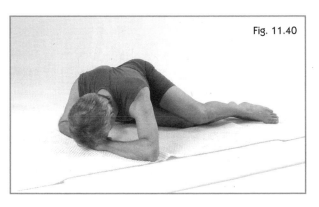

Fig. 11.40

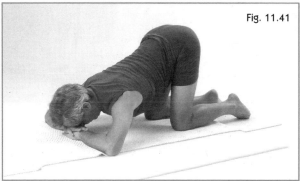

Fig. 11.41

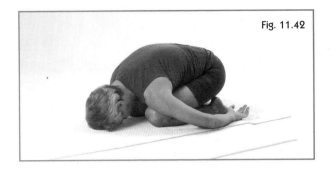

Fig. 11.42

lowering, go back and forth from side to side two more times.

10. Move from the Table pose into Child pose by reaching your sitz bones back to your heels and drawing your arms alongside your body (**fig. 11.42**). Release the weight of your torso onto your thighs. Notice the way your shoulders and ribs feel. Do you notice any difference in the expansion of your torso as you breathe? Observe any pulsing, tingling, or streaming sensations.

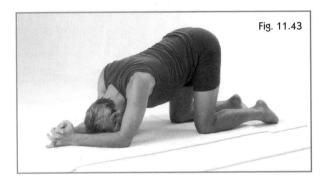

Fig. 11.43

Exploration 2: Puppy Push-ups

1. From the Table pose, lower your elbows to the ground and interlace your fingers. Bring your forehead to the ground and release your chest and sternum to hang (**fig. 11.43**). Begin to deepen your breath; remain connected to the breath as you continue the following exploration.

2. Curl your toes under and press into the balls of your feet, lifting your knees off the ground (**fig. 11.44**). Using your elbows as an anchor for the upper body, take a few tiptoe steps backward and forward. As you become familiar with the dynamics of strength and balance, experiment with walking your toes backward until your hip (**fig. 11.45**). When you tiptoe forward, see how close to your elbows you can come. Experiment with how your head wants to get involved in the movement. As you walk backward, does your head lift off the floor and lengthen away from your shoulders?

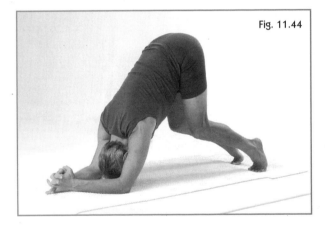

Fig. 11.44

3. When this movement becomes familiar and energizing, play with it. Walk your toes away, lowering the hips to hover above the ground. Keep your feet and elbows in place and lift the tailbone up toward the sky (**fig. 11.46**). Walk your feet in a couple of steps closer and then press into your elbows to lower your sternum out over your

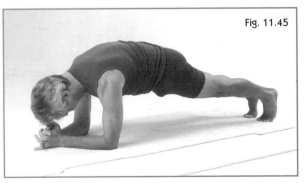

Fig. 11.45

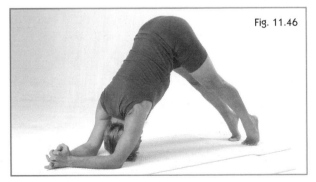

Fig. 11.46

hands (**fig. 11.47**). Use the strength in your shoulders and arms to do a few push-ups, experimenting with the placement of your feet to regulate the amount of stretch you experience

4. When you've reached your comfort zone, lower back into Child pose and enjoy the surging energy moving throughout your body.

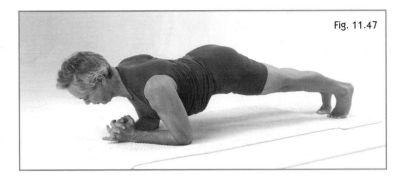

Fig. 11.47

Exploration 3: Donkey Kicks

1. Adjust your hands and knees into a stable Table pose.

2. Inhale and curl your right knee in toward your forehead (**fig. 11.48**). Hold the breath in and notice how the abdominal organs are compressed as you remain curled in this position.

3. Exhale and kick the right heel back and away from you while you simultaneously look forward and bring the back of your head toward your sacrum (**fig. 11.49**).

4. Repeat the movement a few times. Stay aware that the elbows and arms remain upright and that you keep the weight balanced evenly between both arms and shoulders.

5. On the next kick back, keep the leg lengthened behind you. Send the heel further and further away, stretching out of the right hip socket.

6. Keeping your neck and shoulders relaxed and without bending your elbows, bend the right knee and experiment with bringing your right heel to your left buttocks and then your right buttocks (**fig. 11.50**). Find both sides of your buttocks with your right heel. They're back there somewhere. Kick some butt.

7. Lengthen the leg and then bend your elbows and lower your chest to the floor. Keep the right leg lengthened behind you

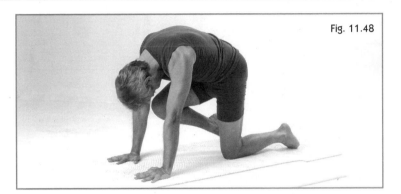

Fig. 11.48

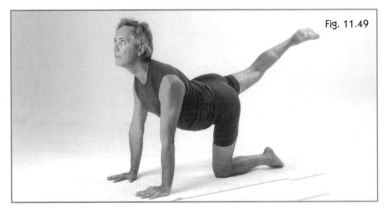

Fig. 11.49

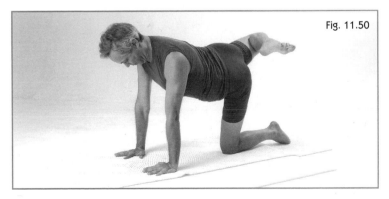

Fig. 11.50

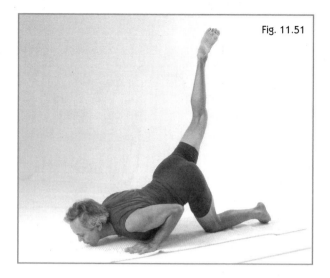

Fig. 11.51

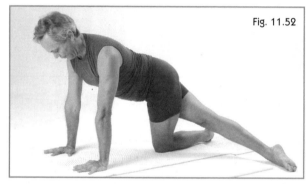

Fig. 11.52

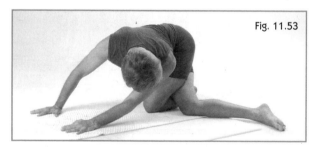

Fig. 11.53

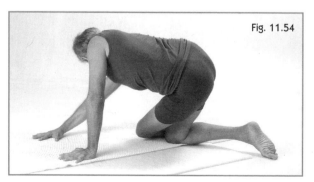

Fig. 11.54

(fig. 11.51). Take a little push-up by pressing into your elbows to raise and lower a few times.

8. Straighten your arms to push your torso up as you lower the right leg to the ground and drag it around behind you to the left side, crossing over the left knee (fig. 11.52). Remaining in this position, bend both knees and turn to look over your left shoulder to see your feet behind you (fig. 11.53). In this phase of the movement it feels very good to let the elbows bend and to exaggerate the rolling motion in the shoulder capsules.

9. Now turn and look over your right shoulder to see your feet behind you (fig. 11.54). Repeat this side-to-side movement, looking over your shoulders and exaggerating the rolling motion in the shoulders.

10. Lengthen the right leg and drag your toes in a semicircle on the floor behind you until your leg comes around and all the way out to your right side (fig. 11.55). Lean into the left hand and arm, lengthening out of the shoulder and straightening the arm. In a sweeping motion, open the right arm up toward the ceiling, following the movement of your hand with your eyes (fig. 11.56).

11. Hold this stretch and experience the sensation of opening across the front side of your chest. If you can remain holding in this position without straining, begin to sweep the arm in full circular rotations in one direction (fig. 11.57), then in the opposite direction. Let your eyes follow the movement of your hand; notice how this movement releases tension in your neck and shoulder.

12. Lower your right hand and arm back into Table pose and bring your right knee underneath you (fig. 11.58). Pause in Table pose and notice the sensations in your body. Observe the difference between the two sides of your body.

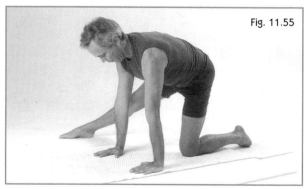

Fig. 11.55

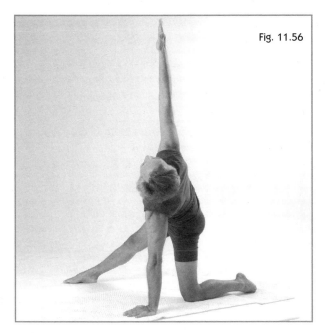

Fig. 11.56

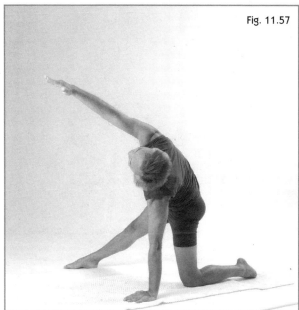

Fig. 11.57

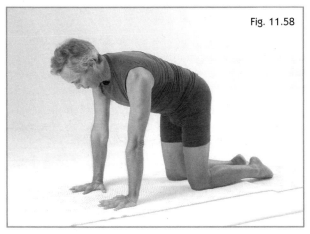

Fig. 11.58

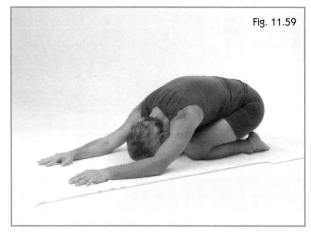

Fig. 11.59

13. Slowly reach your sitz bones back to sit on your heels. Rest here in Child pose before moving to the other side (**fig. 11.59**). Sink into your sensate body to experience the effects of these vigorous and deep stretches.

14. When you are ready to return, press up into Table pose and repeat this sequence on the left side, beginning with curling the left knee in toward your chest. Give yourself permission to follow your urges to invent variations on the new side. Follow the mes-

sages that arise from your body's wisdom about how to use this exploration to tailor the experience to your body's needs.

15. When you are ready, lower back into Child pose. Move to a deeper level of awareness and experience the effects of these vigorous and deep stretches. Release the weight of your torso onto your thighs. How does it feel to bring focused awareness to exploring the strength in your upper body?

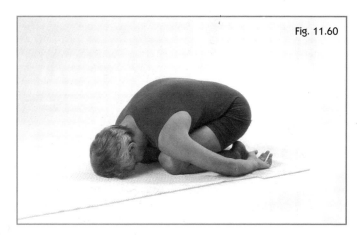

Fig. 11.60

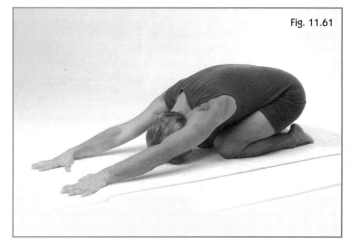

Fig. 11.61

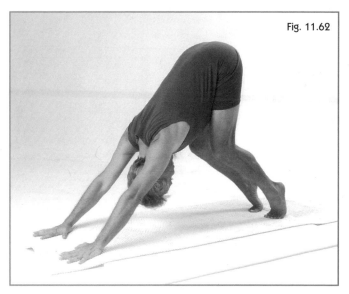

Fig. 11.62

Exploration 4: Downward Dog

1. Come into Child pose, on your knees with your torso resting on your thighs. Bring your arms alongside your body (**fig. 11.60**). Allow the weight of your torso to rest as comfortably on your thighs as possible. Notice any pressure or discomfort in your knees or ankles. After you have made any adjustments that allow you to be in Child pose as comfortably as possible, begin to notice your breathing. Recall how much energy you have experienced through strengthening your arms and legs.

2. Now imagine yourself moving into a pyramid in which the tip of your tailbone forms the apex, with equal pressure down into your arms and legs supporting you. Give yourself permission to move slowly as you enter the following exploration, receiving all of the information that will be passing through your body as sensation. You are now ready to enter Downward Dog.

3. Remaining in Child pose, extend your arms on the floor in front of you. Walk your palms away from you while keeping your shoulders open—down and away from your ears (**fig. 11.61**). Imagine your shoulder blades gliding down the backside of your ribs, the bottom tip of each shoulder blade moving toward the opposite hip pocket. Can you experience how sensing the shoulder blades moving downward in this way allows you to breathe into the backside of your body?

4. A double stretch is occurring as your arms lengthen away from you and your sitz bones pull back to remain anchored on your heels. Open your armpits. Deepen your awareness of the breath by sending the breath into the three chambers of your torso: inhale into your belly, then into your kidneys, and then into your sternum. Exhale, reversing the sequence: release the breath from the sternum, then the kidneys, and finally from the belly. Notice how your attention becomes absorbed in the sound and sensation of your breath.

5. Press into your palms. Curl your toes under and press into the balls of your feet to lift your knees off the ground. Keep your knees bent so that your thighs remain in close contact with your ribs (**fig. 11.62**). How much can you stretch up and out of the soles of your feet?

6. Keeping your heels lifted and your soles stretching, knees bent and in contact with your ribs, draw your awareness to your palms. Fan the fingers into a star, positioning your hands so that the arms are shoulder-width apart. Rotate the crook of your elbows to one another. Spread your shoulder blades apart and send them down the backside of your body toward opposite hip pockets (**fig. 11.63**). Focus your gaze inward toward your navel and then release the weight of your head to hang.

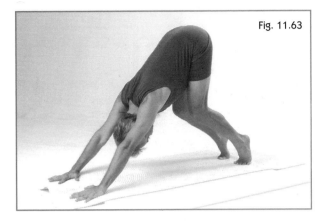

Fig. 11.63

7. Notice how keeping your knees bent and close to your ribs allows you to press into your arms to experiment with your alignment. When you sense your arms are supporting you in a balanced way, send one heel down toward the ground (**fig. 11.64**). Then lift that heel and press the opposite heel toward the ground. Keep your ribs close to your knees as you perform this pedaling motion through the heels.

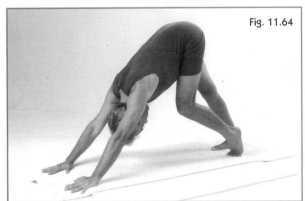

Fig. 11.64

8. Send both heels to the ground and play with shifting your balance so that you feel equal pressure going down into the arms and the legs (**fig. 11.65**). Imagine that you are hanging by your tail, like a monkey hanging from a branch. Take a deep inhale into your belly, your kidneys, and your sternum. Hold that breath in.

9. As you exhale, bend your knees in toward your ribs and lower back down into Child pose (**fig. 11.66**). Allow the weight of your torso to release onto your thighs. Allow your awareness to dissolve into the steady stream of sensation stimulated by this powerful movement.

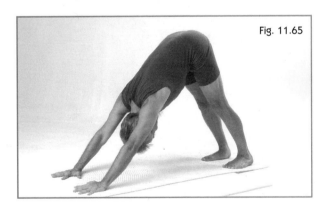

Fig. 11.65

10. Traveling deeper and deeper into relaxation, notice how your whole being opens to receive the effects of balancing the strength of your upper body with your lower body. Notice how gravity moved the fluids of your body from your pelvis through your core, to be received in the bowl of your head. Recall some of the movements in earlier explorations that have prepared you for the experience you have just received. Notice how much of your whole body and mental focus has been engaged in the Downward Dog. Allow yourself to receive all of the information that is coming to you through your sensate body.

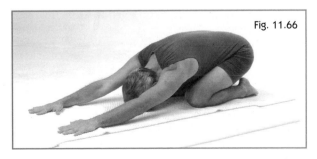

Fig. 11.66

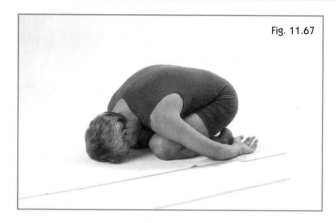

Fig. 11.67

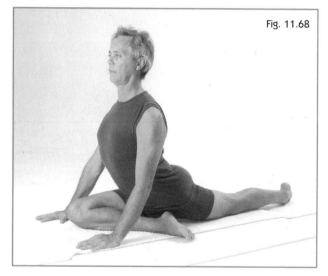

Fig. 11.68

Exploration 5: Pigeon Kicks

1. Come into Child pose, on your knees with your torso resting on your thighs (**fig. 11.67**). Suggest to your mind that this is a time for slowing down and attuning to the sensations that arise within your body. Notice the contact your belly makes with your thighs. Can you sense the abdominal pulse? Notice that your head is lower than your hips and belly. Observe any pulsing, streaming, or tingling sensations as gravity moves the fluids in your body down into the bowl of your head.

2. Begin to slide your palms along the ground and shift your weight forward onto your knees and hands. Adjust your hands and knees into a stable Table pose.

3. Cross your right knee over your left knee and then slide the left leg straight back, lengthening out of the left hip (**fig. 11.68**). This is a classic yoga pose called the Pigeon. Turn to look at your heel (**fig. 11.69**), looking over one shoulder and then the other, allowing the back ankle to roll as you alternate from side to side.

4. Stretch your arms on the ground in front of you and relax the weight of your torso onto the right thigh and leg (**fig. 11.70**). Experience the sensations in the posture as you breathe all the way down into the belly.

5. Curl the toes of the left foot under, digging them into the ground. Slide your hands up beside your shoulders as though you were going to do a push-up (**fig. 11.71**). Take in a deep breath; as you exhale, shift the weight of

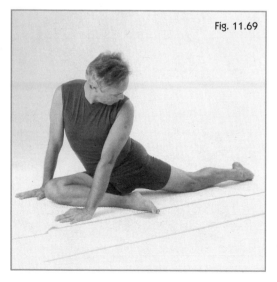

Fig. 11.69

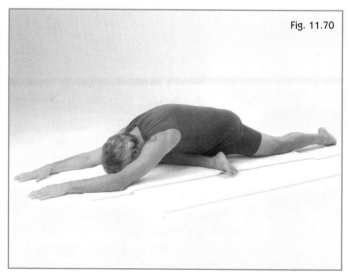

Fig. 11.70

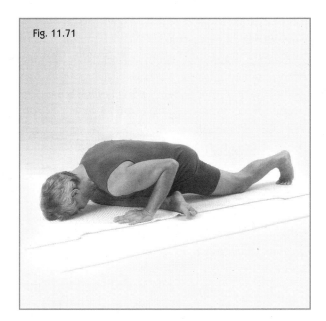

Fig. 11.71

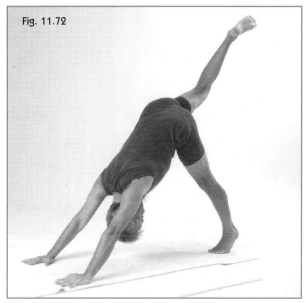

Fig. 11.72

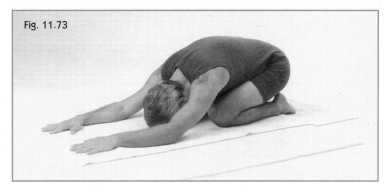

Fig. 11.73

your torso into your hands, straighten your arms, and kick the right heel all the way behind you and up toward the ceiling (**fig. 11.72**). Hold your right leg extended for just a moment and look toward your navel. Notice how you are using the strength in your shoulders and arms to stabilize and balance your body in this position.

6. For the next few breaths move back and forth between Pigeon and Pigeon Kicks, first with your right knee on the floor and then exhaling and kicking the right heel all the way back and up toward the ceiling. Continue until the movement becomes familiar and effortless.

7. Bend both knees and lower down to the floor into Child pose, reaching your sitz bones back to sit on your heels (**fig. 11.73**). Experience the sensations generated in this movement. Allow your breath to return to normal.

8. When you are ready, shift your weight forward onto your knees and hands. Adjust your hands and knees into a stable Table pose.

9. Cross your left knee over your right knee and then slide the right leg straight back, lengthening out of the right hip into

Pigeon pose. Turn to look at your heel looking over one shoulder and then the other, allowing the back ankle to roll as you alternate from side to side.

10. Continue the movement exploration on this side. When you have completed the Pigeon Kicks, bend both knees and lower back down to the floor into Child pose, reaching your sitz bones back to sit on your heels. Allow your breath to return to normal.

11. Move to a deeper level of awareness and experience the effects of these deep stretches. Continue to release the weight of your torso onto your thighs. Notice the way your hips and legs feel. Observe any pulsing, tingling, or streaming sensations.

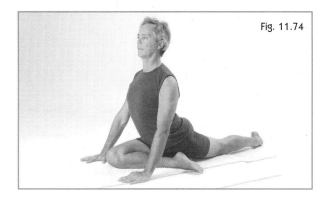

Fig. 11.74

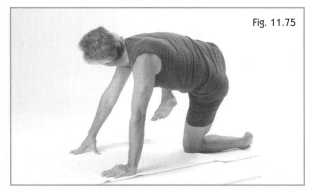

Fig. 11.75

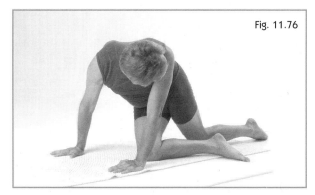

Fig. 11.76

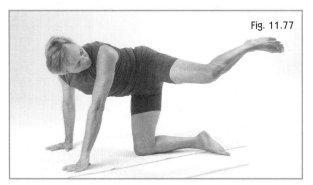

Fig. 11.77

Exploration 6: Pigeon Walk

1. Come into Table pose. Cross the right knee over the left knee and send the left leg behind you into a relaxed Pigeon (**fig. 11.74**). Pause here for a couple of breaths.

2. Bring the knees forward to Table pose. Now cross the left knee over the right knee. Send the right leg back into an easy Pigeon.

3. Over the next few breaths, begin a continuous forward walk by bringing one knee around to cross the other, right over left, then left over right. When this Pigeon Walk becomes familiar, begin to exaggerate the rotation in your hips, making as wide a circle as possible on each side (**fig. 11.75**). Allow your elbows to bend and your upper body to move in rhythmic, dancelike response to the forward walk (**figs. 11.76, 11.77, and 11.78**).

4. When this forward creep has taken you to the edge of your working space, begin to do the Pigeon Walk backward, using the same exaggerations in your whole-body movement. Particularly notice how the head wants to move in response to the movement of the legs and hips.

5. After walking backward and forward a few times, return to Child pose and relax into the sensations. Suggest to your logical mind that you have created new neural bridges between the two sides of your body and between the left and right hemispheres of your brain. Notice any pulsing or streaming sensations, particularly in the space behind your eyes. When you are ready, begin your return.

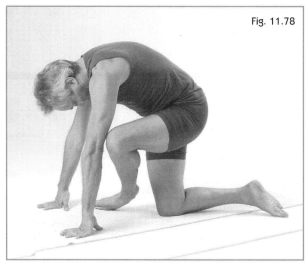

Fig. 11.78

Integration: Pigeon

1. Come into a stable Table pose (**fig. 11.79**).

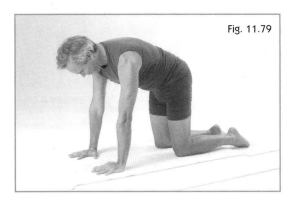

Fig. 11.79

2. Cross your right knee over your left knee, then slide the left leg straight back, lengthening out of the left hip into Pigeon pose (**fig. 11.80**). Take all the time you need to settle into this position. You may want to place a cushion under the right hip to regulate the amount of stretch you receive. Your kneecap or back ankle may also need some extra padding.

3. Once you feel settled, plant your hands on the floor beside you and begin to turn and look over your right shoulder to see the heel of your left foot (**fig. 11.81**). Then turn and look over the left shoulder. Look back and forth, alternating from one shoulder to the other. This movement encourages the hips to open and the whole body to settle. It also sets up a neuromuscular pattern of balancing the two sides of the body by crossing the body's midline.

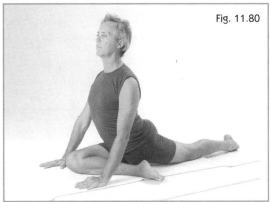

Fig. 11.80

4. Slow down and continue this movement, paying particular attention to the back ankle. Let the ankle roll from the inner ankle to the outer ankle as you look over one shoulder and then the other.

5. Bring your torso to face squarely forward. Notice that your right hip and leg are in position for a seated forward bend; the left hip and leg is in position for a front extension. Inhale progressively into your belly, your kidneys, and then your sternum and notice how this full three-part breath allows you to lengthen from the pubic bone to the sternum.

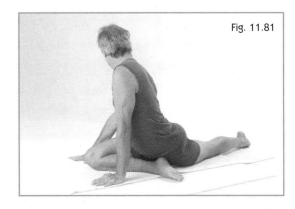

Fig. 11.81

6. Using your hands for balance, press your right knee into the ground and bend at the hinge of your hips. Lengthen through the sternum and imagine that you are going to place your sternum on the floor six feet in front of you (**fig. 11.82**). How much would you have to lengthen in the spine to reach that far with your sternum? Slowly lower the long line of your torso over your right thigh. Use your hands if you need to control the amount of stretch as you lower forward. If you find that you don't need your hands, fold your arms across the small of your back as you lower your torso (**fig. 11.83**).

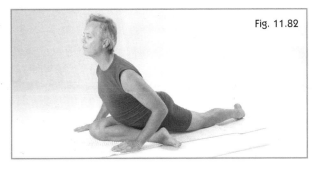

Fig. 11.82

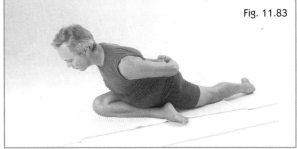

Fig. 11.83

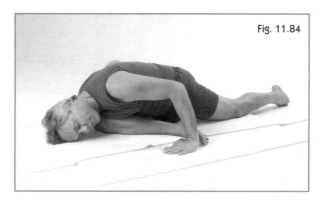

Fig. 11.84

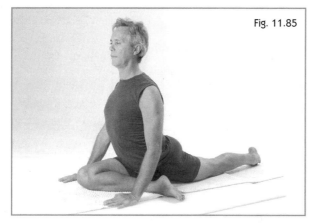

Fig. 11.85

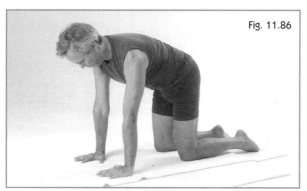

Fig. 11.86

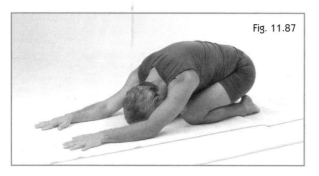

Fig. 11.87

7. When you have folded over the knee, move internally to experience the stretch and all of the sensations that arise in this position. Breathe all the way down into your belly.

8. Remain in this position and notice whether any part of your body is holding on in a protective pattern against the stretch. What happens if you let go of the layers of protection and enter into the actual sensations of the stretch? Notice any emotions or dreamlike images that may arise as you open into Pigeon pose.

9. Roll the muscle of your forehead across the floor (**fig. 11.84**). This releases the "worry" muscle of the brow.

10. Gently and slowly begin to walk your hands and torso back into the upright position (**fig. 11.85**). Pause and notice how your spine is elongated over your pelvis. Then return through Table pose (**fig. 11.86**) into Child pose (**fig. 11.87**). Observe any differences between the two sides of your body. Allow your awareness to receive all of the many sensations that have been stimulated by holding this posture. In this receptive state of deep relaxation, recall any particular emotions or memories that may have surfaced. Acknowledge to your logical mind that it is safe and desirable to experience and release any past holding patterns that no longer serve your whole being. Whatever you have noticed is now released.

11. When you feel ready, slowly transition to the new side by coming into Table pose. Carry out the movements as outlined above on this side. When you finish, slowly and gently walk your hands and torso back into the upright position, returning to Table pose and then to Child pose. Release the weight of your torso onto your thighs. Notice the way your hips and legs feel. Observe the sensations moving through your organism.

12. Remaining in Child pose a little longer, reflect on the explorations that have drawn awareness to the movements your body made spontaneously at a time when you were very young. Notice how much permission you have created for entering deeper levels of your whole being. Witness how you feel when the wisdom of your organism is given the opportunity to communicate through your movement. As you feel ready, stretch and begin your transition into the next events in your day. As you come up to standing, notice how you are moving.

Before Moving On . . .

The inquiries of this chapter have explored the transition from being on your belly to coming onto all fours and differentiating the coordinated bilateral movements of your arms and legs from Table pose. By strengthening the muscles involved in flexing and extending the legs, your body is preparing to enter the standing postures with balance and stability. The transitions from being on your belly to Downward Dog and then to Pigeon require extensive coordination among all segments of the body to maintain balance and stability while remaining flexible enough to adjust to the shifts of balance that these positions require.

With the body wisdom you have developed in these inquiries, you have a solid foundation for exploring the depths of Downward Dog and Pigeon. Because of the way these two postures develop physical strength, stamina, and coordination and are situated at the crossroads for transitioning from being on the ground to standing, they deserve your continued focus, even as you expand to include the wider range of postures that will be introduced in the following chapters. Many yoga traditions hold one or both of these postures as "career postures," meaning that every time you enter the posture it provides fresh learning and insight about how your body is communicating to you from day to day. You can spend a lifetime exploring the subtleties of how your body shifts and opens in ways that impact your alignment by shaping and reshaping the flow of gravity throughout your body.

The coordination you have been developing between the two sides of the body and between the upper and lower body has not been limited to beneficial impacts on your neuromuscular intelligence. In crossing the midline of the body, the coordination of brain-wave activity between the left and right hemispheres of the cerebral cortex is stimulated, generating greater cognitive capacities. The inquiries of the next chapter bring even greater precision to the synchronization of movements that produce both bilateral and cross-lateral efficiency but also bring the cognitive faculties of the intelligent mind into greater contact and communication with the wisdom of the body, creating the possibility for a more powerful, integrated being.

12 Containing the Paradox of Polar Opposites: Individuation through Bilateral Movement

How does opening to the differences in the two sides of the body generate unity consciousness?

YOUR BODY HAS BEEN SHAPED TO FULFILL YOUR INTENTIONS. Pausing to notice the differences that arise between the two sides of your body can reveal very different capacities and information. If we simplistically think that the point of yoga is to work to make the two sides equal, we miss the reality that we are bilateral beings. The inquiries of this chapter allow you to experience these bilateral differences as they are embodied in the whole person that you are.

How do these differences in the two sides of the body arise? Life presents a steady stream of choices. From the yogic perspective, our choices arise from attraction to pleasurable experiences, *raga,* and avoidance of dangerous or unpleasurable experiences, *dvwesha.* These primal impulses are the motivating forces underlying the unfolding development of our organism as a vehicle to fulfill our thirst for self-awareness.

The choices that give shape to our personalities are the sum total of everything that distinguishes us as individuals. Although we are the creatures endowed with infinite capacity to create our lives through our choices, it is difficult to recognize and claim the power that is ours because the present seems so different from our fantasy life. In our most self-confident fantasies, every desire for our life is fulfilled. But the choices we make in "real life" bring consequences that weren't so obvious when we were fantasizing. The body is a walking repository of the consequences of every conscious and unconscious choice we have ever made to fulfill our needs, wants, wishes, desires, dreams, and passions. The body also contains the consequences of our avoidances, phobias, fears, rejections, and intolerances. The inquiries of Self-Awakening Yoga provide an opportunity to slow down and witness our life's creation in this moment with nonjudgmental self-awareness.

The witness is not the judge. The witness is not Dr. Fix-it. In receiving ourselves as we are in the moment, we enter into the paradoxical unity and perfection underlying all of our multidimensional expressions of self.

Nowhere in our experience do polar opposites arise more noticebly than in the way the two sides of our body function. The eyes take in two different views of the same reality and average the difference as one integrated picture. A common pattern is that one eye wants to see everything to the point that it protrudes while the other eye prefers to withdraw. Pose for a portrait and you will want your "good side" in the foreground. What do we mean by having a "good side" and a "bad side"? In one art class experiment each student photographed his or her whole body and then made two prints, one with the negative reversed. We cut the two pictures in half, making one composite of the right side of the body and another composite of the left side.

If both sides of your body looked exactly like your right side (or your left side), what would you look like? To get some idea, hold a hand mirror vertically along the midline of your nose as you look into a wall mirror. Adjust the handheld mirror so you can see what your composite left and right sides look like. In our composite portraits we each saw strong variations, dissimilarities striking enough to reveal two entirely different personalities living in the same body. We saw the sinner and the saint, the master and the slave, beauty and the beast, and every other manifestation of the polarities in our being. Hatha yoga gets its name from observing and honoring these bilateral differences—*ha* ("sun") and *tha* ("moon") refer to the energies of the two sides of the body: masculine and feminine, extroverted and introverted, sun and moon. The list is infinite.

Polar opposites integrate in awareness. By turning up the volume to the differences that exist in our personal, bilateral body, we cultivate the capacity to witness our experience with nonjudgmental self-awareness. Regardless of how you characterize the differences that you notice, there is a place in your being in which the opposites are held in a unifying relationship. One hand may play a supportive role in holding the watermelon while the other hand does the precision work of cutting, but the unifying principle is that the red, dripping, sweet, juicy bite makes it to your mouth. By noticing the special qualities of each side of the body, we inform the whole of its nature. In allowing the differences, we set up a neuromuscular bridge for the two sides to harmonize their functioning more efficiently. In witness consciousness, the differences are perceived in relationship to the whole. This is the essence of yoga—to yoke, to join together.

One of the deepest and earliest self-satisfying experiences of being in a body is that of being rocked. Oscillating between two poles, the counterbalance of opposite movements creates a mesmerizing sense of balance and wholeness. In the first inquiry below, we explore rocking and pendulum swinging to bring awareness to the two sides of the body. These movements increase awareness in the seated yoga postures Butterfly, Lotus, and Tailor Pose. The second inquiry brings us onto our side for locating the outside seams of the body. Using rolling, scissoring, and alternate lifting, the side-stretching movements develop the sense of being at home in the midst of being stretched in two directions. These movements open the body for deeper exploration into the side-bending yoga postures, such as Crescent Moon, Triangle, Half Circle, and Side-Angle Stretch.

In the Magnetic Energy Field Meditation, you can experience how to use your awareness of the magnet field poles of your two sides to generate an energetic womb of regeneration.

Harmonizing Opposite Sides through Perpetual-Motion Rocking

Inquiry: How does rocking from side to side establish a sense of equilibrium?

Equilibrium is often defined as a state of balance among all the forces acting upon the body. Equilibrium is noticeable in your body when you rock slightly to one direction and your body falls back to its original position without losing your center of balance. The closer you are to the ground, the easier it is to remain in a stable state of balance. Conversely, the further your center of gravity moves from the ground, as in standing, the more strength and flexibility is required to maintain balance. The paradoxical effect of rocking while in a seated position, whether rocking backward and forward or swinging from side to side, is that you are training your kinesthetic sense to maintain a state of balance by finding your equilibrium during the movement. In Sitz Bone Rocking, the effects of maintaining your balance on two sides can produce a state of equanimity. When an elephant walks through a village in India, dogs barking and nipping at the elephant's heels cause no pause in the elephant's steady movement forward toward its destination. An elephant knows that with one whack of its swinging trunk, twenty barking dogs will go flying. In a similar way, Finding the Pendulum of the Head and Butterfly Walk generate a sense of taking refuge in the body in the midst of life's demands.

Finding the Pendulum of the Head brings awareness to the way your head moves above your spine, releasing and lengthening the head out of the basket of the shoulders. Shoulder Shrugs and Shoulder Compass provide yet another way to release the arms for circular rotation and cross-lateral swinging in response to moving from your center. Tailor Pose Pendulum opens the torso on each side while you remain grounded in your sitz bones and integrated in your center of being.

Exploration 1: Sitz Bone Rocking

1. Sit in a comfortable position on the ground. Suggest to your logical mind that this is a time for slowing down and attuning to the differences that arise in noticing the two sides of your body. Invite your mental awareness to be present as a non-judgmental witness, simply noticing what you notice. There is nothing to be changed, fixed, or altered in any way. By remaining present to what is, the energy of prana is allowed to flow wherever it is needed for balance.

2. Make any adjustments that help you to settle into the experience. Notice the contact your sitz bones make with the ground. Scan your body to observe the areas that might be using effort to hold you upright. Notice any resistance in your body. Let any resistance be as it is.

3. Moving to a deeper level of awareness, begin to press your sitz bones downward into the ground **(fig. 12.1)**. Does pressing into the sitz bones anchor you to the ground? Do you feel an energetic lifting up through the spine when you exaggerate the press in your sitz bones?

4. Imagine that your head is a helium-filled balloon. Notice how your head hovers above your spine when you breathe into the "balloon" of your head.

5. Slowly open your eyes. Position your feet together in front of you and let your knees drop out to your sides.

6. Rock onto your left sitz bone and lift the right sitz bone and hip slightly off the ground **(fig. 12.2)**. Hold for just long enough to feel the abdominal and hip muscles that are working to keep you lifted.

7. Lower the right sitz bone back down to the ground. Sit for a moment with your eyes closed and sense the difference between the way the two sides of your body contact the ground.

8. Open your eyes and shift the weight of your torso onto the right sitz bone, lifting the left sitz bone and hip slightly off the ground **(fig. 12.3)**. Pause and hold long enough to feel the abdominal and hip muscles that are working to keep you lifted.

9. Lower the left sitz bone back down to the ground. Notice the contact your body makes with the ground now.

10. Alternating from side to side, rock onto one sitz bone and lift the opposite hip and sitz bone off the ground. Use your inhaling

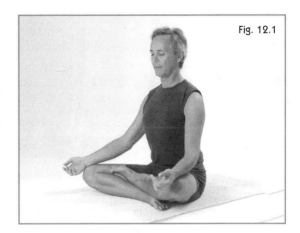

Fig. 12.1

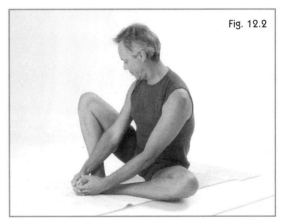

Fig. 12.2

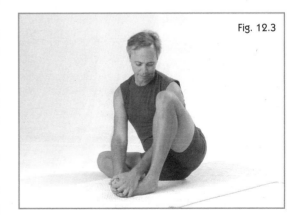

Fig. 12.3

breath to lift; exhale to return to center. Go back and forth from side to side until the rocking momentum propels the movement. **11.** Slow down and bring the movement to stillness. Close your eyes and experience the sensation of contact with the ground. Are there any differences in the way your two sitz bones contact the ground? Observe any pulsing, streaming, or tingling sensations. Observe the position of your head over your spine and body. Does your head feel lighter or does your neck feel longer?

Observe the way your shoulders hang. Do you observe any differences in the way the two sides of your body interact to create balance? Create an image of the way your body looks and feels when your torso is free to rock from one sitz bone to the other. **12.** Begin your return by slowly bringing your palms to your face. Massage the muscles of your eyes, your jaw, and the back of your neck. Open your eyes and notice whether your vision has altered in any way.

Exploration 2: Shoulder Shrugs and Seated Shoulder Compass

1. Sit in a comfortable position on the ground. Rock back and forth from sitz bone to sitz bone as you lift the opposite hip and sitz bone off the ground slightly (**fig. 12.4**). **2.** Bring your legs into a comfortable cross-legged position that you can hold for a few minutes. Notice the way your shoulders are hanging (**fig. 12.5**). **3.** Inhale and shrug both shoulders up toward your ears. Hold the breath in and exaggerate the squeeze. Exhale and completely let go of the weight of your shoulders. Repeat this movement several times, inhaling as you shrug and exhaling as you release. Keep the movement going until you develop a comfortable rhythm and pace for the movement and breath.

4. Bring your shoulders to stillness. Close your eyes and notice the sensations in your shoulders, head, and neck. **5.** Open your eyes. Inhale and bring your right shoulder toward your right ear as you send the left shoulder downward in the direction of your left hip. Exhale, bring both shoulders back to neutral, and then reverse the movement, inhaling as you squeeze your left shoulder toward your left ear and send the right shoulder downward in the direction of your right hip. Exhale and bring both shoulders back to neutral. **6.** For the next several breaths, repeat this movement, squeezing one shoulder toward the ear and the other downward, and then reverse. Continue the movement until you feel a momentum and rhythm take over. **7.** Close your eyes and sit for a moment. Experience the sensation in your shoulders,

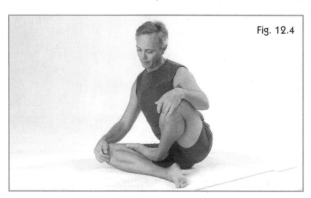

Fig. 12.4

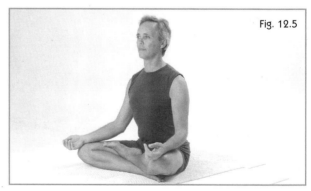

Fig. 12.5

head, and neck. Do your shoulders feel any different from when you began? Observe any pulsing, streaming, or tingling sensations. Observe the position of your head over your spine and body. Does your head feel lighter or does your neck feel longer?

8. Bring your right shoulder up toward your right ear—this is the north pole on an imaginary compass. Keep the right shoulder at the north pole and send the left shoulder downward to the south pole (**fig. 12.6**). Reverse the two shoulders, finding the opposite poles. Repeat this movement several times until it feels familiar and comfortable to you.

9. Send the right shoulder forward toward the wall in front of you—this is east on your compass. Leave the right shoulder forward and send the left shoulder back toward the wall behind you—this is west (**fig. 12.7**). Alternate between east and west a few times.

10. Take the right shoulder into several complete circular rotations, finding each cardinal point along the compass (**fig. 12.8**). Reverse the direction of the circle. Close your eyes and notice the difference in the way the two shoulders are now hanging.

11. Now take the left shoulder into several complete circular rotations, finding every pole along the compass. Reverse the direction of the circle.

12. Set both shoulders at north and begin simultaneous circular rotations all the way around the compass (**fig. 12.9**). Exaggerate the movements as you deepen your breath. Notice how the movement facilitates a deeper level of breathing. Reverse the direction of the circles.

13. Close your eyes and notice the sensations in your shoulders.

14. Now set one shoulder at north and the other at south. Allow the two shoulders to make complete circular rotations all the way around the compass going in opposite directions (**fig. 12.10**). Keep the movement going until it feels familiar

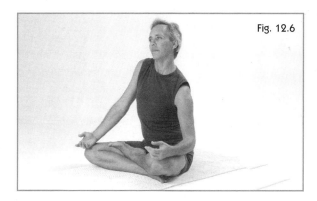

Fig. 12.6

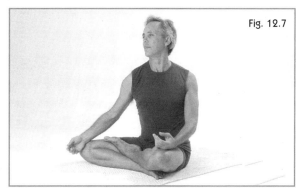

Fig. 12.7

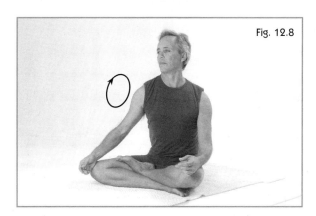

Fig. 12.8

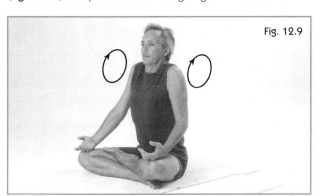

Fig. 12.9

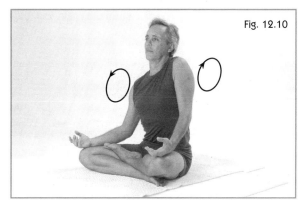

Fig. 12.10

and comfortable. Breathe deeply as you continue. Now reverse the direction of the circular rotations. Experiment with moving a little faster, letting go of the control over the movement and allowing your shoulders to be moved by your breath.

15. Bring the movement to stillness. Close your eyes and sit for a moment. Experience the sensation in your shoulders, head, and neck. Do your shoulders feel any different than when you began? Observe any pulsing, streaming or tingling sensations. Observe the position of your head over your spine and body. Does your head feel lighter or does your neck feel longer? How does moving from one side of your body to the other affect your sense of balance? Do you sense how exploring the differences in the two sides helps to establish equilibrium?

16. Bring your palms to your face and massage the muscles of your eyes, your jaw, and the back of your neck. Open your eyes and notice whether your vision has altered in any way.

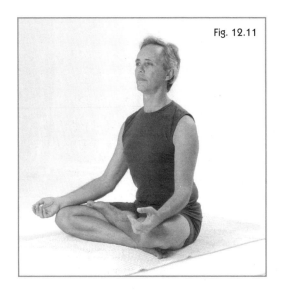

Fig. 12.11

Exploration 3: Finding the Pendulum of the Head

1. Sit in a comfortable cross-legged position, or sit in a chair (**fig. 12.11**). Notice the way your shoulders are hanging.

2. Place an imaginary sponge on your forehead. In a pendulum-like motion, move your head as if you were cleaning a plate glass window with the sponge (**fig. 12.12**). Notice the way your head moves as you embody this image. Let your breath flow freely as you move.

3. Keep the movement going, continuing to internalize the image of a sponge on your forehead, and allow your shoulders to drop away from your ears. As your head moves to the right, let the right shoulder glide down and away from you (**fig. 12.13**). As your head moves to the left, send the left shoulder down and away from you. Experience how the movement in your shoulders affects the movement of your head.

4. Now repeat the movement of your head, but allow the shoulders to squeeze upward toward your ear as the ear comes close (**fig. 12.14**). Alternate from side to side. Let the breath flow throughout the movement.

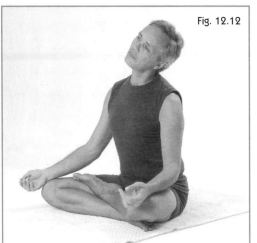

Fig. 12.12

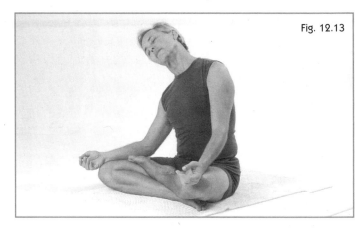

Fig. 12.13

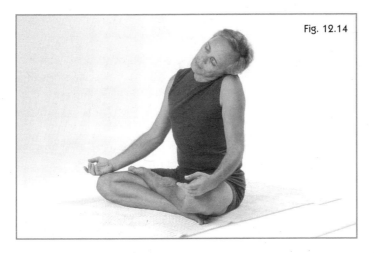

Fig. 12.14

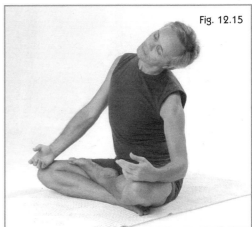

Fig. 12.15

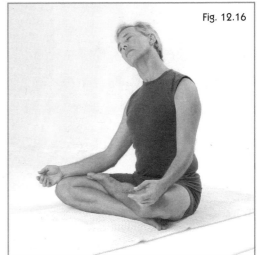

Fig. 12.16

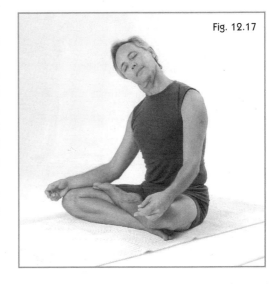

Fig. 12.17

5. Come to stillness and close your eyes. Notice the sensations in your shoulders.

6. Slowly open your eyes. Imagine now that the sponge is placed on the backside of your head; you begin to move the head from side to side. Experience how changing the placement of the sponge changes your awareness and experience of the movement. Continue the movement while you allow the shoulders to drop down and away from the oncoming ear **(fig. 12.15)**.

7. What would it feel like to have a long paintbrush attached to the crown of your head? Lengthen your head to paint an imaginary arc on a domed ceiling above you **(fig. 12.16)**.

8. Imagine now that you have a long beard, like the beard of an Egyptian pharaoh. As your head swings to the right the beard swings out to the left. As your head moves to the left, the beard swings out to the right. Continue the movement and exaggerate the action **(fig. 12.17)**. Can you sense how your movement lengthens your head from the neck, allowing the breath to flow freely?

9. Now combine the images of painting an arc on a domed ceiling with swinging your pharaoh's beard.

10. Bring the movement to stillness. Close your eyes and sit for a moment. Experience the sensation in your shoulders, head, and neck. Observe the position of your head over your spine and body. Does your head feel lighter or does your neck feel longer? How have the explorations of the pendulum movements of your head affected your center of gravity? your sense of balance between the two sides of your body?

11. Bring your palms to your face and massage the muscles of your eyes, your jaw, and the back of your neck. Open your eyes and notice whether your vision has altered in any way.

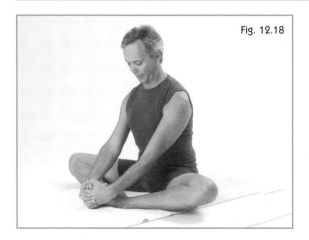

Fig. 12.18

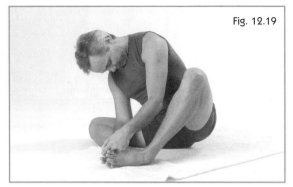

Fig. 12.19

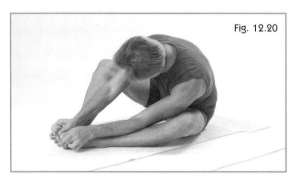

Fig. 12.20

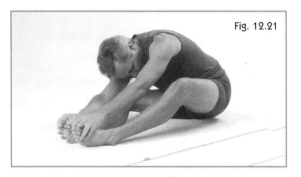

Fig. 12.21

Integration: Butterfly Walk

1. Sit in a comfortable position on the ground. Bring your feet together and let your knees open out to your sides (**fig. 12.18**). Imagine that your open legs are the wings of a butterfly. Do not try to force or push your knees toward the ground. Let them be where they are.

2. Grasp hold of your big toes. Begin to rock from one sitz bone to the other, allowing your head to drop forward and your chin to move toward your chest (**fig. 12.19**). Relax the weight of your shoulders and your jaw, and even let go of the expressions in your face as you continue to rock.

3. Holding on to your toes, begin to walk your sitz bones backward, one sitz bone at the time (**figs. 12.20 and 12.21**). Let the rocking help you reach backward from side to side until your legs begin to lengthen along the ground. Only go back as far as you can go while still holding on to your toes. Keep your head heavy. Think of the weight of your head as a bowling ball hanging between your arms and moving down toward the ground between your legs.

4. After you walk backward to the extent of your stretch, begin to walk forward, sitz bone by sitz bone, until your knees are open to your sides in Butterfly. Repeat this movement walking backward and forward several times until the rhythm and momentum of the movement become familiar and effortless. Use your breath to build the momentum. Each time you walk backward, see if you can walk slightly further, lengthening your legs without releasing your toes. When you walk forward, see how close you can bring your sitz bones toward your heels.

5. Return to Butterfly and release your toes (**fig. 12.22**). Let

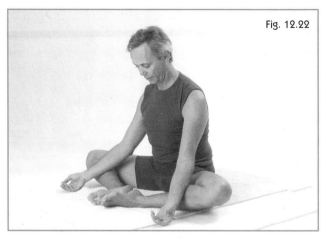

Fig. 12.22

your arms and hands relax in a comfortable position. Close your eyes. Experience the sensation in your groin and hips. Do your hips and inner thighs feel any different than when you began? Are your knees any closer to the ground without attempting to force them down? Observe any pulsing, streaming, or tingling sensations. Observe the position of your head over your spine and body. Does your head feel lighter or does your neck feel longer? What do you notice about how the two sides of your body interact to produce forward and backward movement along the floor? How has the Butterfly Walk affected your sense of balance between the two sides of your body?

Integration: Tailor Pose Pendulum

1. Sit in a comfortable position on the ground. Cross your right ankle over your left ankle in an easy sitting position (**fig. 12.23**). This position is called Tailor pose because it mirrors the way tailors in India sit to do their work.

2. Bring your fingertips to the floor on either side of your legs. Slowly walk the right hand away from you until you can place the right elbow on the floor. Keep your neck and shoulders relaxed as you look down toward your elbow (**fig. 12.24**) and then up toward the sky (**fig. 12.25**). If your elbow doesn't reach the floor, use a cushion to support your elbow.

3. Feel the stretch along the left side of your rib cage. Keep the left sitz bone in contact with the ground to allow a full stretch and to remain grounded throughout the exploration. If you feel like taking a deeper stretch, slowly extend the left arm up toward the sky (**fig. 12.26**) and experience how much more stretch this allows. Breathe deeply into the stretch.

4. Turn your eyes and head to look down at the right elbow and then up toward the left hand. Now reach your left hand all the way over your head to cradle the right side of your head. Point your elbow upward toward the

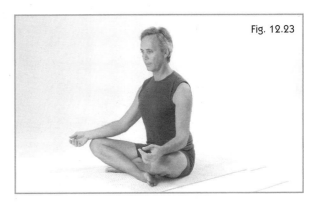

Fig. 12.23

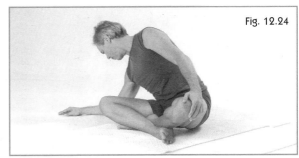

Fig. 12.24

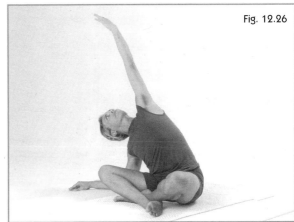

Fig. 12.26

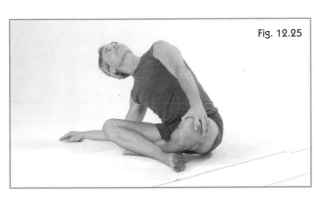

Fig. 12.25

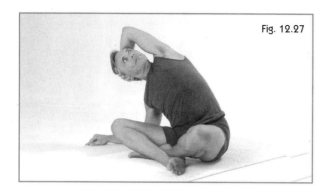

Fig. 12.27

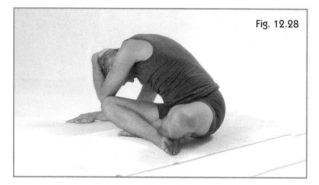

Fig. 12.28

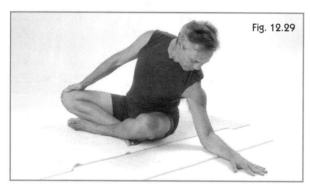

Fig. 12.29

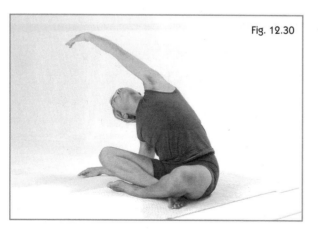

Fig. 12.30

sky (**fig. 12.27**) and then down toward the floor (**fig. 12.28**). Repeat a few times, synchronizing the movement with the breath.

5. When you feel ready to quiet the movement, bring your torso back to the upright position, release your arms to hang at your sides, and sit for a moment. Notice whether the left side of your rib cage feels more open than the right side. Do you notice any difference in the way the ribs on your left side are moving in response to your breath in comparison with the right side? Observe any pulsing, streaming, or tingling sensations wherever they arise in your body.

6. Now cross the left ankle over the right ankle. Bring your fingertips to the floor on either side of your legs. Slowly walk the left hand on the floor away from you until you can place the left elbow on the floor (**fig. 12.29**). Take the sequence of Tailor Pose Pendulum movements over to this side of the body.

7. When you've completed the sequence, bring your torso back to the upright position and sit for a moment. Notice any differences between the two sides of your rib cage. Differences between the two sides of the body are often most keenly felt after explorations that focus on either side of the body. Observe any pulsing, streaming, or tingling sensations wherever they arise in your body.

8. Now slide the right elbow out along the floor and hold just long enough to extend the left arm overhead (**fig. 12.30**). Then return to upright and slide the left elbow along the ground, extending the right arm above your head (**fig. 12.31**).

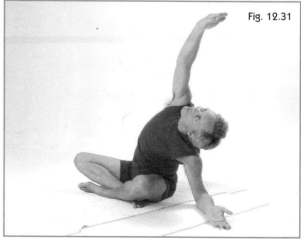

Fig. 12.31

9. Continue this pendulum-like movement from side to side until you feel a rhythm beginning to take over. Breathe fully into each side as you stretch. Notice which ankle is crossed in front and reverse the position of your ankles, bringing the other ankle to the front. Again begin the side to side pendulum movement. Do you notice a difference in the movement when one ankle is crossed in front as compared to the other? Which way feels more open? Can you sense how alternating the pattern of crossing your ankles creates more opportunity to create balance between the two sides of your body? When the movement becomes effortless and free, allow it to begin to slow back down.

10. Let your arms and hands relax in a comfortable position (**fig. 12.32**). Close your eyes. Experience the sensation in your groin and hips and legs. Do your hips and inner thighs feel any different than when you began? Notice the way the sides and back of your rib cage are now moving in response to your breath. Observe any pulsing, streaming, or tingling sensations. Observe the position of your head over your spine and body. Does your head feel lighter or your neck feel longer? Do your legs feel more relaxed on the ground?

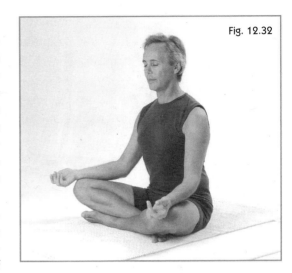

Fig. 12.32

Balancing Strength with Flexibility in Side-Stretching Postures

Inquiry: How does opening and strengthening the upper arm and shoulder muscles and the muscles of the low back create greater flexibility in the sides of the rib cage?

Have you ever seen the statues of the Buddha where he is reclining on his side with his head propped up on his hand and his big belly hanging free? This is a comfortable position you might find yourself in when you are on the beach watching a sunset or on the sofa watching TV. This arrangement provides a relaxed position to explore the outside seam of your body's edges. You will find interesting variations that open your neck and shoulders, your ribs and hips. Allowing gravity to support your body in this position helps you to locate the origin of movement for Side Scissors— opening the hip joint to the side, a movement physiotherapists and kinesiologists call *abduction*. Of all the explorations you've undertaken up to now, you may notice that this one makes a dramatic difference when you compare effects on the two sides of your body.

Elbow Lift directs the flow of prana awakened in the first explorations into a more vigorous movement that strengthens your upper arms and shoulders for the side-stretching yoga postures, such as Triangle, Crescent Moon, Gate, Balancing Angle, and Side Angle Stretch. In addition to opening the sides of the body, these movements strengthen the major low-back muscle, the quadratus lumborum. Balancing strength with flexibility, balancing the low back with the abdominal muscles, allowing each side to develop its potentials are benefits from these inquiries.

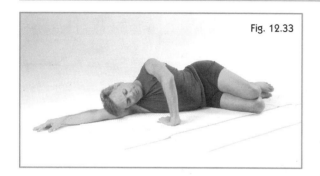

Fig. 12.33

Exploration 1: Reclining Buddha Side Scissors 1

1. Lie on the ground on your right side, your right arm stretched out palm down and your head resting on your arm. Walk your fingertips away from you to fully extend the arm. Bend both knees as though you were positioned to sit on a stool. Stack your knees one on top of the other, ankles one on top of the other. Finally, place your left hand on the floor in front of your torso and use that hand to keep your body from rolling to either side **(fig. 12.33)**.

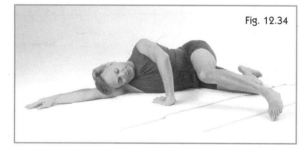

Fig. 12.34

2. Notice how comfortable or uncomfortable your head feels resting on your shoulder. How comfortable is your right shoulder? Do you notice how the right side of your rib cage contacts the ground?

3. On your next inhale, lift the left leg and lower your left foot toward the ground in front of your right leg **(fig. 12.34)** Can you touch the floor with your left foot? If you place the left foot a little further in front of you, can you place your left knee and inner left ankle on the floor? **(fig. 12.35)** Take a few deep breaths and experience what is happening in your hips. Use your left hand on the floor in front of your torso for stability.

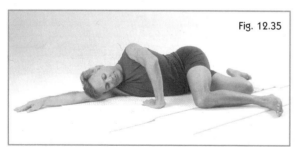

Fig. 12.35

4. On an inhale, lift the left leg and place it behind you, with your foot touching the ground behind the right leg **(fig. 12.36)**. Breathe into the stretch and observe the sensations that arise in this position.

5. Using your left hand for stability, begin to lift the left leg to place it in front of your right leg on the floor, **(fig. 12.37)** then lift it again and place it behind the right leg on the

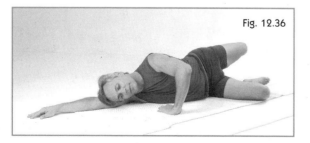

Fig. 12.36

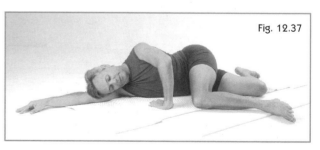

Fig. 12.37

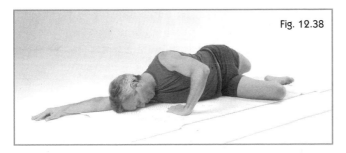

Fig. 12.38

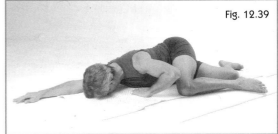

Fig. 12.39

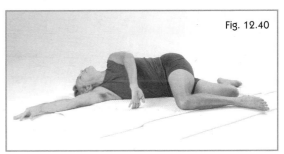

Fig. 12.40

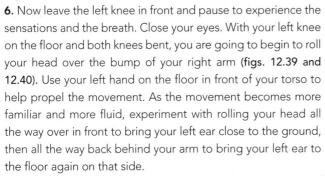

Fig. 12.41

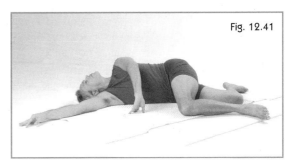

Fig. 12.42

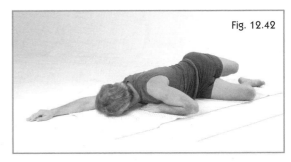

Fig. 12.43

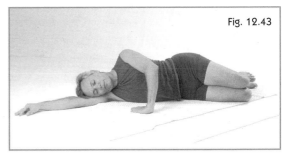

floor behind you (**fig. 12.38**). Repeat this scissor motion a few times, using your inhaling breath to do the lifting and exhaling to lower into the stretch.

6. Now leave the left knee in front and pause to experience the sensations and the breath. Close your eyes. With your left knee on the floor and both knees bent, you are going to begin to roll your head over the bump of your right arm (**figs. 12.39 and 12.40**). Use your left hand on the floor in front of your torso to help propel the movement. As the movement becomes more familiar and more fluid, experiment with rolling your head all the way over in front to bring your left ear close to the ground, then all the way back behind your arm to bring your left ear to the floor again on that side.

7. Repeat the head rolling several times until it becomes effortless and pleasurable to be rolling your head over the bump of your right shoulder. Let your eyes stay closed. Relax your jaw. Relax the muscles of your face and scalp as you roll.

8. Return your head now to rest on your right arm. Notice the effects of this movement in your body. Do you feel any more relaxed or at home in this position than when you began?

9. Now we will put the two movements together. When your head rolls behind you, your left leg with a bent knee lifts and touches the ground in front of you (**fig. 12.41**). When your head rolls in front of the right arm, the left leg reaches to touch the floor behind your right leg (**fig. 12.42**). Repeat this scissor motion until it becomes familiar and effortless.

10. Continue this cross-lateral movement and experiment with the contact your right hip is making with the ground. If you press the right hip slightly into the ground, can you feel how the press helps you to lift the leg and roll your head from your center? Pressing your right hip will help you to establish a fulcrum for the movement.

11. Bring your left leg back on top of your right leg and return your head to rest on your right arm (**fig. 12.43**). Scan your body and notice how your body has spread out to be on your side in this way. Is your head any more comfortable on your shoulder

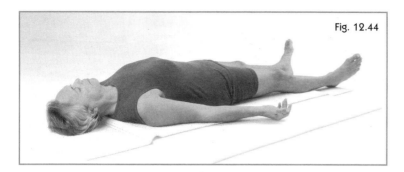

Fig. 12.44

than when you began? Is your shoulder closer to the ground? Notice the movement in your rib cage as you breathe in and out.

12. Slowly roll onto your back and stretch out your legs (**fig. 12.44**). Observe the way your body contacts the ground. Notice the difference between the two sides of your body in the way they contact the ground. Is one side heavier than the other? Do you notice how the right shoulder moves in response to your breath? Does it feel any heavier or more open than the left shoulder? Which side of your body feels longer? Experience any pulsing, streaming, or tingling sensations that arise anywhere in your body.

13. Now roll over onto your left side. Position yourself with your left arm stretched out on the ground, palm facing down and your head resting on your arm. Adjust yourself into the starting position. On your next inhale lift the right leg and lower it to the ground in front of the left leg. Continue your exploration on this side, inventing other movements as your body calls for them.

14. When you have completed your exploration on this second side, slowly roll onto your back and stretch out your legs. Observe the way your body contacts the ground. Notice the difference between the two sides of your body in the way they contact the ground. Do your shoulders feel more open or heavier than when you first began this exploration? Can you sense how your ribs expand out to your sides as you inhale? Notice how the openness in your shoulders is related to the openness in the sides of your rib cage. Experience any pulsing, streaming, or tingling sensations that arise anywhere in your body.

15. Moving to a deeper level of awareness, begin to sense the weight of your bones gliding downward through layers of muscle and tissue in response to the pull of gravity. Notice any changes or effects that occur as you lie on the ground. Particularly notice the way the backside of your rib cage expands against the ground as you inhale and exhale. As you release into deeper and deeper levels of relaxation, allow the two sides of your body to communicate to you. How do the differences in the two sides come into balance in the center of your being?

16. When you are ready slowly begin your return, moving from supine to a seated position to standing. Notice whether you feel taller. How do your shoulders hang? Does your head feel like it is more centered over your body? Take a few steps around and notice the way your feet contact the ground. Notice the way your hips and pelvis move as you walk.

Exploration 2: Reclining Buddha Side Scissors 2

1. Lie on the ground on your right side, your right arm stretched out on the ground, palm down, and your head resting on your arm. Walk your fingertips away from you so that the right arm is fully extended beneath you. Bend your knees and stack them one on top of the other; stack your ankles one on top of the other. Finally, place your left hand on the floor in front of your torso, using that hand to prevent your body from rolling to either side **(fig. 12.45)**. Close your eyes and experience the sensation of being in this posture, stretched out on your right side. Notice the contact your body makes with the ground as it settles.

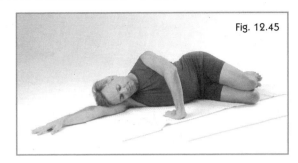

Fig. 12.45

2. Lift your head slightly so that you can reach with your left hand over your head to cup the right side of your head and ear with your left palm. Inhale as you lift your head using your left arm **(fig. 12.46)**. Lower your head down to rest on your right arm. As you rest for a moment, see how much of the weight of your head you can let go into your left palm. In his movement you will be using the strength in your left arm to lift your head while your head remains heavy and passive.

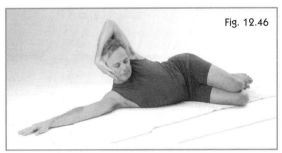

Fig. 12.46

3. On an inhaling breath lift the head, hold for just a moment, and then lower your head back down onto your arm. Repeat this movement several times, experimenting with how much height you can gain without straining or using undue force. Continue until the movement becomes familiar and effortless.

4. Now lift your head, but this time lower your head to the ground in front of your right arm **(fig. 12.47)**. Pause for a moment and experience the sensation of placing your head in this position.

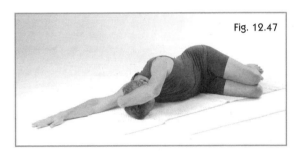

Fig. 12.47

5. Inhale to lift your head; exhale as you lower it now to the ground behind your right arm **(fig. 12.48)**. Pause and experience this position of your head. Lift and lower your head in front of and then behind your right arm for a few repetitions. See how heavy you can let your head be. Notice how much more lift you gain as you continue breathing in and out with the movement.

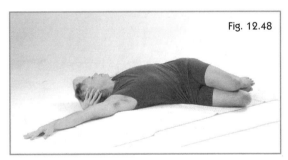

Fig. 12.48

6. In the final phase of this series, lift your head and your left leg at the same time, keeping the left knee bent. Lower the left knee in front of your right leg on the ground as you lower your head behind your right arm **(fig. 12.49)**. Pause for a moment and allow this stretch to become familiar.

7. Inhale as you lift your head and your left leg and reverse the positions, lowering your head in front of your right arm and your left leg behind your right leg **(fig. 12.50)**. Pause for

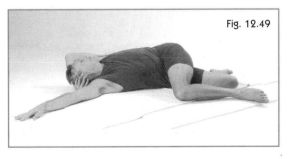

Fig. 12.49

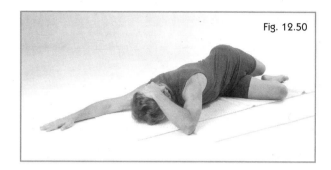

Fig. 12.50

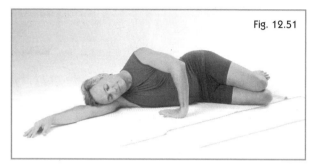

Fig. 12.51

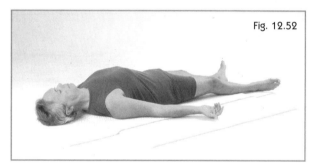

Fig. 12.52

a moment and then begin lifting and lowering your head and leg in this scissors movement.

8. While you continue lifting and lowering your head and leg, experiment with pressing the right hip into the ground as a fulcrum for the movement. The more you press your right hip into the ground, the easier and more effortless it is to lift your leg and head.

9. Put a little speed into the movement and allow the momentum to build as your body opens more deeply.

10. Bring your left leg back on top of your right leg, release your head from the left hand and arm, and return your head to rest

on your right arm **(fig. 12.51)**. Scan your body and notice how your body has spread out to be on your side in this way. Is your head any more comfortable on your shoulder than when you began? Is your shoulder closer to the ground? Notice the movement in your rib cage as you breathe in and out.

11. Slowly roll onto your back and stretch out your legs **(fig. 12.52)**. Observe the way your body contacts the ground. Notice the difference between the two sides of your body in the way they contact the ground. Does one side of your body feel longer than the other? Can you sense how the upper shoulder and neck muscles of your right side have opened? Do you notice how this exploration has opened the right side to move more freely with your breath? Experience any pulsing, streaming, or tingling sensations that arise anywhere in your body.

12. Now roll over onto your left side. Position yourself with your left arm stretched out on the ground, palm down and your head resting on your arm. Recalling the starting position from the first side, position yourself to continue exploring the movements on this side. Allow your body to invent variations that call to you.

13. When you have completed your exploration on this side, slowly roll onto your back and stretch out your legs. Observe the way your body contacts the ground. Notice the difference between the two sides of your body in the way they contact the ground. Experience any pulsing, streaming, or tingling sensations that arise anywhere in your body.

14. Moving to a deeper level of awareness, sense the weight of your bones gliding down through layers of muscle and tissue in response to the pull of gravity. Notice any changes that occur as you lie on the ground. Particularly notice the way the backside of your rib cage expands against the ground as you inhale and exhale. As you release into deeper and deeper levels of relaxation, allow the two sides of your body to communicate to you. How do the differences in the two sides come into balance in the center of your being?

15. When you are ready, slowly begin your return. Moving from a seated position up to standing, notice whether you feel any taller. How do your shoulders hang? Does your head feel like it is more centered over your body? Take a few steps around the room and notice the way your feet contact the ground. Notice the way your hips and pelvis move as you walk.

Exploration 3: Elbow Lift 1

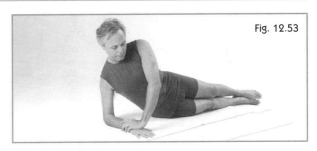

Fig. 12.53

1. Lie on the ground on your right side, your right arm stretched out on the ground, palm down, and your head resting on your arm. Slide your right elbow under your side so that you can lift your torso, allowing your ribs to hang and open like an accordion (**fig. 12.53**).

2. Bend both knees, stacking your knees and ankles. Reach over the top of your left foot with your left hand, grasping the hinge of the toes. Gently stretch the heel out away from you (**fig. 12.54**) and then bend the knee, bringing the foot back (**fig. 12.55**). Feel the stretch across the metatarsal hinge, the ball of the foot.

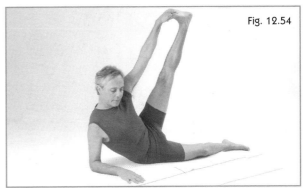

Fig. 12.54

3. Continue stretching and bending your left leg but allow the elbow to cross over the knee so that the knee is to the inside of the elbow on one stretch and is to the outside of the elbow on the next stretch (**fig. 12.56**). Alternate back and forth, bringing the knee inside and outside of the elbow several times. Allow the movement to build, experimenting with stretching the leg further each time.

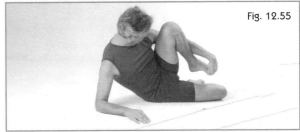

Fig. 12.55

4. Holding your toes with the left leg extended, press down into your right elbow for anchoring and lower your inner ankle toward the ground (**fig. 12.57**). Lift and lower the leg from the ground to upright a few times without letting the inner ankle touch the ground.

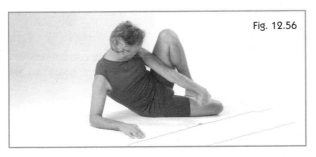

Fig. 12.56

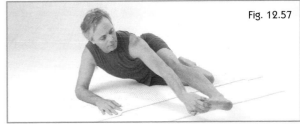

Fig. 12.57

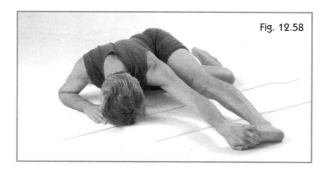

Fig. 12.58

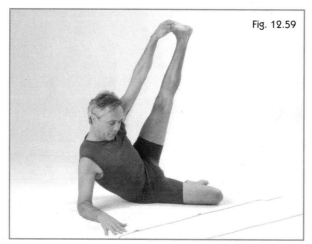

Fig. 12.59

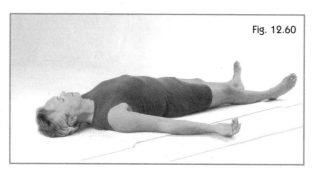

Fig. 12.60

5. Now lower the outstretched leg to the floor and take a few deep breaths (**fig. 12.58**). When you are ready to come up, inhale and press into the right elbow, then exhale to bring the leg upright (**fig. 12.59**). Release the leg and roll onto your back, stretching your arms and legs long (**fig. 12.60**).

6. Can you sense how this exploration has activated different muscle groups? Can you feel how some muscles have received a good stretch while others have been working to support you? Observe how the stabilizing strength of your right side has created a base of support for your left side to explore the flexibility in the hip and shoulder joints. Notice any sensations of pulsing, streaming, or tingling in your body. Observe the difference between the two sides of your body. Do you notice any difference in the movement of your rib cage as you breathe?

7. Now roll over onto your left side. Position yourself with your left arm stretched out on the ground. Bend your knees and grasp the hinge of your right toes and begin the stretch and release on this side. Remember to allow the knee to alternately come inside the elbow and outside the elbow. Allow your head to turn in response to the bending and stretching of your right leg. When you have completed the sequence, release the leg and roll onto your back, stretching out your arms and legs.

8. Notice how the two sides of your body come into balance along your midline. Having alternately stretched and flexed different muscle groups on either side of your body, can you feel how your whole body is now coming into balance? Notice any sensations of pulsing, streaming, or tingling.

9. Moving to a deeper level of awareness, sense the weight of your bones gliding downward through the layers of muscle and tissue in response to the pull of gravity. Receive the effects of this exploration as you lie on the ground. Particularly notice the way the backside of your rib cage expands against the ground as you inhale and exhale.

Exploration 4: Elbow Lift 2

1. Roll onto your right side and bring your right elbow under your right shoulder to prop up your torso so that the right side of your rib cage hangs like a hammock. Play around with the placement of your elbow so that you feel a stable base of support in the arm and shoulder. Lengthen your head and neck up and away from your right shoulder. Maintaining this base of support, stretch out your legs, placing the left leg and ankle on top of the right leg and ankle (**fig. 12.61**). Place your left hand on top of your right wrist. On an inhaling breath, press into the right elbow and lift your right hip off the ground, then lift your entire underside off the ground, all the way down to the ankle (**fig. 12.62**). Exhale as you lower the right hip and leg back down to the ground. Pause for a moment in this resting position (**fig. 12.63**).

2. Before lifting again, consider how this movement is like a one-elbow push-up. Again, take an inhaling breath and press your right elbow into the ground to raise your right hip and right underside off the ground. Stay lifted for a moment and then exhale and lower back down. Repeat this push-up several times until it begins to feel familiar and energizing.

3. After a few repetitions, release your right hip back down to the ground and rest for a moment. Close your eyes and experience how your right arm and shoulder have been working to create the opening along the right side of your body. Notice how this deep side stretch has affected your breathing. If you feel you have come to the limit of your strength at this time, lower down to rest on your back. Pause for a few breaths and then continue the same movement on your left side. If you feel like going a little further and you want to explore additional movements that strengthen and tone the arm and shoulder muscles, continue on with the next instruction.

4. Now inhale and lift again (**fig. 12.64**). Rotate your body as you lower out of the push-up so that when you come down you are seated on your buttocks (**fig. 12.65**). Lift and rotate again to turn toward the floor, lowering your chest (**fig. 12.66**). Continue for a few repetitions, lifting and rotating to feel the full range of strength in the shoulder muscles that are doing the work.

5. Release your elbow and roll onto your back, stretching

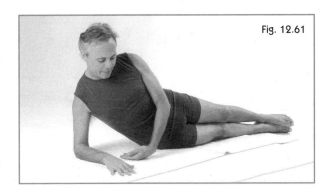
Fig. 12.61

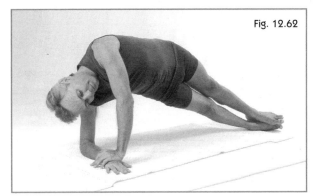
Fig. 12.62

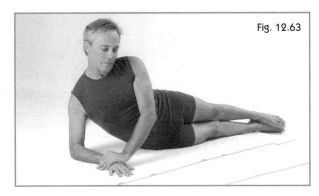
Fig. 12.63

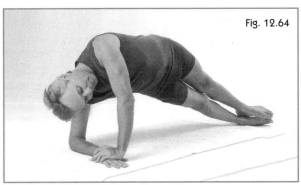
Fig. 12.64

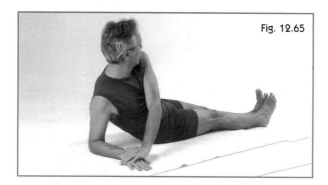

Fig. 12.65

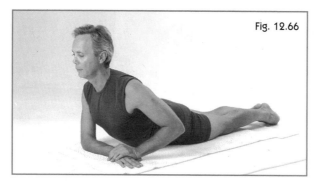

Fig. 12.66

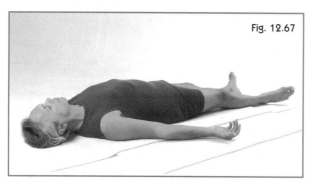

Fig. 12.67

your arms and legs long (**fig. 12.67**). Feel how your right shoulder has been working to lift and support you. Can you sense how different the two sides of your body feel after doing this exploration on one side? Do you notice any difference in the movement of your rib cage from one side to the other as you breathe?

6. Roll onto your left side and bring your left elbow under your left shoulder to prop up your torso so that the left side of your rib cage hangs like a hammock. Play around with the placement of your elbow so that you feel a stable base of support in the arm and shoulder. Lengthen your head and neck up and away from your right shoulder. Maintaining this base of support, stretch out your legs, placing the right leg and ankle on top of the right leg and ankle. Having now set yourself up as you did on the right side, experiment with the elbow lifts on this side. Play with any variations that allow you to experience the dynamics of lifting the entire underside off the ground and rotating to place first the front side and then the backside on the ground. When you have reached your limit, release the elbow and roll onto your back, stretching out your arms and legs.

7. Allow yourself to receive the effects of this powerful set of movements. Notice how much strength has been required to lift the sides of your body off the ground. Can you sense how the two sides of your body cooperate to create both a stable lift and an opening along your sides at the same time? Particularly draw your attention to the contact your low back makes with the floor. Can you sense how the major muscle in the low back, the quadratus lumborum, has been engaged and released through this exploration? How does your low back move in response to your breath? How does the backside of your ribs move with your breath? How do your shoulders move? Remain in this position and then continue on with the following integration, Magnetic Energy Field Meditation.

Integration: Magnetic Energy Field Meditation

1. Lie on the ground on your back and allow your whole body to settle (**fig. 12.68**). Make any adjustments that allow you to be as comfortable as possible. Now is the time to receive the effects of exploring the two sides of your body from many different movement patterns. Suggest to your logical mind that you are now crossing a time boundary to enter the time in which your body actually lives. It is safe, pleasurable, and desirable to expand your awareness to include all dimensions of your experience in the present.

2. Notice your breath and your breathing. Travel to the place in your being where the impulse to inhale and to exhale arise.

3. Spiral into the center of your belly and feel the abdominal pulse growing stronger with every inhaling breath. Inhale warm, glowing energy into your center. Exhale through your backside the past patterns, protections, and limitations that no longer serve your whole being. Exhale them down into the ground. Allow all tension to melt into the ground, like a waterfall.

4. Become aware of the heaviness in your left palm. Allow the palm to be as heavy as it actually is. Can you sense pulsing in the left palm? Imagine that the heavier your left palm becomes on the floor, the lighter your right palm becomes. As the left palm begins to melt down into the ground, your right palm and hand begin to lift off the floor, hovering a few inches (**fig. 12.69**). Allow your breath to lift your right hand, as though you are a marionette and your right hand is being lifted toward the ceiling on the string of your breath. Take as many breaths as you need to float your palm and fingers straight up to the ceiling, then continuing until the back of your right hand

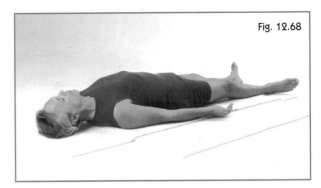

Fig. 12.68

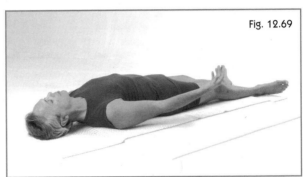

Fig. 12.69

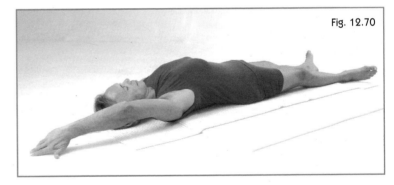

Fig. 12.70

touches the ground above your head.

5. With your left palm heavy and your right palm and fingers and arm stretching away from your head, imagine that your hand is being drawn into the infinite expanse of space beyond your head and beyond your body (**fig. 12.70**). With every inhaling breath, send your kinesthetic sensation into the expanse of space.

6. Experience how your left hand is grounded in the earth and your right arm is

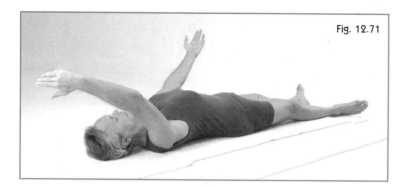

Fig. 12.71

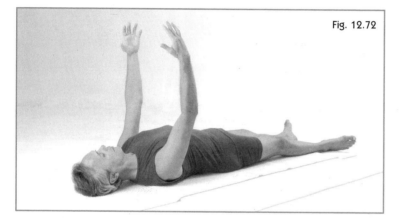

Fig. 12.72

breathe into the space. Allow your awareness to fill all of the space between these two poles.

9. Gradually allow the two palms to be drawn together, like the two poles of a magnet (**fig. 12.72**). Move very slowly and sense the energetic pulsing between your two palms growing more intense as they come closer and closer together but do not touch. When your hands come close to one another but are not touching, notice the strength of the magnetic energy field pulsing between your palms. Allow an imaginary ball of energy to form between the palms. As your hands move in closer, the ball becomes more concentrated. As your palms move slightly further apart, the energy field grows larger.

10. Open your palms wide enough apart to form a sphere that engulfs your entire physical body. Rest your hands and arms on the ground and allow your awareness to become absorbed in the protective, glowing sphere of energy. Imagine that every cell in your body, every layer of your being, is being bathed in this bubble of pure prana.

11. Notice the way you feel when your whole being is absorbed in the nurturing glow of the life force. Receive any messages or guidance that comes to you directly through the wisdom of your organism at this time.

12. In this state of deep regeneration, notice how it feels to be at home in the center of your being. Suggest to your logical mind that you can return to the state of energetic regeneration at any time, under any circumstances, by simply recalling the way you feel in this moment.

13. Slowly begin your return, taking all the time you need to roll into a seated position.

extended into limitless space. Breathe into the entire expanse between being grounded in the earth and open to the heavens at the same time.

7. Slowly begin to allow the two arms and hands to reverse their polarities. The right palm and arm become heavy and start to be pulled by the gravity of earth. Simultaneously, your left palm and hand begin to levitate on the strings of your breath (**fig. 12.71**). At some point in the reversal of polarities in your two arms, sense when they cross. Take as many breaths as you need and move as slowly as you feel like moving.

8. When the palms have opened into the expanse between grounded in the earth and open to the heavens, pause and

Before Moving On . . .

We develop different patterns of movement on the two sides of our bodies, often unconsciously, that allow for specialized, one-sided movements and activities. Playing tennis or golf, cutting vegetables, even holding the telephone to one ear more consistently than to the other—these are some examples from the infinitely long list of specialized ways the two sides of the body are used to fulfill our needs and desires in the moment. The inquiries of this chapter provided wide-ranging ways to explore how the two sides of your body interact to maintain equilibrium.

Starting with exploring the differences in the way your two sitz bones make contact with the ground in Butterfly and how the rocking movement from side to side opens the hip joints and allows for forward and backward scooting, you have observed how the two sides of your body are different, yet work together as a balanced whole. Freeing the side-to-side movement of the head in Pendulum of the Head released the neck and shoulder muscles in a seated position, creating an opening for the deeper and more vigorous explorations of these same muscles that came in the side stretches.

Opening the outside seams of the body in Reclining Buddha and the Elbow Lift series engaged the accordian-like movement of both sides of the back, the rib cage, and the abdominal oblique muscles, allowing for relaxed lateral stretching. Have you noticed that, by exploring these differences and allowing each side to move in the unique way that it moves, your body has begun to shift toward greater balance and equilibrium? In the paradox of the opposition, each side has had the opportunity to learn from the other side. Reflecting on the results of your explorations in this chapter, would you say that opening to the differences in the two sides of the body helps your balance or flexibility? Do you sense that the two sides of your body are more integrated?

By expanding your awareness to include intelligence from both sides of your body, you have opened the possibility for awakening to greater unity among the paradoxical differences that coexist within the wholeness of your consciousness. In developing greater coordination with the bilateral and cross-lateral movements of your body, you have simultaneously stimulated more efficient pathways for expanded cooperation between the cognitive faculties of the right and left hemispheres of the cerebral cortex, encouraging whole-brain thinking. The increase in information and communication flowing among the different aspects of your physical body mirror an expansion in the choices available to you for creating more informed directions in your life as an individual, guided by the knowledge and awareness of your unique differences and strengths.

In the next chapter, we explore the flexibility in the spine that allows for entering the full Spinal Twist. Building on the side-to-side movements of this chapter, the spine now enters movements that facilitate its maximum elongation. You will explore how the opening in your hip joints and legs supports a fuller twist, and how the flexibility introduced into the spine through twisting opens the whole body for bending from the hinge of the hips into the Seated Forward Bend, the posture that induces deep states of introspective awareness.

13 Making the Hero's Journey: Traveling the Time Spiral of the Spinal Twist to Arrive Now in Seated Forward Bend

How does the progression of movement from Hero to Spinal Twist to Seated Forward Bend help me stay grounded in the present while opening to the past and the future?

AN OFTEN-QUOTED AXIOM IN YOGA SCHOOLS STATES THAT a healthy spine is a healthy body. Another variation is "a long spine means a long life." This emphasis on the vertical axis of the spine is more than a physiological metaphor or a health prescription. In bringing awareness to the axis of the spine, we open to the heroic journey of expanded consciousness that the spine not only symbolizes but also makes possible. The spine is the tunneling path through time.

We have seen that the spine has evolved to support the journey from primal organisms in the oceanic darkness to multidimensional beings in quest of vertical ascension into the light. The organismic journey each human being makes from the embryonic stage toward unimpeded, autonomous, balanced movement in every direction plays out in the dialogue between the finiteness of gravity and the infinitude of space. The inquiries in this chapter extend our conversation beyond the physical evolution of the spine, with its neuromuscular and electrochemical structures and functions; it also looks beyond the psychodynamics of an autonomous and individuated complex personality in search of meaning and purpose. The conversation of this chapter begins with the startling discovery that Einstein voiced when he declared that time curves back in on itself. Time and space are paradoxical manifestations of the same phenomenon.

How does the Hero pose get its name? The Hero's journey begins with a summons to enter the moment through inquiring "who am I?" Practicing the As Is principle supports the courage and humility required to accept my experience as it is actually unfolding in the present. The inquiries of Self-Awakening Yoga offer concrete pathways into exploring the present moment, opening lines of communication between the mind and body by focusing awareness on the messages of the body that come through the language of sensation. Along the way, you have the opportunity to notice levels of thoughts, beliefs, and emotions are associated with various sensations that arise through entering different areas of your body.

What can you do when you encounter layers of experience in your being that are unfamiliar and seem to be not of your own creation? These experiences that may arise during your practice of the Self-Awakening Yoga inquiries present an opportunity to practice what I refer to as the As If principle—you may not ever know how or why you created this previously unconscious pattern that is revealed during the practice of your inquiries, but if you assume responsibility in full for the reality that is arising in your field of experience in this moment, you have the choice to experience it *as if* you did create it. As the heroine's and the hero's journey unfolds into unfamiliar territories within the layers of yourself, the "now" you are experiencing in this moment reveals itself to be a continuous, interconnected, simultaneous event with every other "now" in the past, present, and future. Who you are in this moment is not limited to what you can think, feel, or even perceive through your current understanding and awareness. In the journey of self-awakening, everything that arises is a part of who you are. Paradoxically, it may seem that you will always be returning home inside yourself, arriving at the very place from whence you started your journey. The results and benefits of your inquiry are inherent in the act of inquiry itself.

> *We shall not cease from exploration*
> *And the end of all our exploring*
> *Will be to arrive where we started*
> *And know the place for the first time.*
>
> T. S. ELIOT, *FOUR QUARTETS*

From Einstein to Eliot, the twisting, turning road of self-awakening occurs both in the bodily time of sensation and beyond time, in the expanded visions we hold of ourselves that connect us to the meaning and purpose that are the motivating forces behind our quest to discover more of who we are. The time you spend in following the twisting and turning road of self-inquiry is mirrored in the fundamental essence of the Seated Spinal Twist, the posture that supports the flexibility in your spine to open toward both sides. The Seated Spinal Twist begins from Hero pose. As you will discover, Hero gets its name from a special quality of surrender to sensation that the posture itself encourages. Regardless of the degree of flexibility or openness you experience in your hip joints, there are infinite degrees of release that you can experience as you approach this posture. In this series of movements, you may discover that the heroine is not a heroine because she has superhuman qualities or possesses superhuman flexibility. The heroine derives her strength from the humility to accept the reality of her own actual experience, as if it were the result of her own creation. When you begin to open your hips through this inquiry, your body will give you ample opportunity to return to the realities of the sensations that are communicated to you, as you are in this moment.

Recall for a moment how you've progressed through the inquiries that have opened your hips, creating a grounded foundation that enables you to sit comfortably, either directly on the ground or with the support of cushions in Pinwheel, Butterfly, and Pigeon. The openness you experience in the hinge of the hip joints allows a flow of communication between your lower and upper body.

The inquiries of this chapter begin by initiating increased openness in your hip joints in the Hero pose. Opening the hips in this movement series creates further grounding for the sitz bones to be comfortably seated. By sending your roots into the ground of the present in Hero, the spine has a foundation for opening to receive the past in one direction and the future in another direction. Having opened to receive from your connections to the past and the future in Spinal Twist, the movement into Seated Forward Bend invites surrender to a deep dive into the unknown of the Now. Seated Forward Bend is among the most introspective of all yoga postures, inviting you into internal exploration. You may begin to discover that the stress you experience in life about not having enough time begins to dissolve as you allow yourself the time it takes to fully let go into the sensations in your body that arise from being in Seated Forward Bend. The less you do in this pose, the more you enter the realization that inner peace exists beyond time. Regardless of how much time you spend in this posture, touching into the inner stillness that this posture produces will be a source of calmness and relaxed awareness when you return to the events of your everyday world.

The Paradox of Courage and Surrender in Hero Pose

Inquiry: How do open hip joints allow for greater communication between the upper and lower segments of the body?

The hinge between the upper and lower body that is the hip joints is the point of the greatest intersection of energy in the body. When the hips are open, communication passes freely between the information-processing center in the head, the feeling centers in the heart and belly and the doing centers of the hands, down into the lower center of mobility in the legs and feet. Without this free exchange, issues arise that incapacitate our abilities to think creatively and to take appropriate action. Challenging patterns in the hip joints can be revealed and transformed into novel possibilities for movement through explorations into Hero pose. The courage to begin at the point where your body can comfortably sustain the effort of the exploration may require you to elevate your seat to a cushion, a block, or even a chair for creating support in this position. The theme of these explorations into Hero pose is to get comfortable in being where you are in the moment.

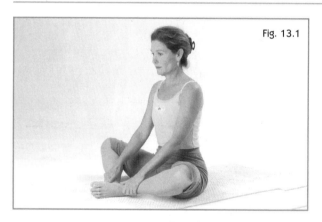

Fig. 13.1

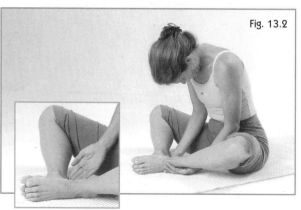

Fig. 13.2

Exploration 1: Butterfly to Hero

1. Sit in a comfortable position on the ground. Bring your feet together and let your knees open out to the sides **(fig. 13.1)**. Imagine that your open legs are the wings of a butterfly. Do not try to force or push your knees toward the ground; let them be where they are. If the stretch is uncomfortable, place a cushion under each thigh to support yourself.

2. Using your hand like a scoop and keeping your thumb next to your index finger, scoop your right hand under your right ankle, letting the outside anklebone rest in the palm of your hand. Scoop your left hand under your left ankle and notice what it feels like to have your ankles and feet resting in the scoop of your palms. Sit in this position and close your eyes. Allow your head to hang forward, your shoulders and your jaw to relax **(fig. 13.2)**. Wait until you experience the sensation of heaviness in the upper body and heaviness of the ankles resting in the palms before you go further. Breathe and relax.

3. Letting your right arm and hand do the work of lifting, lift the right ankle a few inches above the ground and return it back down to the ground. See how heavy you can let the entire left leg and hip remain while your arm does the lifting. Lift and lower a few times.

4. Let your left arm lift your left ankle off of the ground a few inches **(fig. 13.3)** and then return it to the ground. Does any part of your leg want to "help" with the lift? Ask it to remain heavy and to enjoy the ride as you lift and lower the ankle a few times.

5. Now place the back of your right hand on the top of your left ankle. Lift the right ankle off the ground and place it in your right hand **(fig. 13.4)**. Notice how it feels to have your right ankle resting in your right palm, stacked on top of your left ankle. Wait for the sensation of heaviness before you lift the right ankle and return it back down to the ground.

6. Place the back of your left hand on top of your right ankle. Lift the left ankle off the ground and place it in your left hand. Notice how it feels to have your ankles stacked on this side. Does the left side feel in any way different from the right side?

7. Letting your legs remain heavy and letting your arms do the work, alternate back and forth, placing one ankle on top of the other, returning it to the ground, and then placing the other ankle on top. Go back and forth several times and notice whether the lifting gets easier or if the hip joints seem to get more fluid as you go along. Keep the shoulders relaxed. Use your breath to do the lifting.

8. Now begin to reach your ankles a little further up on the opposite calves **(fig. 13.5)**. When this becomes effortless, begin to reach the ankles above the opposite knees.

9. Now lift the right ankle all the way over your left knee and place the right foot on the floor beside your left thigh **(fig. 13.6)**. This is Hero pose. Pause and wait for the relaxation into heaviness. Then lift the ankle and place it back on the ground in Butterfly **(fig. 13.7)**.

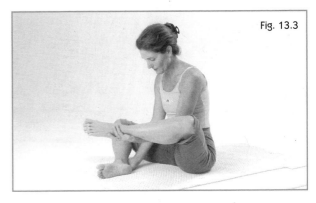

Fig. 13.3

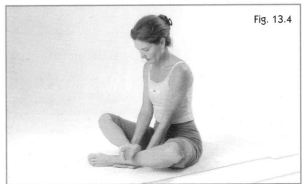

Fig. 13.4

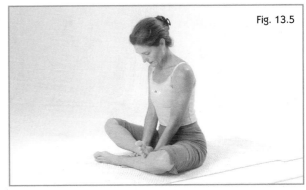

Fig. 13.5

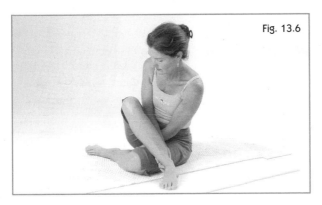

Fig. 13.6

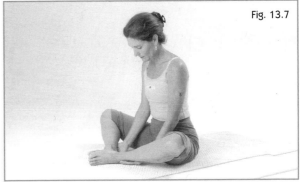

Fig. 13.7

10. Using your left hand like a scoop, slide your left hand under your left ankle and let the outside anklebone rest in the palm of your hand. Wait until you experience the sensation of heaviness in the upper body and heaviness of the ankle resting in your left palm before you go further. Breathe and relax. Now, letting your left arm and hand do the work of lifting, lift the left ankle all the way over your right knee and place the left foot on the floor beside your right thigh into Hero. Notice where you feel the stretch most vividly—is it in your upper or lower knee? in the inner thighs? in the hip joints? in the calves or ankles? Breathe and send relaxation into your lower body, releasing down into the pull of gravity. Return the ankle to the ground in Butterfly.

11. Repeat this sequence a few times, placing one leg across the other into Hero pose on one side and then on the other. Stay relaxed as you lift. Go slowly and experience the sensations as you move. Keep your face and jaw relaxed and continue to breathe fully into the movement.

12. Return both ankles to the ground and release your hands and arms. Let your arms and hands relax in a comfortable position. Close your eyes. Experience the sensation in your groin and hips. Do your hips and inner thighs feel any different than when you began? Are your knees any closer to the ground without attempting to force them down? Did you notice in entering the Hero that the flexibility of one side is different than that of the other side? Observe any pulsing, streaming, or tingling sensations. Observe the position of your head over your spine and body. Does your head feel lighter? Does your neck feel longer?

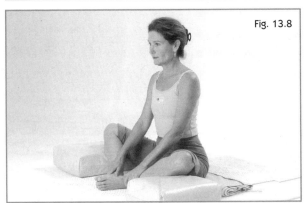

Fig. 13.8

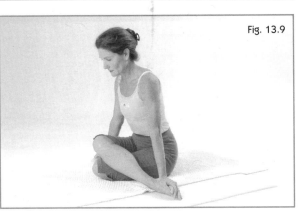

Fig. 13.9

Exploration 2: Hero Lifts and Simple Twist

1. Sit in Butterfly pose. Place cushions under your knees for support. If you find your spine rounding, sit on a folded blanket, a cushion, or a block **(fig. 13.8)**. Elevating your hips in the seated positions helps you to remain grounded in your sitz bones.

2. Lift your right leg, crossing it over the left into Hero pose. Sit with your palms resting on the soles of your feet **(fig. 13.9)**. Close your eyes and relax into the sensation in your lower body. Can you sense a pulsation in the soles of your feet against the palms of your hands? This position creates a current of energy that moves through your body like a figure 8.

3. Press your palms into your feet and lift your hips off the ground. Experiment with walking your feet a little further apart from your hips **(fig. 13.10)**. Lower your hips back down to sit on the floor or cushion. Repeat this lift and release several times, experiencing the sensation of using the strength in your arms to raise the upper body.

4. The next time you lift, stay up and shift your hips over to bump the right heel, then lift and bump your hips against the left heel **(fig. 13.11)**. This is a pendulum-like motion, with the hips bumping back and forth from one heel to the next.

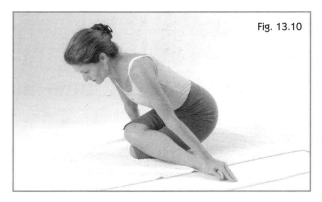

Fig. 13.10

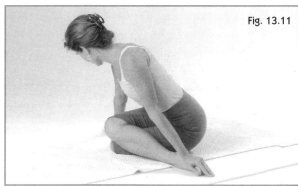

Fig. 13.11

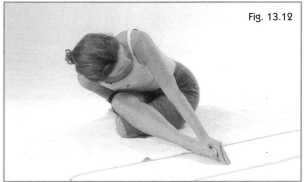

Fig. 13.12

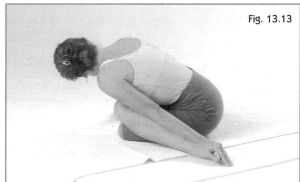

Fig. 13.13

5. Stay lifted and twist slightly, bringing the right shoulder toward the left foot, then twist bringing the left shoulder toward the right foot (**fig. 13.12**). This twisting motion is similar to the side-to-side motion a coffee grinder makes.

6. Repeat this twisting movement from side to side several times. Begin to look with your eyes in the direction of the twist and notice how focusing your gaze takes you deeper into the twist (**fig. 13.13**). Use the exhaling breath to twist a little further in each direction.

7. Lower the buttocks back to sit on the ground or cushion. Interlace your fingers between your toes (**fig. 13.14**). Notice the interesting sensations of having all of your digits interlaced in this way. Close your eyes and experience the effects of being in Hero pose on this side of your body.

8. Open your eyes and stretch both legs long on the ground. Notice the difference in the way the two legs contact the ground. Now repeat the Hero Lifts and Twist on the other side.

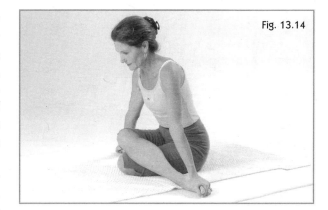

Fig. 13.14

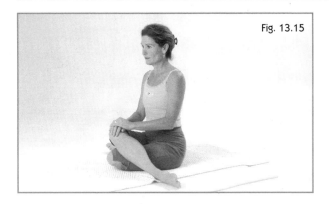

Fig. 13.15

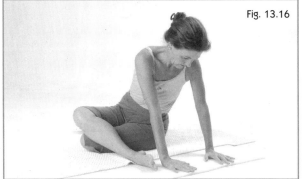

Fig. 13.16

Integration: Hero Whirlwind

1. Sit in Hero pose with your right knee over your left leg. Elevate your hips by sitting on a cushion or block to regulate the amount of pressure in the stretch. Place both hands on your right knee **(fig. 13.15)**.

2. Slowly walk your hands down your right shin, ankle, and foot until both hands are on the ground over to your left side **(fig. 13.16)**. Using the floor for support, lean into your hands and begin to walk them around you to the back. Your feet are going to turn in place as you lift your hips off the ground and allow your body to follow the circular movement along the floor behind you **(fig. 13.17)**.

3. Continue walking the hands all the way around to the other side **(fig. 13.18)** and back to the front. **(fig. 13.19)**. When you are facing the same direction as you started, bend both knees and sit back down into Hero pose. Your legs are now crossed in the opposite position, with the left knee over the right knee **(fig. 13.20)**.

4. Place both hands on your left knee. Using your hands on the floor for support, begin to walk down the length of your left leg and ankle toward the floor on your right side.

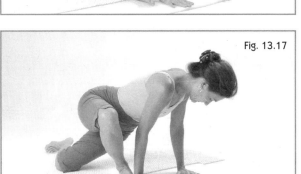

Fig. 13.17

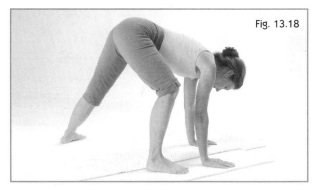

Fig. 13.18

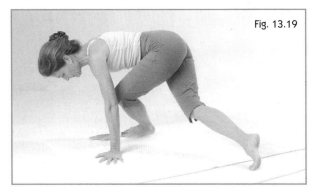

Fig. 13.19

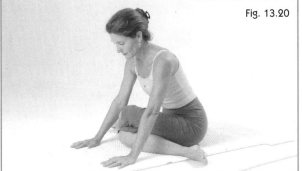

Fig. 13.20

Lean into your hands and begin to walk them on the floor around behind you. Your feet are going to turn in place as you lift your hips off the ground and allow your body to follow the circular movement along the floor behind you.

5. Continue walking the hands all the way around to the other side and back to the front. When you are facing the same direction as you started, bend both knees and sit back down into Hero pose. Your legs are now crossed with the right knee over the left knee.

6. Repeat this movement, alternating sides, until the movement becomes familiar and effortless. When it becomes easier, see what happens when you put a little speed into the movement. Can you make the turn without keeping your hands on the floor for support? The faster you go, the easier it is to do the movement without using your hands. Consider the image of a whirlwind turning you from side to side.

7. Let the movement bring you into stillness. Come back to Butterfly pose. Allow your arms and hands to relax in a comfortable position. Close your eyes. Experience the sensation in your groin and hips and legs. Do your hips and inner thighs feel any different than when you began? Are your knees any closer to the ground than when you started? Check this without attempting to force them down. Can you sense how the openness in your hip joints allows for more balanced communication between your upper and lower body? Observe any pulsing, streaming, or tingling sensations. Observe the position of your head over your spine and body. Does your head feel lighter or does your neck feel longer? Do your legs feel more relaxed on the ground?

Integration: Pose of Tranquillity

1. Sit in Hero pose with your right knee crossed over your left leg. Elevate your hips by sitting on a cushion or block. Rest your palms on the soles of your feet (**fig. 13.21**).

2. Close your eyes and relax into the sensations arising in your lower body. Moving to a deeper level of awareness, notice how your mood begins to shift as you focus on the contact of palms to soles. Can you sense a pulsation in the soles of your feet against the palms of your hands? When your hands are contacting your soles in this position, you are creating a natural magnetic polarity. Using your hands to direct the flow of prana in this way is called creating a *mudra*; the word *mudra* means "gesture." The name of this mudra is Pose of Tranquillity. Relaxing into this position creates a current of energy that moves through your body like a figure 8. As the pulsing becomes stronger, allow your body to sway with the energetic flow.

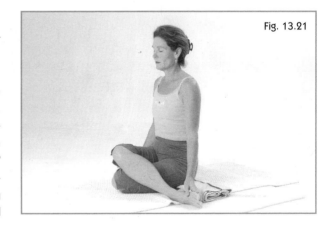

Fig. 13.21

3. Release your legs from this side and slowly transition into the Pose of Tranquility on the other side, placing your left knee over your right leg. As you bring your palms to the soles of your feet and begin to enter deeper levels of relaxed awareness, notice how quickly and deeply your whole being becomes absorbed in the pulsation of prana.

4. Suggest to your logical mind that you can return to the feelings of being absorbed in the flow of prana at any time under any circumstances in life by recalling the sensations that are coursing through your body in this moment. Notice how your body is continuously generating the flow of prana throughout every dimension of your being.

5. When you are ready, slowly begin your return. Stretch out your legs and allow your body to be moved by the urgings of prana. See what movements want to happen through you in this moment.

Spinal Twists

Inquiry: How does my body enter the spinal twists?

The physiological event of entering a spinal twist induces many dynamics that are easily observed. Opening the hips in Hero provides a foundation of support that allows the whole spine to elongate and rotate into the twist. Twisting has the effect of toning and hydrating the intervertebral discs while also stimulating the flow of fresh blood and oxygen to all motor nerves that branch from the spinal cord. The deep massaging action in the abdomen stimulates digestion, improves peristalsis and elimination, and decongests the kidneys, liver, gallbladder, spleen, and pancreas. With so many of the core organ systems receiving an infusion of energy, it is easy to appreciate how relaxing into sensations while entering the spinal twist boosts our sense of well-being. Anchoring in the present allows for the freedom to turn generously toward the past and the future by integrating thoughts, movements, and feelings along the axis of the spine. Many of these effects are obvious during the posture, but the deeper inquiry opens in the stillness after releasing the movement. Here is an opportunity to follow the spiraling movement internally and receive what is opening.

In a less serious vein, Chubby Checkers said it this way, "Come on baby, let's do the twist." Chubby's rock and roll chant caused an evolutionary movement in the 1960s in which people of all generations from all around the planet began an inquiry into the spinal twist. His dancing version of the twist became a way to "get with the times."

Exploration: Knee-Down Twist

1. Lie down on the ground. Bend your right knee and place your right foot on your left thigh above the kneecap **(fig. 13.22)**. Gently press down on the thigh with the right foot. Experiment with how much you can let go of any holding in the left leg as you press downward. Send the left heel out along the floor.

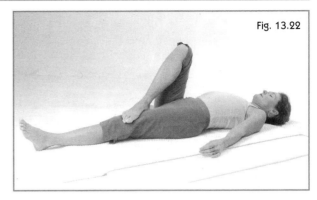

Fig. 13.22

2. Extend your left arm straight out from your shoulder on the floor. Bring your left hand up to grasp the knob of your right knee firmly. In a gradual rocking movement, bring the knee over to your left side and back. Keep your foot firmly planted on the thigh while you let the rocking movement get larger and larger. Allow your head to roll in opposite the direction of your knee **(fig. 13.23)**. Send the right shoulder blade down the backside of your body, toward your hip pocket.

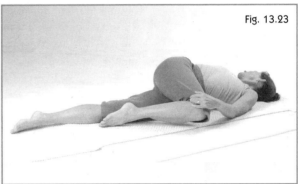

Fig. 13.23

3. Stay in this position for several breaths. Make any small adjustments in this position that allow your left hip to remain comfortably on the ground. Roll your head back and forth, looking from ear to ear. Use long, slow breathing to assist in deepening into the twist.

4. Suggest to yourself that there are infinite degrees of release as you hold the twist and breathe into the entire length of your spine. Before releasing, extend out through the left heel one last time.

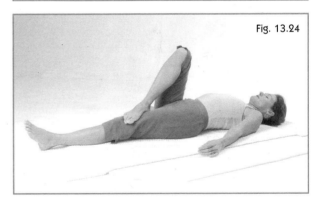

Fig. 13.24

5. Slowly release the twist **(fig. 13.24)**, bringing your right knee up and then stretching the right leg on the ground. Close your eyes and experience the difference between the two sides of your body. Observe any pulsing, streaming, or tingling sensations in your body.

6. Moving now to the other side, bend your left knee and place your left foot on your right thigh above the kneecap. Gently press down on the thigh with the left foot. Experiment with how much you can let go of any holding in the right leg as you press downward. Extend your left arm straight out from your shoulder on the floor. Bring your right hand up to grasp the knob of your left knee firmly. Send the right heel out along the floor **(fig. 13.25)**.

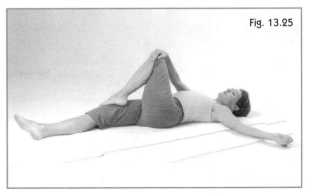

Fig. 13.25

7. In a gradual rocking movement, bring the knee over to your right side and back. Keep your foot firmly planted on the thigh while you let the rocking movement get larger and larger. Allow your head to roll in the opposite direction

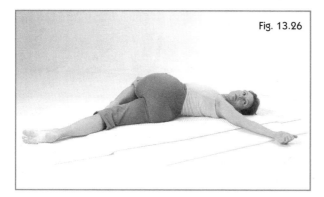

Fig. 13.26

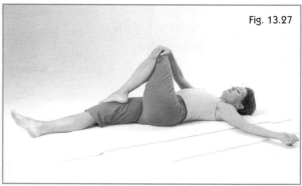

Fig. 13.27

of your knee (**fig. 13.26**). Roll your head back and forth, looking at the place on the ground where your ear would touch. Continue your exploration of the spinal twist on this side.

8. Slowly release the twist, bringing your left knee up (**fig. 13.27**) and stretching the left leg along the ground. Close your eyes and experience any pulsing, streaming, or tingling sensations in your body. Allow your breath to flow in and out without attempting to control or inhibit the breath in any way. Notice any surges of energy moving up and down the spine.

9. Notice any changes or effects that occur as you lie on the ground. Particularly notice the curves beneath your neck and low back. Are they closer to the ground than when you began? How do your shoulders contact the ground? Do you notice a sense of more of your spine and rib cage being on the ground than when you first began this exploration?

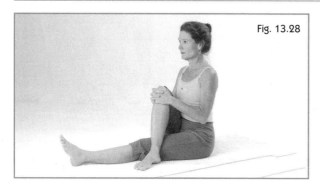

Fig. 13.28

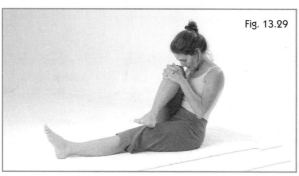

Fig. 13.29

Integration: Seated Spinal Twist

1. Sit in a comfortable position on the ground. Extend both legs long in front of you. Pick up the right foot and cross it over your extended left leg, placing the foot on the floor to the side of your left thigh. The closer you can bring your right foot toward your left hip, the more comfortable you will be in this position.

2. Interlace your fingers in the nonhabitual way (see Integration: Spiraling Up to Sitting, page 166) and cup the knob of your right knee in your palms (**fig. 13.28**). Close your eyes and experience the sensation of holding your right knee in your hands. Allow your shoulders and arms to remain relaxed and heavy. Notice the contact your sitz bones make with the ground.

3. Keeping your fingers interlaced, lift your right knee toward your chest and give yourself a good squeeze. Rock back onto your sacrum and slightly curl your spine as you squeeze the knee (**fig. 13.29**).

4. Keeping your fingers interlaced but turning your palms away from you, press the knee down against the lower extended leg (fig. 13.30). Press and release a few times until you get the sense of allowing pressure to build.

5. Now alternate the movement between squeezing your right knee in toward your chest and then pressing the right knee down onto the left leg. Use your breath and allow a rolling rhythm to build in the spine. As you press the knee down each time, let the torso roll out over the knee, as in the Dolphin movement (fig. 13.31). Experience what is happening in the hinge of your hips. Notice how the lower leg is being supported to release toward the ground.

6. Open your palms to the ceiling, as if you were holding a platter in your hands. Put an imaginary ten pounds of weight onto the platter. What would you hold—oranges, shoes, seashells? With your imaginary weight, begin to bend at the hinge of the hips and lengthen your torso over your thighs to place the platter on the ground in front of you (fig. 13.32). Using your exhaling breaths to lengthen and lower further, move to your natural extension (fig. 13.33).

7. Release the imaginary tray and lower your palms to rest on your extended lower leg (fig. 13.34). Do not use your hands or upper body strength to pull or to force yourself down toward your thigh. Allow the natural weight of your torso to hang. Release the weight of your head and shoulders to hang.

8. Breathe into the sensations of the stretch in the lower leg. Rock from sitz bone to sitz bone. See if the rocking allows you to release any of the pressure you may feel in the legs.

9. Slowly release the forward bend by lengthening through the sternum and crown and then walking your hands back up to your right knee (fig. 13.35).

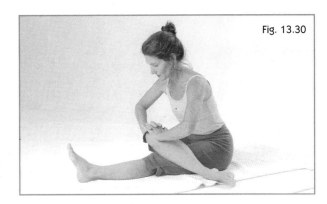

Fig. 13.30

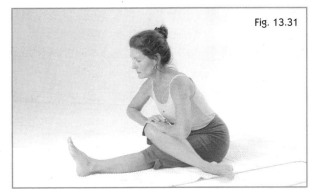

Fig. 13.31

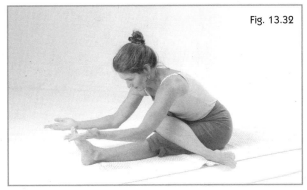

Fig. 13.32

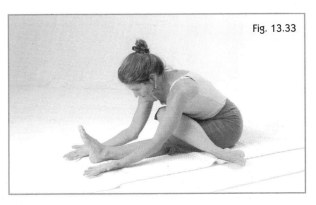

Fig. 13.33

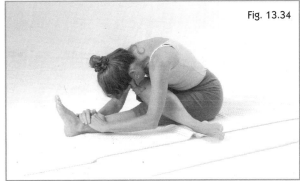

Fig. 13.34

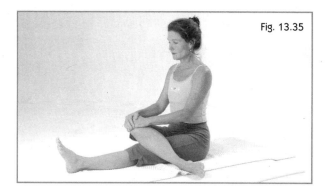

Fig. 13.35

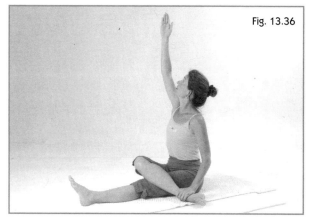

Fig. 13.36

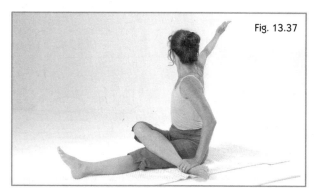

Fig. 13.37

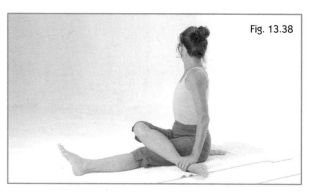

Fig. 13.38

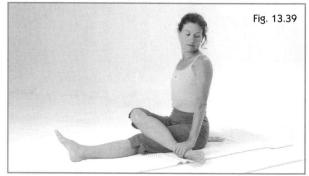

Fig. 13.39

10. Hold the right foot with your left hand and extend your right hand to the ceiling. Lengthen from the little finger side of your arm as you open the right side of your body. Shift your gaze up to see the airborne hand (**fig. 13.36**). On your next exhaling breath lean into your sitz bones and begin to sweep your arm around behind you, following the movement with your eyes (**fig. 13.37**).

11. Plant your hand on the floor behind you, walking the heel of your palm in as close to the base of your spine as is comfortable. Lean back into the supporting arm as you roll your right shoulder down and away from you (**fig. 13.38**).

12. Following your gaze, elongate through the neck and look with your eyes from one shoulder to the other (**fig. 13.39**), allowing the deepening of your breath all the way down into your belly to help you twist a little further each time you exhale.

13. You have placed your body in a supported position to begin deep three-part breathing into the length of your spine. Exhale all of the breath, following the exhale to the point where your navel moves in toward your spine. Inhale into the lower belly, then into the kidneys, and finally the sternum. Soften your gaze over the right shoulder. At the top of your inhaling breath, tuck the chin slightly and hold the breath in. Then release the exhale from the sternum, then the kidneys, and finally from the lower belly. Continue to hold the twist for another five cycles of three-part breathing.

14. Slowly begin your return by lengthening your right arm, sweeping an arc overhead and following your hand with your eyes (**fig. 13.40**). Rest your palm on your lap. With your eyes closed, sit for a moment and experience the sensations of being in this position.

15. Open your eyes, uncross your right leg, and extend both legs on the ground. Close your eyes and experience the difference between the two legs. Does one leg feel longer than the other? Does one hip, buttock, and thigh feel closer to the ground than the other? Do you notice any difference in the way the two sides of your ribs move with your breath? When you feel ready to transition to the other side, slowly open the window of your eyes.

16. Pick up the left foot and cross it over your extended right leg, placing the foot on the floor to the side of your right thigh. Recalling the details of this movement from the first side, begin to enter your exploration of the Spinal Twist to this side.

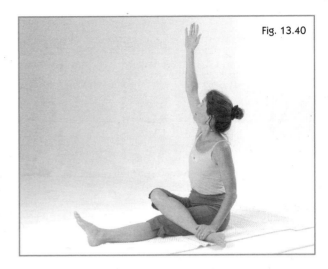

Fig. 13.40

Balancing the Upper and Lower Body in Seated Forward Bend

Inquiry: How do we channel awakened energy from whole-body movement into introspection?

All seated postures are forward bends. Even when sitting in a chair the spine and legs are at a right angle, pivoting at the hinge of the hips. Making adjustments that bring your sitz bones to the ground and elongate the spine dramatically affect the quality of your experience of energy flowing throughout the open channel of your body. For example, it requires a lot of work to hold yourself up in a position in which the spine is hunched and you're rolled back onto your buttocks and sacrum rather than sitting upright on your sitz bones. Increasing the flexibility of the hinge of the hips and toning the abdominal muscles to support the spine allows for relaxed, effortless sitting and opens the communication lines between the upper and lower body

The first exploration below, Basketball Knees, helps to release the hamstring muscles in the back of your thighs. Hara Walk brings energy to the abdominals for supporting the spine. Half Tortoise and Tortoise open the hinge of the hips. When you are ready to relax into Seated Forward Bend, your awareness will be drawn like a magnet into the deep reservoir of inner stillness and tranquility. The posture itself produces a circuit of prana that cycles from the crown of your head through the soles of your feet. In the deep tranquillity arises a clear mind that can bring steady concentration to any point of focus you choose.

The key to opening into these powerful energetic effects lies in one word—

relaxation. If you are not comfortable or supported in the posture your attention will be drawn toward managing discomfort. At the beginning of the instructions for Seated Forward Bend are some special directions for creating support. You will be guided through a dynamic phase of entering the Forward Bend and then into a regenerative phase in which you hold the pose.

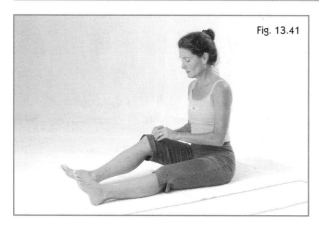

Fig. 13.41

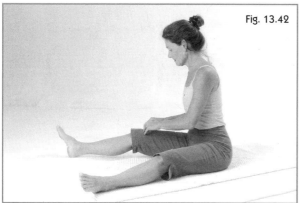

Fig. 13.42

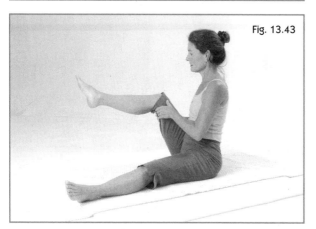

Fig. 13.43

Exploration 1: Basketball Knees

1. Here is a fun way to begin opening your legs. Come into an easy seated position with your legs extended. Place both of your hands on your right knee and begin to press into your knee as if you were dribbling a basketball (**fig. 13.41**). If you let go in your leg, the back of your knee will relax into a slight bounce. Play with this movement a bit; when you get the hang of it, your whole leg will move in response to the bouncing basketball knee.

2. Dribble the ball down court by allowing your knee to travel out to your side and back in toward the midline (**fig. 13.42**). If you lift the knee toward your chest, you can take a jump shot, sending the heel and then the leg back down to the ground in front of you (**fig. 13.43**).

3. Pause for a moment and feel the difference in the way your two legs contact the floor. Do you notice how the hamstrings and calf muscles have released? When you are ready, move to the other leg. As you get more playful with this exploration, you may want to move your hands along to different positions on your thigh as the contact point.

4. Now dribble both knees at the same time. Get a little outrageous and allow the legs to separate and then come back together. Experience what wants to happen as you let go of your legs in this way.

5. Return to stillness. Allow your eyes to close and experience the release that is happening your legs. Has your mood altered from playing with your legs in this way?

Exploration 2: Sitz Bone Hara Walk

1. From an easy seated position on the ground, extend both legs. Send the heels away from you, which will have the effect of bringing the backs of your legs in closer contact with the ground (**fig. 13.44**). Rock from side to side and find the contact your sitz bones make with the ground. This movement is a way to energize your abdominal muscles by walking from your sitz bones. It is also called the bun warmer, which should give you some idea as to how you are about to move.

2. Make fists and extend your arms over your legs. Inhale to lift one sitz bone and leg (**fig. 13.45**); as you exhale, send the whole leg forward, stretching through the heel to land this leg about an inch past its partner.

3. Perform the same movement on the opposite leg. On your exhaling breath, begin to make the sound "h-a-a-a-a-a-a-a," which activates your belly center. You can throw a punch with your fists and arms to help you propel forward (**fig. 13.46**). Reaching one leg and then the other while punching and scooting by the sitz bones, you will begin to travel across the floor.

4. Pick up the pace until you feel as though you are moving from your hara. You will know you are in the ballpark with the energetics of this movement when your forward walk starts to glide your underwear up in a bundle. Before getting too bundled, begin to walk backward, using the same dynamics of sitz bone walking and hara punching.

5. Go back and forth a few times until all seriousness has vaporized and you are having some big fun with the movement.

6. Relax. Let go of the movement and flop back on the ground (**fig. 13.47**). Without trying to control your breath, allow your breathing to gush in and out. As the breath normalizes, allow your eyes to close and begin to notice the pulsing in your abdomen. Notice how you have been using the core muscles of your lower abdomen to power your whole-body movement. Notice how you have been in a seated forward bend for this whole time, using movement and breath to open your body into the position.

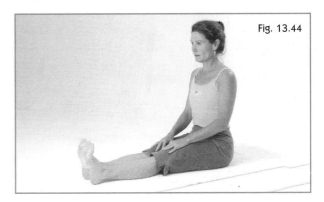

Fig. 13.44

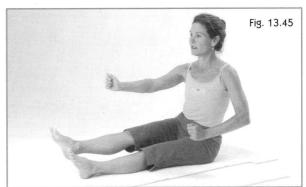

Fig. 13.45

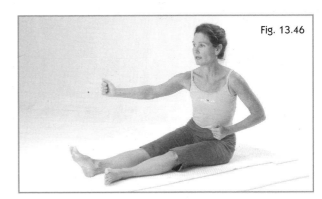

Fig. 13.46

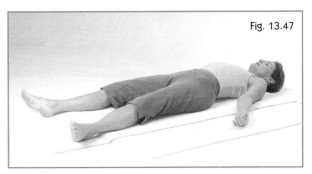

Fig. 13.47

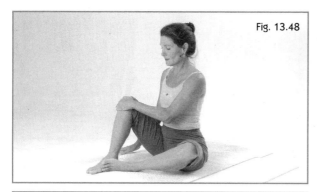

Fig. 13.48

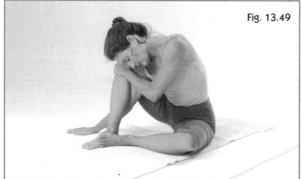

Fig. 13.49

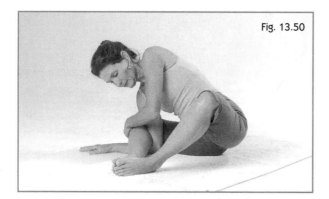

Fig. 13.50

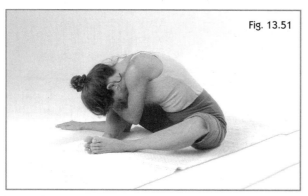

Fig. 13.51

Exploration 3: Tortoise

1. Sit in a comfortable position on the ground. Bring your right knee upright, placing your right foot on the floor. Allow your left knee to be bent and relaxed out to your left side on the floor. Grasp the knob of your right knee with your left hand **(fig. 13.48)**.

2. Thread your right hand under your right knee and slide your right hand along the floor out to your right side. Lower your right ear on top of your left hand and rest the weight of your head on your upright knee **(fig. 13.49)**. Using your right hand on the floor as an anchor, begin to rock your body from one sitz bone to the other, back and forth. Let the rocking create relaxation in your body as you hold this interesting position **(fig. 13.50)**.

3. Lower your head toward the floor and reach the right hand a little further out on the floor to your right **(fig. 13.51)**. Experiment with how much of your right shoulder you can get underneath the bridge of your right knee. Again, as you reach a comfortable stretch, begin to rock and release any tension in your neck, jaw, or face. Let your head hang heavy. The heavier your head is, the more your shoulder will tuck under your knee.

4. Now reach your right hand all the way around your right hip, placing your palm on or close to your right hip pocket. Lower your head and rock into the position.

5. Release your right knee with your left hand and reach your left hand all the way around behind your left side **(fig. 13.52)**. See if your hands can hold on to each other or make contact. If they do not touch, you can hold on to a sock so you feel the contact of your hands together behind your back. Lower your head once again and begin to rock into this stretch **(fig. 13.53)**.

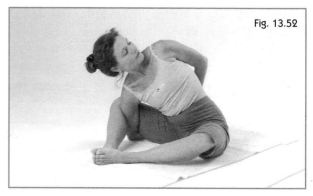

Fig. 13.52

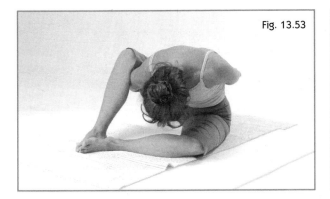

Fig. 13.53

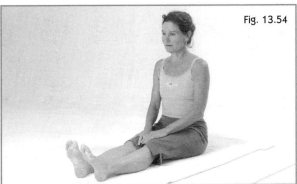

Fig. 13.54

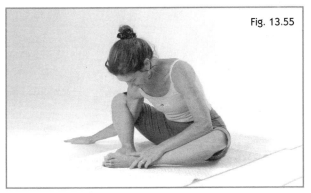

Fig. 13.55

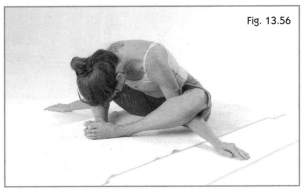

Fig. 13.56

6. Release your hands and arms, stretch both legs long, and notice the difference between the two sides of your body **(fig. 13.54)**. When you are ready, repeat this sequence of movements on the left side. Feel free to invent variations that help you to explore the opening in your hips.

7. Release your hands and arms, stretch out both legs, and notice the effects.

8. Moving to a deeper level of awareness, begin to press your sitz bones downward into the ground. Does pressing into the sitz bones anchor you to the ground? Do you feel an energetic lift through the spine when you exaggerate the press in your sitz bones?

9. Imagine that your head is a helium-filled balloon. Notice how your head hovers above your spine when you breathe into the balloon of your head.

10. Now we will move into Tortoise pose. Bring both knees upright, placing your feet on the ground. Thread your right hand under your right knee and slide your right hand along the floor out to your right side **(fig. 13.55)**. Thread your left hand under your left knee and slide your left hand along the floor out to your left side **(fig. 13.56)**. Lower your head and your torso as low to the ground as is comfortable and begin to walk your hands further and further apart **(fig. 13.57)**. When you reach a comfortable stretch, begin to breathe and to rock, releasing any strain or tension as you hold the stretch. Keep your head as heavy as possible. With your arms peeking out from under your knees, do you get an idea of why this pose is called the Tortoise?

11. Begin to walk your heels out, lengthening your legs and noticing how the weight of your knees begins to bring your arms lower to the ground **(fig. 13.58)**. Do not overstretch, but allow yourself to walk your legs out as far as they can go without straining. From sitz bone to sitz bone, allow

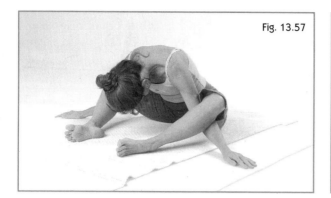

Fig. 13.57

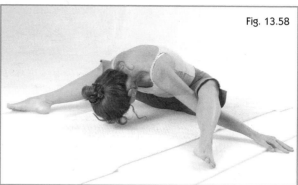

Fig. 13.58

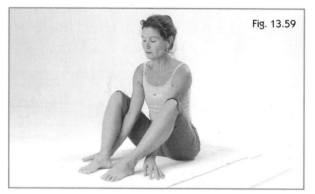

Fig. 13.59

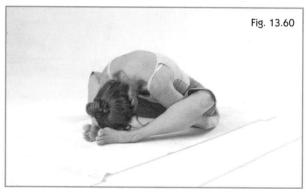

Fig. 13.60

your breath to take your torso closer and closer to the ground.

12. When you are ready to come up, walk your heels back in until your knees are once again upright and the soles of your feet are on the ground (**fig. 13.59**). Just for fun, reach both hands under both knees and see if your hands can make contact with each other behind your back (**fig. 13.60**). However far you go into the stretch, hold for just a moment. Relax your head, rock, and breathe.

13. Release your hands and arms, stretch both legs long, and lie on your back. Observe the effects of this stretch deep in the hip and shoulder. Do you notice any pulsing, streaming, or tingling sensations? Allow your breath to flow in and out without attempting to control or inhibit it in any way.

Integration: Seated Forward Bend

1. Here is a set of special instructions for supporting your body in this integration pose.

- Sit at the edge of a folded blanket to elevate your hips two to three inches off the ground.
- Place a rolled towel beneath your knees to avoid overstretching.
- Place a folded towel under your heels or ankles for padding.
- Place a bolster or stack of pillows between your torso and thighs for use during the surrender phase (see step 3).
- Caution: Do not use a strap around your feet to pull you into the posture. Use your abdominal strength to lengthen your spine, then allow gravity—not your upper body strength—to bring your torso over your thighs.

2. Sit on the ground with the support of the padding as out-lined above (**fig. 13.61**). Using your hands, roll the flesh of your buttocks apart, allowing your sitz bones to come in contact with the blanket on which you sit. Again, use your hands to roll your thighs inward toward each other, sug-gesting to the muscles through your touch that the inner thighs roll inward for the Forward Bend (**fig. 13.62**).

3. Lengthen through your heels, allowing them to move toward the wall in front of you. Rest your hands on your legs or to your sides. Allow your eyes to close and notice the attention to details that has brought you into this pre-cise preparation. Now you can relax all the fussiness and begin to slow down and enter the time in which your body lives. Suggest to your logical mind that you are entering a posture that allows you to stimulate a flow of sensation that can induce a deep state of clarity, focus, and concentration.

4. Notice the way you are breathing. Begin to relax more fully into the sensation of your breath. Deepen your breath, entering the three-part breath by inhaling into your belly, then your kidneys, and finally into your ster-num. Exhale in the reverse sequence. With every inhaling breath, imagine the torso lengthening from the sitz bones to the crown. With every exhaling breath, notice how your sitz bones press into the ground, the muscles of your pelvic floor squeeze upward, and your chest, ribs, and shoulders soften and relax.

5. Place a bolster or a stack of cushions on your thighs. On your next full exhalation, fold your arms behind your low back and release the shoulders away from your ears (**fig. 13.63**). Pause in this position, noticing how having your arms behind you allows you to center your head over your spine, your spine grounded in the sitz bones. Imagine your head is floating above your spine, hovering like a helium-filled balloon.

6. Keeping the three-part breath going, think of a string being attached to your sternum. As you exhale, squeeze the lower abdominals and begin to lengthen the sternum toward the wall in front of you (**fig. 13.64**).

7. Moving in gradual increments, notice how lengthening through the sternum allows you to bend from the hinge of your hips. As your torso moves further forward, your but-tock muscles roll open and your tailbone lifts out behind you. Your inner thighs roll inward and your heels lengthen away from you. Your head remains a long extension of your

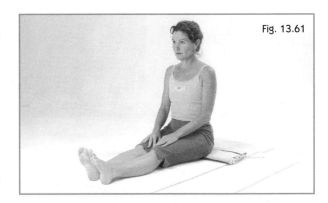

Fig. 13.61

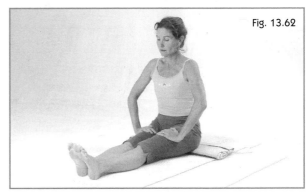

Fig. 13.62

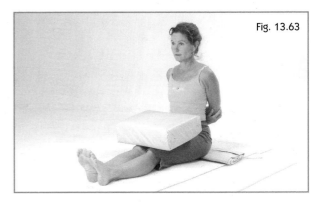

Fig. 13.63

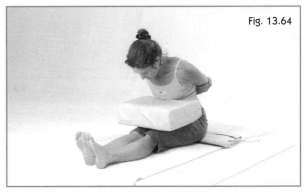

Fig. 13.64

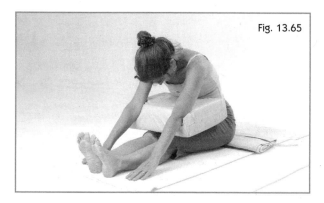

Fig. 13.65

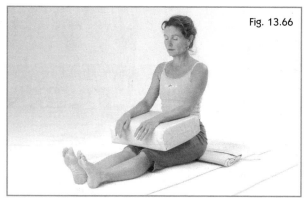

Fig. 13.66

spine with your chin slightly tucked, the back of your neck remaining long.

8. Entering deeper levels of concentration, allow your awareness to travel sequentially into every part of your body.

9. When you have reached the full length of your spine, with your torso elongated over your thighs, release your arms from behind your back. Sweep your palms along the floor and lower your torso over the bolster (**fig. 13.65**). If the bolster is wide enough to support your arms, reach your arms over the bolster. Otherwise let your elbows drop down toward the ground and release the weight of your torso over the bolster.

10. As you settle the weight of your torso over the bolster, make any microadjustments that allow you to enter the regenerative phase in Forward Bend. Bring awareness to the three-part breath; with every exhale release the weight of your head, your shoulders, your ribs, and your abdomen into infinite degrees of relaxation. Notice the sensations that pulse through your body. Allow your awareness to ride the waves of calm, steady sensation. As discomfort arises, make any adjustments that return you to the place of serenity and peace in the center of your being. Surrender into the wisdom of your organism as every dimension of your being is bathed in prana.

11. Allow yourself to receive from every dimension of your universe, becoming integrated and at peace in your center. Suggest to your logical mind that you will be returning with the knowledge and wisdom of being at home and at peace in your center.

12. Gradually begin your return by deepening your breath. Pressing into the sitz bones and lengthening through the crown of your head, begin to reach through the sternum to lift the long line of your spine back into the upright Seated Forward Bend (**fig. 13.66**). Allow your shoulders, arms, and hands to glide, hanging heavy and remaining relaxed as you return to sitting.

13. Remain with your eyes closed and experience the natural support of your torso. Notice where you have gone inside yourself. Notice the way you feel when all expressions have melted from your face and you are at home in your center.

14. When you feel ready, allow the windows of your eyes to slowly open. Receive the world into your center. Allow your body to move and stretch, letting emerge any sounds that come with your movement. Find any movement or posture your body is calling for that will provide a counterstretch and will move energy into your limbs.

15. What possibilities are now open for you to walk into a new future generated from accessing all dimensions of your being?

Before Moving On . . .

The inquiries of this chapter have presented movements that open the hip joints for entering Hero, Seated Spinal Twist, and Seated Forward Bend in such a way that you can follow the sensations that arise into deeper explorations of your inner connection to time. Lodged in the core muscles of your body are residual layers of stress that are imposed upon the body when your ordinary state of mind is operating from an urgency around time—that there is not enough time to do everything that needs to be done. In this mode, the body unconsciously becomes a slave to fulfill our ever-growing to-do lists. Entering these postures requires slowing down into the time it takes to feel the sensations that arise in the hips and legs, the spine, the shoulders and neck. The twist offers an opportunity to stay grounded in the sitz bones and pelvis while turning toward the past in one direction and toward the future in another. In Seated Forward Bend you have the opportunity to slow down, to spiral inward to the core of your inner self for even greater introspection into the experience of the present moment. Being willing to slow down to the time in which your body lives is nothing short of a hero's and a heroine's journey.

The traveler is heroic from the very beginning of this journey into self-awakening. The courage to inquire into the nature of your inner experience begins in the state of mystery as to what will be revealed. And yet, all that is revealed along the journey are reflections of who you already are. The intention when entering the inquiries of Self-Awakening Yoga is the expansion of consciousness through becoming aware of your body's own wisdom. In concluding the inquiries of this chapter, you have traveled through a comprehensive network of explorations that have included every part of your body, each revealing an interconnection of patterns that remind your organism of its natural freedom to move. While the movements have been releasing inefficient neuromuscular habits and restoring balanced working relationships among the various segments of your physical body, the intelligence of your organism has been simultaneously communicating directly to your mental perceptions of self through the language of sensation. Awareness of sensation has the effect of amplifying and intensifying the actual movement of energy or prana throughout your body. Prana is the name used for the aspect of this energy that is intelligent and that stimulates the evolutionary impulse in all forms of life. In recognizing the presence of this intelligent force at work in your body, you have expanded your consciousness to include the wisdom that is guiding the unfolding of your organism, the same wisdom that is guiding the unfolding of the universe. In this expansion of the perceptions you hold about who you are, you have the opportunity to witness that the wisdom of the macrocosm is encoded in the microcosm of your world.

All of the inquiries to this point, culminating in Hero, Seated Spinal Twist, and

Seated Forward Bend of this chapter, have allowed you to maintain close bodily contact with the ground, enabling you to explore the support of the ground beneath you. Maintaining this low center of gravity provides a safe and supported way to rediscover the working relationships of your body's movement. Staying close to the ground enables you to retrace the development of your organism from infancy to maturation and to strengthen and balance all of the muscular patterns that interact to maintain your balance in a standing position. The benefits of your inquiries have hopefully made some noticeable differences in your standing postures as you have progressed through these chapters. The miraculous event of standing is the outcome of the learning your organism has undergone in its journey from being bound to the earth on belly or back to coming all the way up into Standing Mountain pose.

In the next chapter we explore Standing Mountain pose. The results of all of the inquiries to this point are now interacting to aid you in the discovery of how you can maintain an upright, balanced standing position, with your weight distributed evenly along the axis of your spine.

14 The Miraculous Journey to Standing in Now, the Open Moment

What are the possibilities for walking into a new future generated from expanding consciousness to include the body's own wisdom?

STANDING ON YOUR OWN TWO FEET OPENS NEW POSSIBILITIES for exploring the world. After growing through the stages of pushing off the ground from crawling or pulling up with helping hands, at long last we come to standing. Our physical structure supports us in becoming autonomous, enabling us to draw from our potential to participate more fully in the dance of life.

In this chapter we explore Standing Mountain pose and its variations. Now that you are standing, how do the dynamics you have been exploring interact to help you maintain a posture that is relaxed and naturally comfortable for you and yet stable and balanced on two feet and legs? How does the upright and elongated vertical axis of your spine maintain balanced equilibrium with the weight passing through the length of your body?

The inquiries of this chapter begin with exploring the triangular base of support built into the design of the feet. Locating this base of support allows you to explore the way gravity transfers throughout the musculoskeletal system and the corresponding rebound of energy that moves upward through the body. Interacting with the phenomenon of gravity has given shape to your movement: from being on your back, then your belly, then front extending, forward bending, twisting, crawling, pushing, pulling, and scooting. Now the funded wisdom from all of the inquiries to this point come into play as you shift your orientation to finding your center of gravity in standing.

When you are established in your center of gravity, sinking your roots into the earth, you can move anywhere and yet be at home. Standing in Mountain pose with all of its variations, or balancing on one leg in Tree, or stepping forward into the Runner's Stretch, or engaging the world as the Warrior, your yoga practice can always take you to greater depths when awareness of your foundation in the feet, legs, and pelvis is active and alive. Following these inquiries into the way you stand will enhance your ability to incarnate into your body more fully, to bring more conscious awareness into witnessing the innate wisdom of your unique organism.

Finding a Leg to Stand On

Inquiry: How does leg strength produce confidence and self-determination?

The ability to stand represents a victory over the compelling forces of gravity and inertia. The self-determination required to find one's footing as an infant is a quality that the inner self now has for developing the skills to move forth into the world. Hara Shakedown and Release opens the flow of energy throughout your whole body, setting your physical and mental clocks to present time. Exploring how your feet work enables you to establish a strong foundation for natural alignment through your entire body. Balancing on one leg clarifies the work that each leg contributes to supporting a grounded, balanced stance. The Squatting Hara Breath brings energy and strength into the legs and integrates the lower body with upper body strength, centered in the belly.

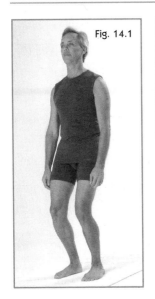

Fig. 14.1

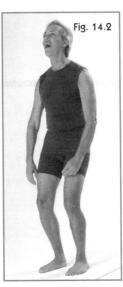

Fig. 14.2

Exploration 1: Hara Shakedown and Release

1. Stand with your feet a comfortable distance apart. Bend at the knees slightly, lowering your center of gravity. With your arms and shoulders hanging loosely at your sides, begin to pulse up and down **(fig. 14.1)**.

2. As the momentum begins to build, pulse more vigorously. Open your jaw and allow any sound to come out.

3. Allow the movement to build until the entire body gets involved. Release control over the movement and see what wants to happen **(fig. 14.2)**. The longer you stay in the experience, the deeper the release will be when you come to stillness.

4. Allow the movement to subside. Close your eyes and notice the sensations pulsing through your body. Can you feel energy pulsing from the soles of your feet up through the crown? Notice how it feels to release your body to find its natural alignment.

Exploration 2: Everything about the Feet

1. Come to a standing position. Lift the toes and fan them apart (**fig. 14.3**). Notice how easy or difficult it is to place each toe on the ground individually.

2. Sit so you can cradle one foot in your lap. Holding the foot with both hands, press your thumbs along the line of the arch, pressing very firmly (**fig. 14.4**). You'll know you are pressing in the right place with the right pressure when your big toe dances as you press.

3. Now firmly grip the ball joint of the big toe in one hand and the ball joint of the second toe in the other hand and vigorously separate them back and forth (**fig. 14.5**). Move to the ball joints of the second and third toes. Repeat the back-and-forth movement, progressing to the last set of ball joints.

4. Now stand on both feet and notice the difference between the two feet. Does one foot feel more alive, more grounded. Do you have more spring in your step on that foot?

5. Take a few steps and notice the difference between the two feet. Observe how much difference you can make in the sense of aliveness in your foot with such little effort. Lift and fan the toes apart—is it easier on the foot you've massaged?

6. Sit down and repeat the back-and-forth movement on the other foot, then stand and take a few steps. Notice the effects.

7. Now we'll locate the triangular base of support in your feet. Stand with your feet directly under your hips and parallel to one another. Shift your weight from the heels to the balls of the feet (**figs. 14.6 and 14.7**). Exaggerate the shifting, noticing that muscles work harder to compensate for the shifting from forward to back.

8. Slowly return to stillness, finding the balance point between the heels and the balls of the feet.

9. Lift your toes and fan them apart, reaching the little toes toward the horizon and the big toes in toward the midline of your body (**fig. 14.8**). With your toes lifted, can you sense the ball joints of your big and little toes forming the base of the triangle, with the ball of your heel as the apex?

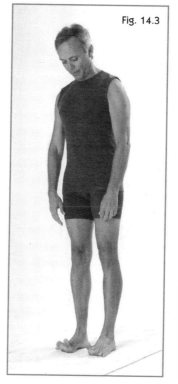

Fig. 14.3

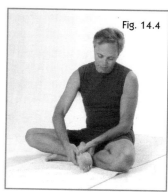

Fig. 14.4

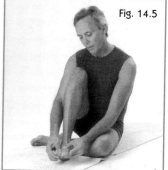

Fig. 14.5

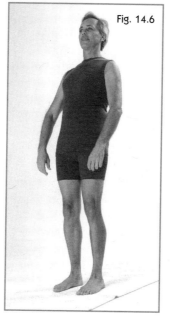

Fig. 14.6

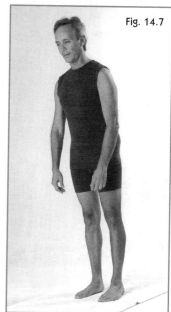

Fig. 14.7

Notice how the arch is lifted when you keep your toes lifted. Experience the sensation of standing on the triangular base of support in each foot

10. To exaggerate the sensation of the triangular base of support we will lower the heel into "negative space." Stand on a ½-inch block or book, the balls of the feet on the prop and your heels firmly contacting the ground (**fig. 14.9**). Repeat the Hara Release movement from the previous explorations (**fig. 14.10**).

11. Come to stillness and experience the sensations in your feet. With your eyes closed, carefully take two steps backward off the block. Standing still, notice the sensations in your feet. Are they more enlivened? Do you feel grounded? Has your center of gravity shifted to the balance point between heel and toes?

12. Take a few steps around and experience the sensations in your feet. Notice how much easier it might be to locate the triangular base of support in your feet.

13. To locate and open the metatarsal hinge of the toes, begin by lifting and fanning the toes. Notice much effort is required to place each toe on the ground individually. Anchor your hands on your hips. Shift your weight onto your left foot. Curl the toes of the right foot downward, applying a moderate amount of pressure (**fig. 14.11**). Notice the sensations as you explore varying amounts of pressure and angles relative to the floor.

14. Now curl only the right big toe, with the other toes remaining stretched (**fig. 14.12**). Then curl the toes under with the big toe stretched (**fig. 14.13**).

15. Release the right foot and notice any differences in sensation between the two feet. Does one foot feel more grounded?

16. Now repeat the toe curls on your left foot.

17. Standing still, notice the sensations in your feet. Have your feet grown more enlivened? Do you feel more grounded? Take a few steps around and experience the sensations in your feet. Notice how much easier it is to locate the triangular base of support.

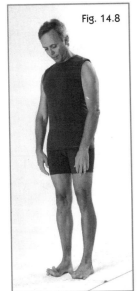

Fig. 14.8

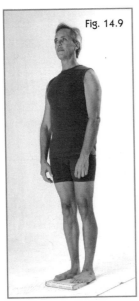

Fig. 14.9

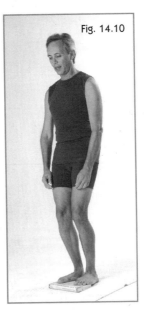

Fig. 14.10

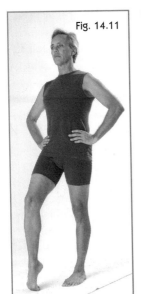

Fig. 14.11

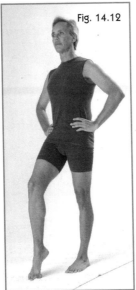

Fig. 14.12

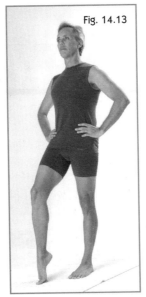

Fig. 14.13

Exploration 3: Balancing on One Leg

1. Stand with your feet parallel. Shift your weight from side to side (**fig. 14.14**), imagining grains of sand drifting from one leg to the other, filling the hollow tubes of your legs all the way down into the feet and toes.

2. Imagine roots growing down from the center of your foot into the earth. Let the roots penetrate down to the center of the earth. Draw earth's energy back up through the feet and into the legs. In this moment you are rooted, grounded.

3. Imagine all of the sand grains shifting to fill the right foot and leg. When you feel grounded, lift the left foot, gradually bringing it to rest on the inside of your right ankle or calf. Softly focus your gaze on the ground about ten feet in front of you (**fig. 14.15**).

4. Notice how long you are able to remain balanced on one foot, feeling rooted like a tree.

5. Repeat on the opposite foot.

6. Standing still now, notice the sensations in your feet. Have your feet grown more enlivened? Do you feel more grounded?

7. Take a few steps around and experience the sensation in your feet. Notice how much easier it is to locate the triangular base of support.

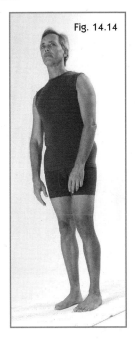

Fig. 14.14

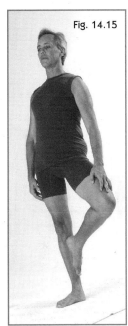

Fig. 14.15

Awakening the Nervous System with the Sound of Z

It is easy to bring an overabundance of mental energy into your practice when you want to incorporate all of the details of a movement. When you want to clear out your mind and activate more sensation in your standing postures, add this sounding exercise at the beginning, in the middle, or at the end of your practice. Make sure that you feel grounded in your feet, legs, and pelvis, then soften your knees by slightly bending them and lowering your center of gravity. Take a deep breath in and begin a long, slow exhalation while making the continuous sound "z-z-z-z-z-z-z-z-z."

Just making this sound begins to simulate the nervous system. If you want to add even more sensation to the experience, allow your hands and arms to shiver in response to the sound. You can repeat this sounding exercise for as many times as you want, allowing the sound to get longer and louder depending on how much of your exhaling breath you put into the sound. When you come to stillness, notice any pulsing, streaming, or tingling sensations arising throughout your body and nervous system.

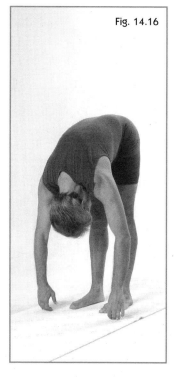

Fig. 14.16

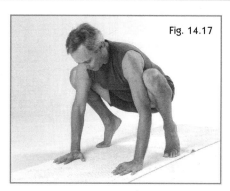

Fig. 14.17

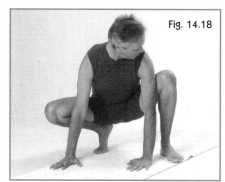

Fig. 14.18

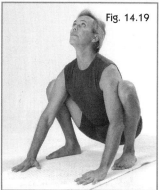

Fig. 14.19

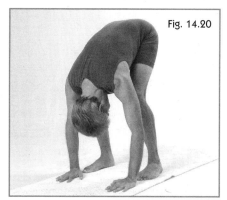

Fig. 14.20

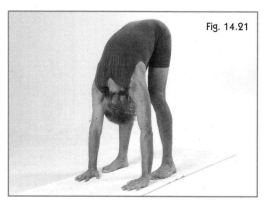

Fig. 14.21

Integration: Squatting Hara Breath

1. Effortless standing happens when your feet and legs are open and energized. To begin the Squatting Hara Breath, bend from the hinge of your hips, allowing your torso and arms to hang. Release the weight of your head to hang. Notice how close your torso comes to your thighs without using force (**fig. 14.16**).

2. Now walk your feet apart wider than your hips. Bend your knees into a squat. Use your hands on the floor for balance and to regulate the amount of pressure you feel in your knees. Allow your heels to come off the floor (**fig. 14.17**).

3. Turn your head to look over your left shoulder, allowing the left heel to come toward the floor while you stretch up and out of the arch of the supporting right foot (**fig. 14.18**).

4. Now turn to look over the right shoulder, bringing the right heel toward the floor and stretching out of the left arch and sole.

5. Letting your breath accompany the movement, turn from side to side, finding a rhythm and pace that allows you to explore the rotation in your hips, the bend in the hinge of your hips, and how your feet alternately flex and extend.

6. Return to center in your squatting position. Notice whether both of your heels come closer to the ground than when you started. Inhale as you look up and allow the back of your head to move toward your sacrum (**fig. 14.19**). Exhale as you lower your gaze to look between your legs (**fig. 14.20**). Press into your feet and lift your sitz bones toward the ceiling (**fig. 14.21**). Notice how this allows for lengthening through your legs.

7. Inhale and return to the squat, looking upward. Exhale, making the sound "h-a-a-a-a-a" as you lower your gaze to look between your legs, press into your feet, and lengthen your sitz bones to the ceiling.

8. Now you have all the pieces for practicing the Squatting Hara Breath. Continue this movement, allowing the momentum to build and the heat generated in your belly to release and energize your legs.

9. After eight to ten repetitions of the Squatting Hara Breath, return to standing. Allow your eyes to close. Release all control over your breath and breathing. When your breath begins to normalize, return to breathing though your nose. Experience the sensations pulsing through your body. Imagine that roots are extending from the soles of your feet down into the ground. Drawing energy up through your feet and legs, allow the pulsing in your belly to travel up through your spine and out through the crown of your head. Expand your kinesthetic awareness to fill the entire space of your body, from your feet to your crown. How does it feel to have your legs and feet supporting your whole body?

10. When you are ready, allow the windows of your eyes to open and receive the world down into your center. Notice the way you are connected to the world around you.

Balancing Resolute Determination with Lightheartedness

Inquiry: How do I access the body's sense of humor?

To fulfill your heart's desire, you need the freedom to interact with the situations and events of your life with dexterity and strength. With the legs firmly established as support for the upper body, energy from the belly now moves into the heart and out into the limbs, allowing the arms and hands to explore the tasks of holding on and letting go. Releasing the shoulders is key to moving energy from the belly, through the heart, and into the arms and hands for lighthearted, passionate engagement with the world. Butterfly and Moth Hands is a playful way to use the body's weight to release unconscious holding patterns in the shoulder and arms, as well as to move prana into the hands for enhancing our capacity to manifest. Pulling Onions exaggerates the rotation in the shoulder capsules that allows the shoulders to support but not to needlessly carry inappropriate responsibility. Swinging Buckets patterns the arms and shoulders to work in synchronized harmony with the spine. Breath of Joy integrates upper body freedom with lower body strength.

Exploration 1: Butterfly and Moth Hands

1. Come to a relaxed standing position. With your eyes closed, notice the way your two arms are hanging at your sides. Beginning with your dominant arm and hand, allow your hand to move as though you were flicking water off your fingertips (**fig. 14.22**). Let this movement originate from deep in your belly rather than your shoulder; let the movement be as effortless as possible.

2. Imagine that the same hand becomes a butterfly. Let the bones of the hand move vigorously, in the way a butterfly moves, taking the arm along with it. Move through as much of the space around your body as you can. Let your

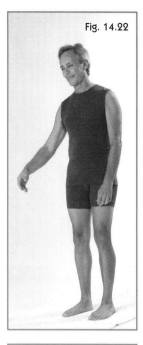

Fig. 14.22

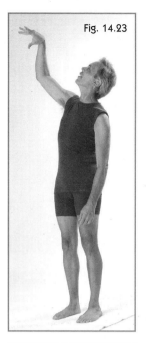

Fig. 14.23

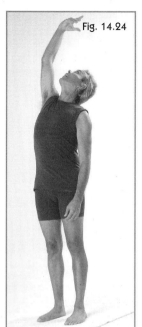

Fig. 14.24

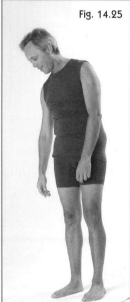

Fig. 14.25

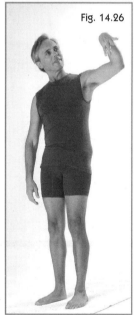

Fig. 14.26

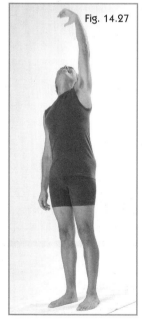

Fig. 14.27

tingling, or streaming sensations? Do you sense any difference in the length and the kinds of sensations of the two arms? Open your eyes and notice whether your vision has altered in any way.

4. Now repeat with the nondominant arm and hand, first flicking water and then allowing the hand to move as a moth moves (**fig. 14.26**). Unlike a butterfly, a moth never knows where it will flutter to next. Because this is your nondominant arm, it may be more challenging to let go of the control over your movement; therefore, embodying the movement of a moth, rather than a butterfly, should help in loosening control. Does the dominant arm and hand creep up to "help" the nondominant hand? After all, that hand couldn't possibly do something on its own without the dominant side assisting . . . at least so it would seem.

5. Flutter the hand up to the sky, take a deep breath in, and look in the direction of the stretch (**fig. 14.27**). Exhale as you release the arm to float back down to your side. Closing your eyes, once again witness the sensations arising in the hand and arm. Can you sense how energy is moving from the core of your belly up through your heart and down into the arms and hands? Notice the way your arms hang when they are free to release inappropriate responsibility for making things happen.

6. When you open your eyes, notice whether your vision has altered in any way.

eyes follow the movement of your butterfly hand (**fig. 14.23**). Eventually let the butterfly flutter up to the sky above you (**fig. 14.24**). Take in a deep breath and hold for just a moment. Then exhale and release the arm down to your side (**fig. 14.25**).

3. Close your eyes and notice the sensations streaming through your hand and arm. Do you feel any pulsing,

Exploration 2: Pulling Onions

1. Come to a comfortable standing position. Bend your knees slightly to lower your center of gravity. Make easy fists and draw your hands close to your hips (**fig. 14.28**). In front of you is a wall of green onions growing with the tops toward you. Reach your right hand in front of you, slowly opening the hand to take hold of the tops of a bunch of onions. After your grab on to the onions, exaggerate the twisting action in your wrist and shoulder (**fig. 14.29**). Exhale and pull the fist back to your side (**figs. 14.30 and 14.31**). Working with the same hand, repeat this reaching and grabbing several times, inhaling as you reach and exhaling the sound "h-a-a-a-a-a-a" as you exhale to your side and exaggerate the twisting and rolling action in your wrist and shoulder.

2. As the speed builds, begin to reach overhead to pull onions down from the ceiling to your side (**figs. 14.32 and 14.33**) making the same sound on your exhale breath.

3. Slow the movement down to stillness, close your eyes, and notice the sensations generated from this movement and breath. Note any differences between the two sides of your body.

4. Open your eyes and repeat

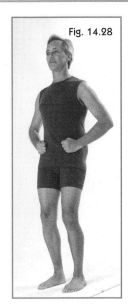

Fig. 14.28

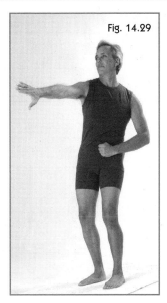

Fig. 14.29

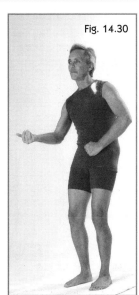

Fig. 14.30

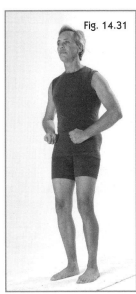

Fig. 14.31

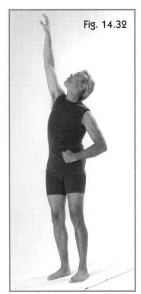

Fig. 14.32

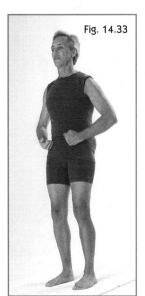

Fig. 14.33

the same action with the left hand and arm. First pull onions from a wall in front of you, then transition to pulling onions down to your side from the ceiling.

5. For the final phase of this exploration, pull onions using both hands at the same time, first pulling the onions from the wall in front of you (**fig. 14.34**) and

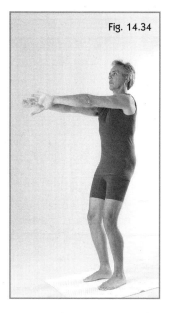

Fig. 14.34

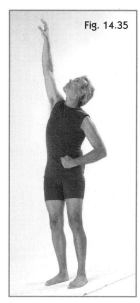

Fig. 14.35

then transitioning to pulling the onions from the ceiling (**fig. 14.35**).

6. Slow the movement down to stillness. Allow your breath to normalize. Notice the sensations that arise with this vigorous movement and breath. Particularly notice any warmth accumulating in the shoulders. How does it feel to release the holding in your shoulders, arms, and hands?

7. When you are ready, allow your eyes to open and receive the world through the window of your eyes.

Exploration 3: Swinging Buckets

1. Come to a comfortable standing position. Bend your knees slightly to lower your center of gravity (**fig. 14.36**). Notice how your arms feel hanging at your sides. Bend your knees a bit further and reach down to pick up a bucket with your right hand (**fig. 14.37**). Imagine there are eight potatoes in the bucket, and that the bucket weighs a few pounds. Gradually begin to swing the bucket forward and backward, bending your knees as the bucket swings past them. Let your eyes and head follow the movement by looking at the imaginary bucket (**fig. 14.38**).

2. Let the movement gradually build, inhaling on the upward swings and exhaling on the downward swings. Eventually allow the bucket to swing all the way around in a circle in your full range of motion (**figs. 14.39 and 14.40**). Remember to watch the movement of the bucket with your eyes to protect your neck.

3. Slow the movement and reverse the direction of the circle, inhaling on the upward swings and exhaling on the downward swings.

4. Slow the movement down to stillness and notice the difference in sensation between the two arms. Does one arm feel longer? How does it feel to have this much energy streaming through your right hand, arm, and shoulder? Can you sense how the sensations begin to spread from this arm and shoulder throughout your body?

5. Now repeat to the opposite side, starting with the swing back and forth and building

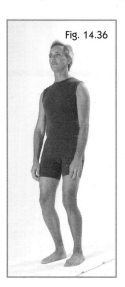

Fig. 14.36

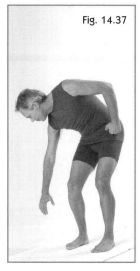

Fig. 14.37

to the arm circles in both directions. Allow your arm to be carried by your breath. When you feel ready, slow the movement down and return to stillness. Allow your breath to flow in and out without controlling its flow. When your breathing normalizes, experience how energy is moving through your left arm and shoulder. Can you sense how you are able to feel the natural weight and length of both arms as a result of these movements? How have your shoulders released? Do you feel any taller than when you first began?

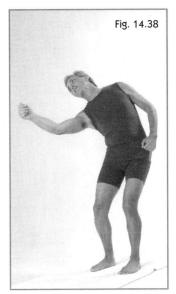
Fig. 14.38

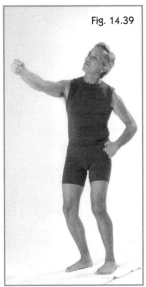
Fig. 14.39

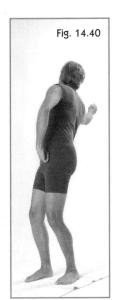
Fig. 14.40

Exploration 4: Monkey Breath

1. Step your feet apart wider than your hips. Bend at the knees slightly, keeping your center of gravity low (**fig. 14.41**).

2. Slowly slide the left arm down the outside of the left leg as you simultaneously slide the right hand up the right side of your rib cage, toward the armpit. Using the whole surface of your right hand, massage the ribs on your right side, sensing the bones beneath your flesh (**fig. 14.42**). Knead the muscles between the right hip and ribs. Experience how much pleasure you can discover by massaging your side when it is open in this way.

3. Turn your head to look down at your left foot (**fig. 14.43**), then turn your head and look up over your right shoulder as you bring yourself to upright by sliding your left hand back up your left leg and returning your right hand down to your side.

4. Stand for a moment and experience the difference in the way your ribs move with the breath, noting any differences between your two sides (**fig. 14.44**).

5. Now shift to the other side and repeat the movement, massaging the ribs on your left side and finding the bones and muscles of your left hip as your right hand and arm press into your right leg, supporting your torso. Rotate your head down to look at your right foot. As you rotate the head up to look over the left

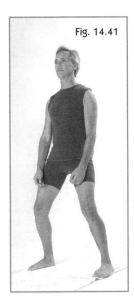
Fig. 14.41

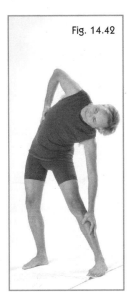
Fig. 14.42

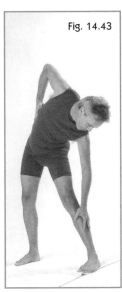
Fig. 14.43

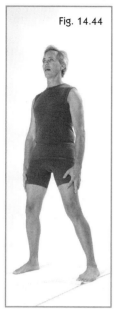

Fig. 14.44

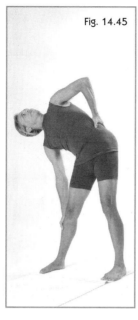

Fig. 14.45

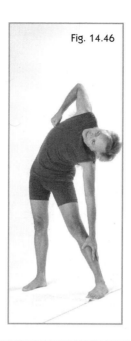

Fig. 14.46

shoulder (**fig. 14.45**), return to upright.

6. Now perform the movement from side to side, making an easy fist that moves up into your armpit on each side (**fig. 14.46**). Find the rhythm of the movement with your breath: exhale through an open mouth, making the sound "h-a-a-a-a-a-a" as you go down and inhaling as you return to upright.

7. Allow the movement and breath to build, picking up the pace when you feel balanced. Notice that this side-to-side action resembles a monkey's movement.

8. Gradually slow the movement down and return to upright. Close your eyes and notice the sensations streaming through your body. Allow your breath to normalize.

Integration: Breath of Joy

1. Stand with your feet a comfortable distance apart. Bend your knees slightly, lowering your center of gravity. In an easy, sweeping motion, inhale and bring your hands up to your shoulders (**fig. 14.47**). Massage your shoulders, taking handfuls of tension and throw that tension down to the ground (**fig. 14.48**). Again, reach up and take handfuls of whatever "shoulds" are sitting on your shoulders. Bending at the knees, throw those "shoulds" down to the ground.

2. Gradually allow this movement of reaching the arms up and swinging them down to build until the whole head, neck, shoulders, and torso get involved in the swinging of the body (**figs. 14.49 and 14.50**). Inhale as you come up and exhale as you sweep back down. Pay attention to allowing the knees to bend each time you swing downward.

3. Continue this movement at an easy pace, increasing the speed when you feel grounded.

4. Slow the movement to stillness. Allow your breath to normalize. Notice the sensations streaming through your body. Do you sense a whole-body aliveness? Do you feel more grounded than when you began?

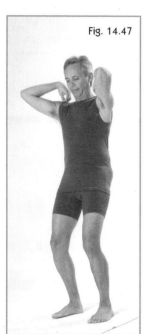

Fig. 14.47

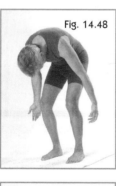

Fig. 14.48

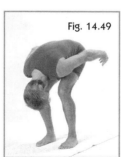

Fig. 14.49

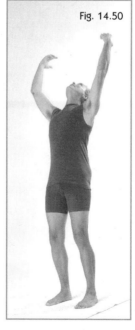

Fig. 14.50

Walking through Life with the Strength of a Lion and the Heart of a Lamb

Inquiry: How do quiet strength and perseverance nurture my intentions?

Being able to stand in a relaxed, balanced way and experience energy moving through the body requires the integration of upper- and lower-body strength, as we have been exploring. To carry those same effortless qualities into walking and lunging forward brings the challenge of a center of gravity that is continuously shifting without losing the strength and support of the upper and lower body. Abdominal strength allows for the low back to stay relaxed and mobile during all movements but particularly during movement when the body is carried by the legs.

When the abdominals are not receiving clear signals about their role in movement, the low back winds up having to do not only the work of mobilizing the hips and pelvis but also of supporting the weight of the upper body, developing a pattern in which the low back shortens with each forward step rather than lengthening for greater mobility and balance in the stride. Place your hands on your low back and take a few steps around to notice how your low back responds to each shift of your weight with a forward step. Can you sense how the back participates?

The following explorations will provide a greater sense of how to release the low back while walking, running, or lunging. Cat Tilt/Dog Tilt clarifies the muscular action in a neutral pelvis. Heel Kick Walk opens the low back for forward walking. Puppy Dog Legs opens the front sides of the hips, releasing the iliopsoas muscles and freeing the pelvis for pendulum-like motion. Forward Lunge integrates the full flexibility of the pelvis and legs while remaining grounded in the center of gravity.

Exploration 1: Cat Tilt/Dog Tilt

1. Do you remember an earlier exploration where you came to all fours in Table pose and then found Cat Tilt by rounding your spine, as if to stand the fur all along the back side of your spine? The Dog Tilt happened by moving the back of your head toward your sacrum, lengthening the front side of your body from the pubic bone to the sternum. Now we find the same movements in standing.

2. Stand comfortably, your feet parallel and positioned directly under your hip sockets. Lift and fan your toes, locating the triangular base of support in your feet (**fig. 14.51**). Bring one palm to your low back and one palm to your low abdomen. Imagine a downward-moving escalator that lengthens the low back from the belt line to the tip of your tailbone; slide your back hand down to the tip of the tailbone a few times, anchoring this downward sensation with sliding friction massage.

3. Now the escalator moves upward from your pubic bone to your navel; support from the pubic bone to the navel is an upward movement in the muscles. Use the

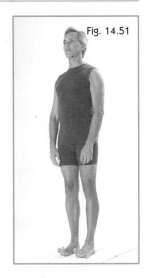

Fig. 14.51

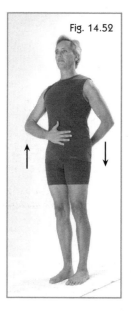

Fig. 14.52

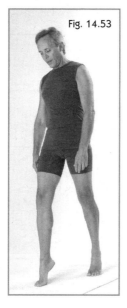

Fig. 14.53

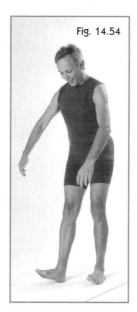

Fig. 14.54

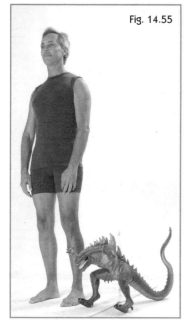

Fig. 14.55

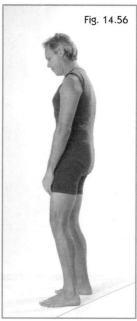

Fig. 14.56

legs to support the long line of the upper torso to the crown of the head.

5. Just for fun, walk around on the forward balls of your feet, as though you are in very high-heeled shoes (**fig. 14.53**). Can you feel how this distorts your center of gravity by shortening the entire backside of your body and the low back while thrusting the chest forward? Given that the bowl of the pelvis cradles your core energy and strength, how would this extreme Dog tilt affect your expression of life energy were you to hold this pattern for life?

6. Now walk on the ball of your heels, keeping your metatarsal balls (the "balls of the feet") off the ground (**fig. 14.54**). Can you feel how this throws your center of gravity backward, shortening the front side of your body? Do you find that you have to throw your head forward to counterbalance this backward pull? How would this extreme Cat Tilt affect your expression of life energy were you to hold *this* pattern for life?

7. Now return to a neutral pelvis, allowing your center of gravity to drop down into the bowl of the pelvis. Imagine that you have a long, thick dinosaur tail hanging from the tip of your tailbone. The tail is so heavy that it lengthens the sacrum and tailbone down toward the ground, dragging on the ground between your inner anklebones (**fig. 14.55**). Take a few steps around with this imaginary weight hanging from the tip of your tailbone (**fig. 14.56**). Can you sense how the pelvis stays under your spine for support?

8. Return to stillness. Stand with your eyes closed and sense the bowl of your pelvis as a cradle for supporting all of your movement and activity in the world, supplying nurturing strength for all of your expressions.

upward-sliding hand to communicate the direction of support the lower abdominals provide for the upper body.

4. This time, sliding both hands simultaneously, find a circle of moving energy—up the front and down the back (**fig. 14.52**)—that brings the pelvis into a supportive foundational position for drawing energy up from the

Exploration 2: Heel Kick Walk

1. Come to a comfortable standing position. Lift and fan your toes, locating the triangular base of support in your feet **(fig. 14.57)**. Shift your weight onto your left leg and foot. Imagine a soda can on the ground in front of you; remaining grounded in the left leg, use your right heel to kick the can **(fig. 14.58)**. Remaining in place, continue kicking the can with the right heel—this is an easy kick that emphasizes lengthening the low back as you kick. To emphasize the length in your low back, feel how sending the heel stretches out the backside of your leg. Repeat the kick several times.

2. Come to stillness and notice any differences in your sense of the length of each leg.

3. Now create a stable base of support in the right foot and leg as you repeat the swinging kick from the heel of your left leg. Invent a way to do this kick that allows you to lengthen out of the low back as you kick, rather than arching or shortening the lower back **(fig. 14.59)**.

4. Now you are ready to put both sides together for the Heel Kick Walk. Walk around a large space, putting a heel kick into every forward step. Exaggerate the Heel Kick, walking very fast at first. Now slow down and make the heel kick so subtle that you could be walking down the street and no one would notice that you are performing the Heel Kick Walk **(fig. 14.60)**.

5. Putting this heel kick into your walk retrains the muscles of the low back to lengthen—rather than shorten—as step. If you are a jogger or a runner, experiment with incorporating this awareness into your stride and notice how much energy comes into your body as you open the pelvis by releasing the length in your low back for forward mobility.

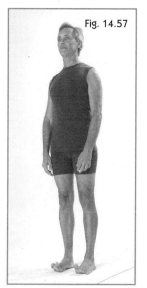

Fig. 14.57

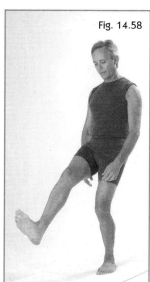

Fig. 14.58

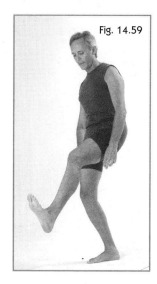

Fig. 14.59

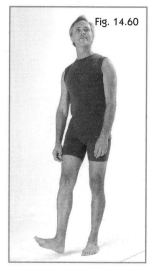

Fig. 14.60

Exploration 3: Puppy Dog Legs

1. Come to a comfortable standing position. Lift and fan your toes, locating the triangular base of support in your feet **(fig. 14.61)**. Shift your weight onto your left leg. Remaining stable and grounded in your left foot and leg, imagine a puppy is biting on the back right cuff of your trousers. Extend the right leg behind you and give a little kicking movement to shake the puppy off (but don't harm the puppy!) **(fig. 14.62)**. Make this kick in such a way that you allow the weight of the bones of your right leg to lengthen the leg out of the hip socket. Notice how the front surface of your right thigh lengthens as you kick behind you.

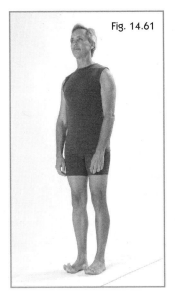

Fig. 14.61

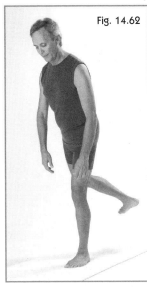

Fig. 14.62

2. Now repeat this kicking motion with the left leg.

3. When you have finished kicking each leg individually, alternate back and forth between one leg and the other, giving a kick that you can feel all the way up into your hip socket.

4. Allow your eyes to close and sense how the front of your hips have opened, allowing the line from your pubic bone to your sternum to lengthen. Relax into your breath and enjoy the sensations of energy moving though your open hips and pelvis.

Integration: Standing Mountain

1. Come into a comfortable standing position, your feet parallel and centered directly beneath your hip joints. Lift and fan your toes, locating the triangular base of support in your feet. Soften your gaze. Allow your eyes to bring an easy focus to a point along the horizon. Receive the world through the window of your eyes, remaining centered in the bowl of your pelvis.

2. Release into rhythmic three-part breathing, inhaling first into the bowl of the pelvis, then into the kidneys, and finally into the sternum. Hold the breath in for a moment, allowing the ribs, shoulders, and arms to relax into that holding. As you exhale release the sternum, then the kidneys, and then squeeze the abdominals and lift the pelvic floor muscles. Repeat this breath rhythm for four cycles, establishing awareness of the pattern of breathing that will continue throughout this practice of Standing Mountain pose.

3. Focus your awareness in the bowl of your pelvis. As you send energy down the back side of your legs, elongating your lower back, experience how you can send roots down through your feet into the ground.

4. Now draw energy up through these roots. The energy travels up the front side of your legs, lifting your kneecaps and thighs; from there draw energy up through the inner thighs and pubic bone to your navel. Imagine that nothing can move you off your ground, your place on the earth.

5. Experience the bowl of your pelvis as the foundation from which the spine naturally elongates. Like an infinitely expanding vertical rod, imagine how the axis of the spine in the core of your body extends upward through your neck and head and continues to expand into the infinite space above you. As the spine elongates the sternum moves inward, allowing the ribs to hang and the collarbones to separate.

6. Release your jaw and tongue. Allow all expressions to melt from your face. Again, soften your gaze and deepen your breath.

7. Following the upward surging path of energy, draw your awareness up through the soles of your feet—feel your shinbones and kneecaps lifting, your inner thighs moving up and into the pubic bone, and the pelvic floor and lower abdominals lifting while the sternum softens inward and the head releases to hover above your spine (**fig. 14.63**).

8. Following the downward surging path of energy, draw your awareness down the back of your neck and shoulders. Imagine the shoulder blades gliding down the backside of your rib cage toward opposite hip pockets. Release the weight of your arms to hang as energy moves down the inner arms, through your palms and down the little-finger sides of your hands. Your tailbone hangs like a pendulum as energy moves down the hamstrings and the back of your calves, through the soles of your feet and down toward the center of the earth.

9. For the next few breaths, sink your roots down through layers of ground, through underground streams and caverns, to penetrate the liquid molten heat in the core of the earth. Draw this warmth upward through your feet and legs, fueling the glowing, pulsing belly center. Traveling up through the core of your spine, filling your head and streaming up and out through the top of your head, your entire organism is rooted in the center of the earth while glowing and lengthening upward, like a volcano, into the infinite space above you.

10. Allow your eyes to close and let your vision spiral inward to the center of your being. Experience the sensation of being the mountain: grounded, eternal, and at home in your place on the earth, being all of who you are in relation to the world around you. You are the mountain, effortlessly still and rooted in all of life unfolding.

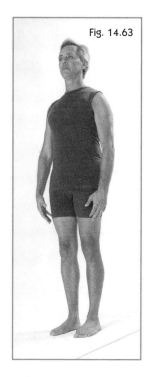

Fig. 14.63

Integration: Warrior Lunge

1. Enter the experience of Mountain pose. Recall the movement of energy as you send your awareness from your feet upward through the core of your body to your crown and downward through the shoulders and arms, the pelvis and legs. Travel the cycle of energy that connects you to this moment as the mountain.

2. Open your eyes and softly focus your gaze at a point along the horizon. Receive the world into your center through your gaze. Imagine that you are about to courageously send your energy into the world. All the forces of the universe are lining up to support your intentions. All obstacles to fulfilling your intentions are being dissolved in this moment, opening up a tunnel of safe passage.

3. Exhale all of your breath as you send the little finger side of your arms and hands downward toward the center of the earth. Inhale as you rotate your palms upward, lifting your arms to shoulder height and lengthening your arms away from your shoulders (**fig. 14.64**). Pause here and take as many breaths as you need to relax into the length across the beam of your shoulders. Roll the shoulders down and back, releasing the shoulder capsules. Soften the sternum inward and allow the ribs to hang.

4. Exhale all of the breath as you slowly extend your arms upward

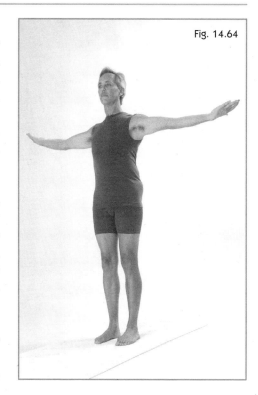

Fig. 14.64

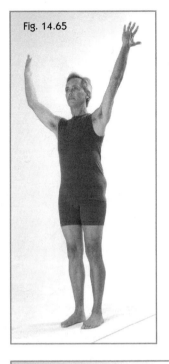

Fig. 14.65

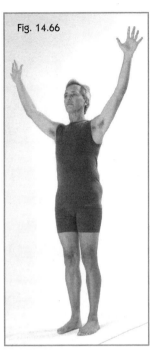

Fig. 14.66

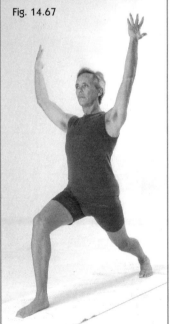

Fig. 14.67

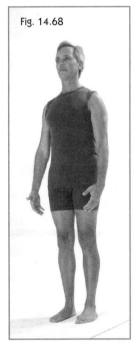

Fig. 14.68

toward the heavens, your shoulders rolling down away from your ears and your shoulder blades sliding down the backside of your ribs toward the opposite hip pockets (**fig. 14.65**).

5. When your arms have reached a comfortable extension above your head, pause and breathe into the entire length of your body. Like an arrow, you are sharpening your intentions in preparation for launching forth. Allow your energy to build as you hold this extended Mountain pose.

6. Take a deep inhaling breath. Hold the breath in. On an exhaling breath, float your arms back down through an ocean of space around you (**fig. 14.66**). As your arms float downward to your sides, experience a simultaneous surge of energy upward through the core of your body.

7. Preparing now for the Warrior Lunge, soften your gaze and exhale all of your breath. As you inhale, lunge the right foot forward, planting the foot a few steps out in front of your body. As you lunge the foot forward and your center of gravity shifts to balance between your two legs, simultaneously allow your arms to lengthen upward, as in the extended Mountain (**fig. 14.67**). Pause and find your balance in Warrior Lunge. Walk your right heel so that it is positioned directly under your knee.

8. Take a deep breath in. On the exhale, step your right foot back into Mountain pose and lower your arms to your sides (**fig. 14.68**). Close your eyes and experience the energy that arises when you have the freedom to lunge forward into the unknown.

9. Pause for a moment and bring your awareness back to full, relaxed breathing. Recall the image of standing in Mountain pose. Suggest to your logical mind that you are now about to enter a new experience and will receive different information from your left side than you have just received from your right side. When you are ready, repeat the Warrior Lunge, stepping the left foot forward (**fig. 14.69**).

10. Now alternate back and forth between lunging with the right foot forward, returning to Mountain, and then lunging with the left foot forward. Return to Mountain pose between each lunge. Each time you lunge forward, pay attention to aligning the heel under your front knee. See what happens when you step further forward. Find your maximum stride without causing strain when you return back up to Mountain.

11. When you have completed your inquiry into the Warrior Lunge on both sides, stand in a relaxed, natural Mountain pose and receive the effects of your movement. What are the possibilities for walking into a new future as you stand in now, the open moment? How does centering your awareness in Mountain pose produce confidence and self-determination? Is it possible to balance between resolute determination and playful lightheartedness at the same time? How do you wish to direct your lion-hearted strength?

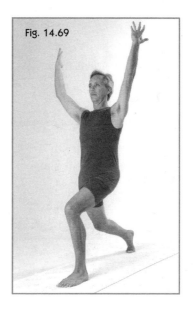

Fig. 14.69

Before Moving On . . .

Through the inquiries of Self-Awakening Yoga you have been building a bridge of communication between the mind and body by steadily focusing your awareness on the sensations that arise in your body, informing you of the wisdom inherent in your physical experience. Developing your capacity to witness sensations and the resulting awakening of bodily intelligence that is liberated when the evolutionary energy of prana is free to act upon your physical body simultaneously strengthens your ability to witness the corresponding self-perceptions and the images you hold of yourself and your potentials. Your capacity to witness your physical, mental, and emotional experience as an interrelated whole is none other than your journey home to the center of yourself. Witnessing is your capacity to transition from moment to moment, from one life experience to another, while remaining grounded in your body. Although we are infinitely greater than the merely physical body, our journey to expanded consciousness has begun by listening to the wisdom of the body.

Establishing functional communication and an integrated relationship between your mind and body is a good foundation for continuing your learning throughout your lifetime. What may happen beyond the ultimate release of your body is concealed in the Great Mystery. What is apparent from an integrated consciousness that includes bodily wisdom is that the wisdom of the body is interconnected to the evolutionary life force of prana in its eternal, infinite, creative power.

Witness consciousness is dream walking between the observable concrete world of our own creation and the subtle world of intentionality that, as our consciousness expands, is forever rewriting the genetic code for our future. There are no boundaries between what exists and what is possible when we awaken to the power of prana as an active force in our lives. Witnessing your actual experience is the doorway to releasing the same creative force that births new stars, planets, and galaxies, all unexpected and unpredictable new forms of existence, to work within the tangible domain of your body in the present moment.

Moses came across a burning bush in the desert. He was perplexed that the fire did not consume the bush. When he came close to observe the dazzling and mysterious phenomenon, he heard a voice that he recognized as the voice of Jehovah saying, "Moses, take off your shoes. The ground on which you stand is holy." Taking off his shoes in surrender to the commandment, Moses soon found himself transfixed, standing barefooted before the illumined manifestation. In the process of surrendering to the mysterious guidance, he received reassurance of his place of leadership in the world, inspiration for continuing his difficult journey, and courage to make difficult decisions that lay ahead of him. Though the wisdom of the body rarely speaks to us in such bold language, we are each capable of cultivating our awareness of inborn, inherent wisdom. It is interesting that Moses was asked to remove his shoes to experience the holiness of the ground on which he stood. The standing postures of this chapter have invited you to "take off your shoes" and to feel the ground beneath your feet.

As you cultivate respect for your body as your partner in awakening to the dance of life, every bodily gesture, every physical action, every mudra of the body can become an opportunity for evoking a creative interaction among the diverse domains of your experience. Expanding your consciousness to include the wisdom of your body evolves and transfigures your consciousness of the one inside who witnesses your multidimensional selves at play. From the perspective of traditional yogic understanding, this union of body-mind experience with witness consciousness is *samadhi,* "balanced, ecstatic knowing."

How does witnessing the connection of your mind and body experience lead to samadhi? The thread of connection unfolds in this way. *Ecstasy* and *experience* come from the same root word: *ek,* or *ex,* means "outside"; *stasis* means "to stand." Therefore, *ecstasy* translates as "to stand outside oneself," or in other words, "to witness." The syllable *peri,* in *experience,* means "to pass through." In this chain of understanding, the word *experience* thus means "to go beyond or outside of oneself, passing through to a place where one has never been."

The next chapter guides you into experiences that place you in direct communication with the wisdom of prana as a source for guiding your yoga practice. Having given yourself so fully to opening your body to the movement of prana, you are now ready to allow prana to guide you into places inside yourself where you may never have been before.

15 The Practice of Flowing with Life's Unfolding Mystery

How can the spirit of inquiry be continuously nurtured through a personal yoga practice?

THE INQUIRIES OF SELF-AWAKENING YOGA DRAW FROM commonly shared roots of many varieties of yoga traditions practiced in both the East and West today, but they are not limited to traditional forms or interpretations of yoga. In keeping with the spirit of the early shamanic yogis, who were the original artists and scientists of yoga, the inquiries of Self-Awakening Yoga expand to include many doorways and practices that intend and produce an integration of body, mind, and spirit.

Yoga has its origins in shamanic practices that emerged out of the ancient religious culture of India. The early yogis were quintessential scientists, men and women engaging in experiments into the nature and content of their personal inner experience. Often shunned or persecuted for the threat their freedom posed to the religious and social norms of the times, yoga practices evolved independent of Hindu culture, and often in secret. Prior to written texts such as that of Yogi Patanjali, yoga teachers created codes out of Hindu terminology and philosophical principles as a means for teaching their students while at the same time hiding the powers of the practice from those who were suspicious about the aims of yoga.

Yogic principles developed in this carefully guarded climate, empowering its practitioners to reject the rigidly structured religious culture and caste systems of Hinduism in early India. The body of knowledge known today as yoga resulted from the clandestine meetings of these early practitioners, who would gather in forests and caves and share the results of their experiments and experiences with one another. Recurring experiences among the practitioners accrued through centuries and became the traditions of yoga that were carefully passed down by the early masters.

Because yoga instruction is now universally available and is often presented in group or classroom settings by a teacher, yoga appears to be an external physical experience that can be learned just like any other subject. But the original teachings of yoga were carefully guarded secrets passed on by the guru to only the closest students who committed their full attention to the practice of yoga. From the perspective of the original yoga shamans, a person could potentially damage her or his intuitive connection to inner wisdom by unconsciously participating in a culture or religious society. Substituting technique for conscious awareness has a dumbing effect on our delicate inner guidance mechanisms. By devoting your life energy to preserving the prescribed boundaries of a group—especially fundamentalist groups, which organize around formulaic and impersonalized practices of yoga—you can easily displace trust in your ability to know and to act upon what is right for you. Without the personal power to travel into your own highest source of counsel and guidance within, you are at the mercy of the person who conveys the most pervasive and convincing influence, authority, and control.

Perhaps the biggest magic in the early shamanic development of yoga was the way the yogis discovered the importance of awakening to deeper levels of consciousness, sitting in their true source of power while living in the middle of ordinary human life. The early yogis discovered a pathway into one's own experience to find the power to fulfill the deeper urges for self-knowledge. While immersed in profound states of introspection and trancelike meditation, yogis discovered that the physical body would undergo movements, postures, and breathing patterns that purified and strengthened the body and produced internal mental and emotional states of great tranquillity, bliss, and insight. Such introspective inquires form the basis of Self-Awakening Yoga.

The term *asana* means "to sit or rest in the seat of the self." Because many asanas are traditionally known by the names of animals—such as Cobra pose, Lion, Eagle, and Tortoise—it would seem that the yogis observed animals and attempted to return to primal states of evolution by imitating the behavior or posture of the creature. But asanas actually emerged out of deep states of meditation in which prana moved the body into particular positions that were simultaneously and independently discovered and then corroborated from one yogi to another. In Self-Awakening Yoga, we take the perspective that the postures are archetypes encoded in the development of the neuromuscular system in the human body, and that every individual embodies the urge to discover the hidden potentials implicit within the patterning of his or her own organism.

Originally the asanas were not taught as yoga. Internal awareness was the focus of yoga, a focus out of which the postures were certain to arise. In the popular yoga trends of today, postures are taught as yoga. On the contrary, the true power of yoga is the process by which you, as an individual, use the postures or other existential experiences as a means for entering into an authentic relationship with the multidimensional aspects of your entire being. By acknowledging these early roots and shamanic origins of yoga you can claim permission and draw the inspiration required to move beyond ritualistic and traditional forms of yoga, to inquire, experiment, and enter into direct interaction with your own experience. Engaged in your own genuine inquiry into self through yoga, you can serve as a potent guide to help others to listen for the voice of their own inner wisdom. One of the extraordinary results of your practice is your ability to accept others with tender and humble positive regard and to witness the issues and archetypes that we hold in common as developing, evolving human beings. The results of your yoga inquiry actually contribute to and further the continuing evolution of yoga itself. You are a yogi.

The inquiries of this chapter focus on integrating the knowledge and insight you have harvested through your journey by creating a personal practice that provides a perpetual opening for your continued attunement to the wisdom of prana. The energy to be awakened through your yoga practice is best accessed through a form that suits your personality, interests, and needs. By establishing a practice that feels like home base, you are free to open into greater depths of inquiry. A personal practice taken on for the purpose of self-awakening is called *sadhana*. In the Bhagavad Gita, Krishna teaches his yoga student Arjuna that it is better to perform one's own spiritual practice imperfectly than to perfectly imitate the practice of another. It is your divine birthright to explore and to discover the yoga practice that gives you access to the great unfolding mysteries in your life.

Yogi Patanjali gives two criteria for establishing a regular yoga practice. These criteria work together like the banks of a river, allowing the flow of creative energy to move in a direction you intend to go. *Abhyasa,* or "resolute determination," provides a ground of commitment for your continued growth. When you make a wholehearted commitment to a practice that you choose, you are liberated from the fluctuations of indecision. You know what you have chosen to do and you organize your life to fulfill that commitment. Commitment to your practice does not mean that you will be perfect.

Vairagya, or "non-attachment to the results of your practice," comprises the other riverbank; it opens the doorway for accepting yourself regardless of the results. Making a commitment to use your practice as a way to see yourself includes both the times when your practice happens effortlessly and the times you may fall off. Falling off is just as much a part of the practice as sticking to it. Committing to your practice does not mean that the results will show up as you envision. Therefore, cultivating the attitude of nonattachment allows you to continuously enter the mystery by surrendering the results to the wisdom of your organism. When you willfully make the best choice for yourself, taking into account all of your awareness up to this point in your life, you are then free to let the results unfold as a guiding grace in your life.

The inquiries that follow are suggestions for a variety of yoga flows that can help you develop ideas for crafting a practice that is right for you. These inquiries cover a wide range of energetic dynamics. You may want to use one inquiry or a combination of inquiries for a while to get a feeling for how they suit your needs. You do not have to choose one practice for the rest of your life. As you change your practice will need to change as well. When you are grounded in your own connection to inner wisdom, it is valuable to explore many yoga classes from different teachers as a way to continue expanding the possibilities for inner growth.

A yoga flow, or *vinyasa,* such as those you are about to experience, is somewhat like a choreographed dance. A vinyasa is a sequence of yoga postures connected by transitional movements. Your yoga practice becomes one long sequence of movements that unfolds as a meditation in motion. Angel Wings Breath is a simple flow that coordinates breath with movement. Salutation to the Child moves your spine in all six basic directions and allows you an armature to add any of the movements from the preceding inquiries into your flow. The Sun Salutation is the most familiar flow of postures; Sun Salutation allows you to bring in the elements of speed and cardiovascular exertion, which build physical strength. Prana Flow is slow and meditative, combining rhythmic, ocean-sounding breathing with spontaneous movement to interact with the subtle forces of prana as it moves through your body. This form of moving meditation begins by transitioning from willful control over your postures and movement into unprompted intuitive movements that begin in your hands, like a prayer dance, and then expand to include the spontaneous movement of your whole body.

The form of your practice will evolve from experimenting with insights that arise from continuously asking yourself the question, "What am I passionate about?" As you well know, there is no "right" way to practice your yoga. What will make your practice a constant source of energetic regeneration is that you are passionate about the emerging results that mirror your continuously expanding self awareness.

Integrative Flow 1: Angel Wings Breath

How can I invite effortless meditative awareness through movement?

As its name suggests, this flow allows you to open your whole being to the benevolent flow of prana. After the first couple of repetitions you will not have to think about what you're doing, because you'll have focused your physical and mental energies by synchronizing your breath with the movement. This flow quickly induces a meditative state of awareness as the mind becomes absorbed in the sound of the breath and the sensations of prana, allowing the intelligence of your organism to dance.

Flow: Angel Wings Breath

1. Begin in a comfortable standing position (**fig. 15.1**). Close your eyes and notice how quickly and deeply your awareness travels to the center of your being in the center of your body. Step your feet slightly wider apart than your hips. Soften your knees and deliberately let the weight of your torso sink into the strength of your legs (**fig. 15.2**). Can you allow your feet and legs to support the weight of your upper body? Notice how releasing down into gravity creates a simultaneous upward-moving surge of energy through the core of your body and out through the top of your head.

2. Create an intention for yourself to be present to all dimensions of your being during this practice. Release any responsibility to make anything happen. Suggest to your logical mind that this is a time to allow the wisdom of prana to guide your experience.

3. Bring your palms together in front of your pubic bone, fingertips pointing down. Softly bend in the knees. Exhale your breath as you release your shoulders to roll down and back (**fig. 15.3**).

4. In one long, slow, deliberate inhaling breath, press into your feet to straighten your legs while simultaneously rotating the palms upward and inward until the fingertips are pressing into your sternum (**fig. 15.4**).

5. Maintain a relaxed but firm

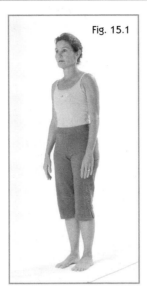

Fig. 15.1

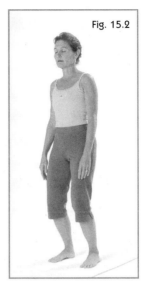

Fig. 15.2

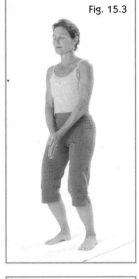

Fig. 15.3

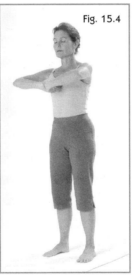

Fig. 15.4

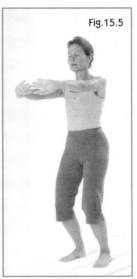

Fig.15.5

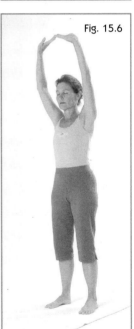

Fig. 15.6

pressure between your palms as you exhale from your heart and begin to slowly soften your knees and extend your palms in front of your body at shoulder height (**fig. 15.5**).

6. Inhaling, begin to extend your open palms above your head into temple position, middle fingertips slightly touching. Allow your arms to come in line with your ears (**fig. 15.6**).

7. On one long, slow, deliberate exhaling breath, open the palms and sweep the arms in semicircular

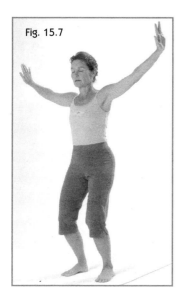

Fig. 15.7

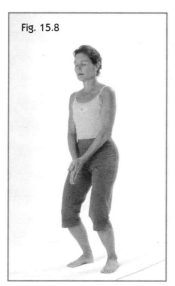

Fig. 15.8

arcs, as though you are spreading your angel wings to fill the entire space around you (**fig. 15.7**). As your arms are floating downward toward your sides near the end of the exhaling breath, allow the knees to soften, as you bring your hands together in prayer position pointing downward in front of your pubic bone (**fig. 15.8**). Press the palms together to squeeze all of the breath out.

8. Take an inhalation, then begin one long exhaling breath as you repeat the sequence of movements—pressing your palms together at the pubic bone with the fingertips pointing downward and pressing into your feet to straighten the legs as you rotate the fingertips upward and inward toward the heart. Exhaling, soften the knees as you extend the palms forward at shoulder height, then continue with an inhalation, sweeping the palms overhead into temple position. Hold the breath in for a moment, then sweep the arms along your sides as you exhale and extend your angel wings to fill the space around you. At the

end of the circular sweep, bring your hands into prayer position at the pubic bone for continuing into the next round of Angel Wings Breath.

9. Over the next few repetitions, relax into the timing of this movement in such a way that you can fully exhale and inhale, taking each breath to your maximum comfort level. As a way of deepening the trance-inducing concentration on sensations, you can repeat this movement with your eyes closed and your awareness focused internally. To begin bringing more prana into your practice, pause for a few seconds at the end of every inhalation and exhalation.

10. When this flow becomes effortless and mindless, allow your body to be moved by the flow of breath and prana. Stay in this meditation-in-motion for as long as you can remain engaged in witnessing the flow of internal experiences that begin to emerge.

11. You may feel drawn to enter into a spontaneous dance of movement that engages your whole body. Or you may wish to slow the repetitions down to ever more deliberate mudras. Wherever the practice takes you, allow the experience to slowly bring you into a position for meditation or relaxation. In this stillness, receive the effects of your practice, allowing every level of your self to integrate in the center of your being.

12. Offer your gratitude for the opportunity to release into the regenerative, creative force of prana moving through you. Notice how the wisdom of your organism is communicating its messages to you in this moment.

13. When you are ready, begin your return, carrying with you the effects of your practice.

Integrative Flow 2: Salutation to the Child

How does meditative awareness arise through synchronizing breath with full-body counterbalancing movement?

At the heart of this posture flow is Child pose. As you might recall from previous explorations, the fetal position allows you to curl back into the center of your being and deeply connect to your source of nurturance in the belly. The beauty of repeating this yoga flow is that it provides multiple opportunities for branching into front-extension postures, such as Sphinx, Cobra, and Kneeling Forward Lunge, or into the crawling postures from Table pose, or into the seated postures, such as Pinwheel, Seated Forward Bend, or Spinal Twist. You can use the structure of the flow to vary your practice according to the messages you receive from your body. This flow also provides a counterbalancing sequence of positions that take you from standing down to the ground and back up again to standing.

Flow: Salutation to the Child

1. Begin by creating an intention to open to the many dimensions of your being that may arise during your practice. What feelings do you have about contacting and honoring the pure and eternally present child within you?

2. Come into a comfortable standing position **(fig. 15.9)**. Adjusting your feet into Mountain pose alignment, with your feet parallel and directly under your hips, notice the connection you have with the ground. Deepen your breath as you locate the triangular base of support in your feet. Softly focus your gaze, drawing your concentration into your belly center.

3. Exhale and allow the little-finger side of your hands to be drawn down toward the center of the earth **(fig. 15.10)**. As you inhale, spread your arms outward toward the horizons **(fig. 15.11)**, then sweep them upward toward the heavens **(fig. 15.12)**. Take

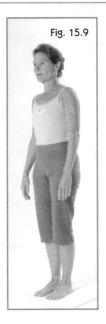

Fig. 15.9

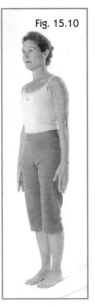

Fig. 15.10

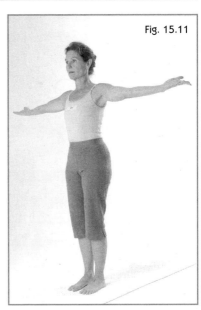

Fig. 15.11

as many breaths as you need as you allow the upward-surging energy in your spine to lengthen your torso and your arms above your shoulders. As the torso and arms expand, your shoulders roll down and back.

4. Hold the next inhaling breath for a moment, then bend from the hinge of your hips, sweeping

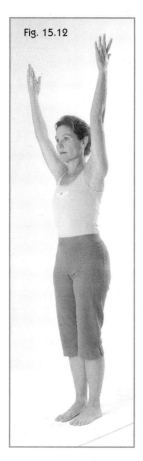

Fig. 15.12

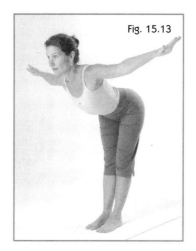

Fig. 15.13

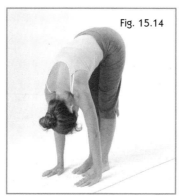

Fig. 15.14

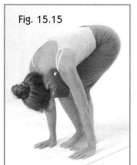

Fig. 15.15

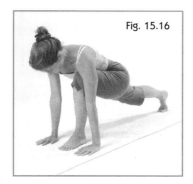

Fig. 15.16

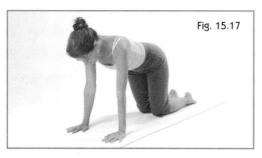

Fig. 15.17

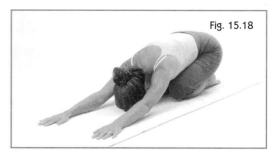

Fig. 15.18

your arms out to your sides and lowering your torso toward your thighs (**fig. 15.13**). As your torso lowers, open the "book" of your buttocks and focus your gaze forward, then toward the floor in front of you, then to your feet and your legs. Finally, with your arms hanging at your sides, look upward and in toward your navel (**fig. 15.14**).

5. Hanging from the hinge of your hips in the Standing Forward Bend, soften the back of your knees and shift your weight to release the pressure in your hamstrings and thighs. Release the weight of your head, your jaw, and your eyes into the downward pull of gravity. Stay here for as many full inhalations and exhalations as you desire, noticing the infinite degrees of release that occur as you relax into the pose. Lengthen from the tip of your tailbone to the crown of your head as you let the strength in your legs create relaxation in the torso.

6. Bend at the knees and lower your torso onto your thighs. Sink a little lower into your legs, allowing the weight of your torso to melt into the support of your legs (**fig. 15.15**). Place your hands on either side of your feet and take a giant step backward with your right foot into Runner's Stretch.

7. Take as much time as you need to adjust your forward knee so that it is centered over the ball of the heel. Send the back heel away from you; this lengthens the back leg and allows you to drop down into your center of gravity (**fig. 15.16**). Notice how you can stretch through the back heel while at the same time lengthening upward through the torso and the crown.

8. Drop the back knee to the ground and bring the left knee alongside the right knee (**fig. 15.17**), then reach your sitz bones back to sit on your heels as you lower your torso onto your thighs into Child pose (**fig.**

15.18). Walk your hands away from your shoulders and spread your palms while you roll the shoulders open and breathe into the backside of your body. Then release your armpits and arms to hang (**fig. 15.19**).

9. Remain in Child pose as you focus awareness on releasing your belly down into deeper relaxation onto your thighs. Make any adjustments that allow you to enter a state of relaxed awareness of the sensations and feeling that arise while you hold Child pose.

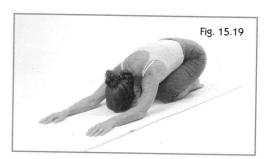

Fig. 15.19

10. Now press into your hands, peel your sternum off your thighs, and glide up into Table pose (**fig. 15.20**). Spread your fingers and adjust your palms so they are directly under your shoulders. Exhale fully as you round the spine into Cat Tilt and look inward toward your navel (**fig. 15.21**). Hold the breath out for a moment as you suck the navel up and in toward the spine.

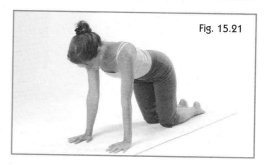

Fig. 15.20

11. Inhaling, press into your palms, roll your shoulders away from your ears, and lengthen the back of your head toward your sacrum into the Dog Tilt (**fig. 15.22**). Exhale into Cat Tilt and inhale into Dog Tilt four or five times, allowing for deeper sensations to arise each time you repeat the counterbalancing stretches in your spine.

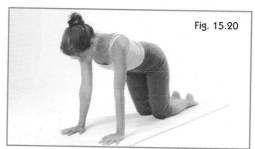

Fig. 15.21

12. Now curl your toes under, press into your palms, and lift your sitz bones and tailbone toward the sky into Downward Dog (**fig. 15.23**). Keep your knees bent and your torso in contact with your thighs as you locate the strength in your arms and shoulders to lengthen your whole spine. With the back of your neck remaining relaxed, stretch the soles of your feet. Alternately lengthen one heel and then the other toward the ground (**fig. 15.24**), until you feel ready to send both heels toward the ground at the same time (**fig. 15.25**).

13. Remain in Downward Dog as you cycle your awareness from the elongation in your spine to the length through your heels and the backs of your legs to the strength in your palms, arms, and shoulders.

14. When you are ready, bend both knees. As you exhale, step the right foot forward between your hands, adjusting the front

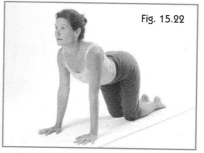

Fig. 15.22

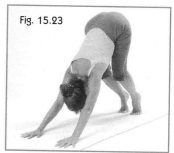

Fig. 15.23

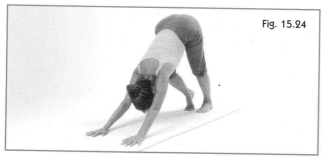

Fig. 15.24

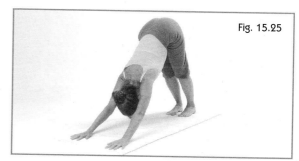

Fig. 15.25

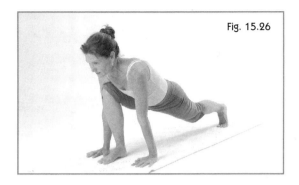

Fig. 15.26

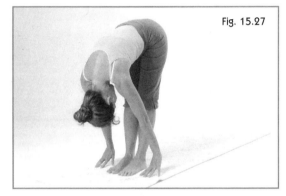

Fig. 15.27

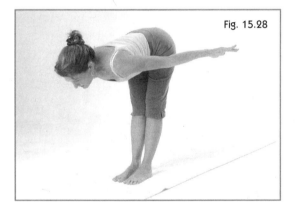

Fig. 15.28

knee to center over the ball of your heel. Send the left heel away from you, lengthening the back leg away from you. Sink into the bowl of your pelvis and elongate through your torso and crown (**fig. 15.26**).

15. Exhaling, step the left foot forward alongside the right (**fig. 15.27**). As you hang in Standing Forward Bend, keep your knees slightly bent and release the weight of your torso to hang, lengthening from the tip of your tailbone through the crown of your head.

16. On an inhaling breath, press into your feet, spread your arms open to your sides, and peel your torso upward off your thighs (**fig. 15.28**). Continue lengthening the long line of your spine upward into Mountain pose, your arms extending upward toward the heavens (**fig. 15.29**). Pause and relax into your breath as you allow your gaze to softly focus toward the horizon and your shoulders to roll downward and back. Experience the surge of energy that streams upward from the center of the earth through the arches in your feet, upward through the core of your body and out through the crown of your head.

17. Allow your gaze to soften as you hold extended Mountain pose. Hold an inhaling breath, then rotate your wrists with the palms facing downward and allow your arms to float down through an ocean of energy (**fig. 15.30**). As the arms float to your sides, prana streams up through the core of your body.

18. Stand in Mountain pose for as long as you desire, then begin the Salutation to the Child again, this time stepping the

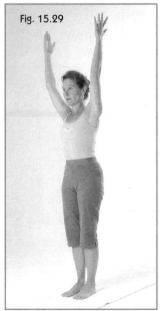

Fig. 15.29

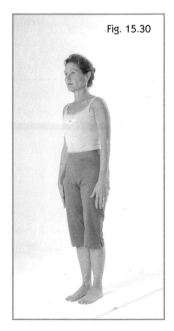

Fig. 15.30

left leg back into Runner's Stretch. Continue through this flow of postures for as many times as you wish, noticing how each repetition enhances the flow of prana throughout your body. From Table pose you may want to move into a front extension, such as Sphinx, Iguana, or Frog. Another direction might take you into Pigeon, Hero, Spinal Twist, and Seated Forward Bend. Take this opportunity to allow your body to communicate to you what would feel balancing and energizing in this moment.

19. When you are ready to complete your practice, choose one of the relaxation inquiries from chapter 10 to deepen your contact with the movement of prana awakened in your practice. End your practice by offering gratitude to your logical mind for creating this important time for integrating the many dimensions of your being.

Integrative Flow 3: Salutation to the Sun

How does movement invite meditative awareness?

The Sun Salutation is a way to generate body heat as you energize the solar plexus in your body's center. There are many versions of this traditional vinyasa. The posture flow you are about to experience channels the radiant heat from your core throughout your whole body. While the original flow emerged as a way to both generate and honor the solar battery within your body, it is also used as a way to honor the forces of external nature symbolized by the sun. You may wish to practice this flow outdoors in the fresh air where you can see the sun; otherwise, visualize the sun when you are practicing indoors.

Synchronizing your movements with your breath greatly enhances the invigorating effects of stimulating circulation, digestion, and elimination, and helps to massage and tone all of the vital organs and glands in the body. The dance of counterbalancing stretches characteristic of this vinyasa invigorates the muscles and joints, enhancing strength, flexibility, and general physical fitness. On an internal level, repeating this flow deepens concentration and is a means for cultivating mental clarity and peace of mind.

It is most helpful to begin your repetitions of this sequence slowly, drawing your awareness to the internal sensations and effects. As concentration deepens and your breath begins to flow you can enter into a dynamic pace that allows the intelligence of your organism to take over. When you are ready to slow down, it is beneficial to hold each of the postures for several inhalations and exhalations as a way to more intentionally direct the flow of prana into the areas of your body that are affected.

As with the Salutation to the Child, you can use this flow as an armature to bring other standing and balancing postures into your practice: try adding Triangle pose,

Warrior, Tree, Eagle, King of Dancers, or Standing Yoga Mudra. Or you can move from Downward Dog into any of the floor postures you might wish to include, such as Hero pose, Pigeon, Seated Spinal Twist, or Seated Forward Bend. Toward the end of your flow you may wish to include some inversions, such as Bridge, Half Shoulderstand, or Plow.

Before you end your practice, allow yourself some time to enter into a spontaneous flow in which you let your organism be moved by the awakened flow of prana in your body. Transitioning from the more willful postures of the Sun Salutation into your own prana flow will maximize the external physical effects and create a bridge for experiencing and integrating the internal results throughout all dimensions of your being.

Flow: Salutation to the Sun

1. Begin by creating an intention to open to the many dimensions of your being that may arise during your practice. What feelings do you have about contacting and honoring the warm, glowing energy of the sun present in the center of your belly?

2. Come into a relaxed standing position. Adjusting your feet into Mountain alignment, with your feet parallel and directly under your hips **(fig. 15.31)**, notice the connection you have to the ground. Deepen your breath as you locate the triangular base of support in your feet. Softly focus your gaze, drawing your concentration into your belly center.

3. Exhale and bring your palms together in prayer position in front of your heart. Press the palms as you roll your shoulders down and back and lengthen your torso upward from the bowl of your pelvis **(fig. 15.32)**. As you inhale, send your palms upward toward the heavens **(fig. 15.33)**.

4. Tuck your chin slightly and press the hip

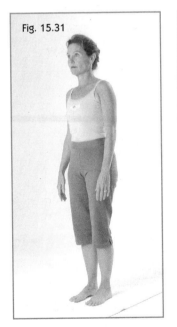

Fig. 15.31

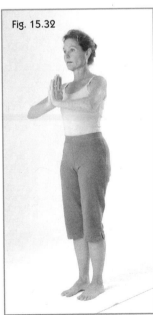

Fig. 15.32

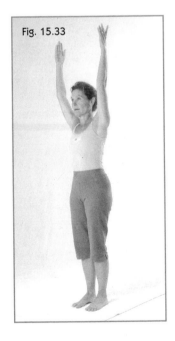

Fig. 15.33

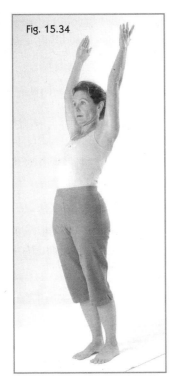

Fig. 15.34

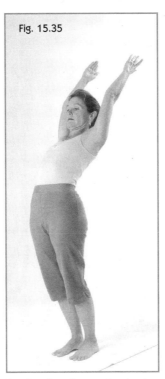

Fig. 15.35

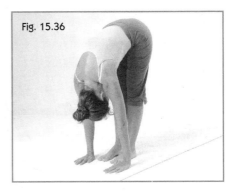

Fig. 15.36

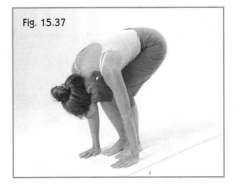

Fig. 15.37

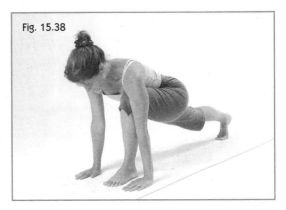

Fig. 15.38

bones forward to lengthen the front side of your body (**fig. 15.34**). Take as many breaths as you need as you allow the upward surging energy in your spine to lengthen the line from your pubic bone to your sternum, arching you backward (**fig. 15.35**). As the torso and arms lengthen, your shoulders roll down and back.

5. Hold the next inhaling breath for a moment, then bend from the hinge of your hips, sweeping your arms out to your sides and lowering your torso toward your thighs (**fig. 15.36**). As your torso lowers, open the book of your buttocks and focus your gaze forward, then toward the floor in front of you, then to your feet and your legs. As your arms hang to your sides, look upward and in toward your navel.

6. Hanging from the hinge of your hips in the Standing Forward Bend, soften the back of your knees and shift your weight to release the pressure in your hamstrings and thighs. Release the weight of your head, your jaw and your eyes into the downward pull of gravity. Stay here for as many full inhalations and exhalations as you desire, noticing the infinite degrees of release that occur as you relax into the holding. Lengthen from the tip of your tailbone to your crown as you let the strength in your legs create relaxation in the torso.

7. Bend at the knees and lower your torso onto your thighs (**fig. 15.37**). Sink a little lower into your legs, allowing the weight of your torso to melt into the support of your legs. Place your hands on either side of your feet and take a giant step backward with your right foot into Runner's Stretch (**fig. 15.38**).

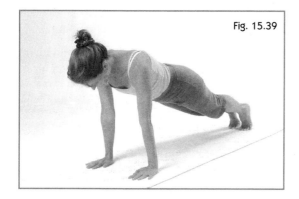

Fig. 15.39

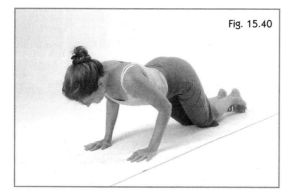

Fig. 15.40

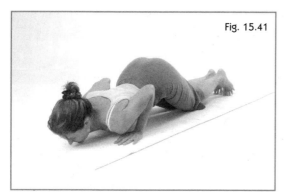

Fig. 15.41

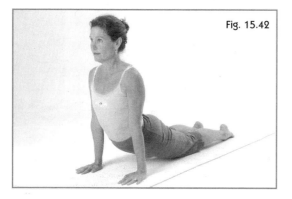

Fig. 15.42

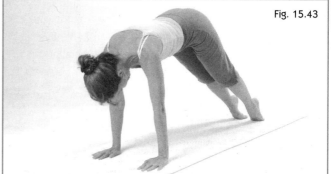

Fig. 15.43

8. Take as much time as you need to adjust your forward knee so that it is centered over the ball of the heel. Send the back heel away from you, which lengthens the back leg and allows you to drop down into your center of gravity. Notice how you can stretch through the back heel while lengthening upward through the torso and crown at the same time.

9. On an exhaling breath, stretch your left leg back into Plank, adjusting your palms directly under your shoulders and rolling your shoulders away from your ears **(fig. 15.39)**. Focus your gaze toward the ground in front of you to lengthen the back of your neck. Take as many breaths as you need as you hold this position. Continue lengthening your entire body, maintaining a long line by stretching up out of the soles of your feet and pressing the heels away from you as you lengthen the front side of your body from the pubic bone to the sternum. Take a deep inhaling breath and hold it in.

10. Exhale and lower your knees to the ground **(fig. 15.40)**. Inhale fully, then exhale and bend your elbows in close to your ribs and bring your sternum and forehead close to the ground while your hips remain elevated in Caterpillar **(fig. 15.41)**. Remain in this position for two full inhalations and exhalations.

11. Inhale and press into your palms, rolling onto the tops of your feet. As you press into the tops of your feet and your hands, extend the front side of your body into Upward Dog **(fig. 15.42)**. Experiment with keeping the hips off the ground as you lengthen the legs behind you while extending from the pubic bone through the sternum and the crown of your head. The shoulders roll down and back away from your ears and the arms remain in contact with the ribs. You may need to keep your knees on the ground and your elbows bent to stay in the posture for two full inhalations and exhalations.

12. Exhale and press into your palms as you roll over your toes to curl them under **(fig. 15.43)**. Lift your tailbone to the sky and take a couple of baby steps forward to adjust your feet to enter into

Downward Dog (fig. 15.44). While holding this posture, bend your knees in toward your ribs and stretch up out of the soles of your feet. Keep the knees bent as you find the strength in your arms by pressing into the palms and rolling your shoulders open away from your ears. Let your head hang to keep the back of your neck long and relaxed. Alternately lengthen the legs by sending the heel of one foot toward the ground, (fig. 15.45) then send the other heel toward the ground, continuing back and forth until you are ready to send both heels toward the ground at the same time (fig. 15.46). As you hold this position, deepen your breath and experience how pressing equally into your palms and your feet allows you to lengthen the torso and the legs upward to the apex of the hip hinge.

13. Remain in Downward Dog as you cycle your awareness from the elongation in your spine to the length through the lengthening of your heels and the backs of your legs to the strength in your palms, arms, and shoulders.

14. When you are ready to come out of Downward Dog, bend both knees (fig. 15.47). As you exhale, step the right foot forward between your hands (fig. 15.48). Adjust the front knee to be center over the ball of your heel, then step the left foot forward alongside the right (fig. 15.49). As you

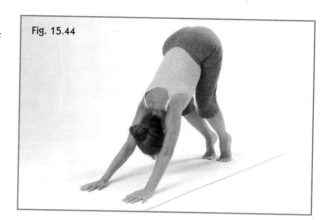
Fig. 15.44

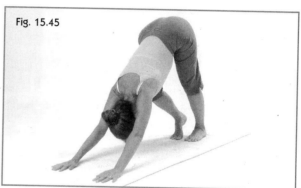
Fig. 15.45

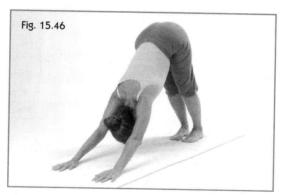
Fig. 15.46

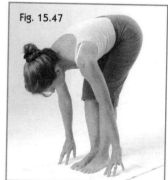
Fig. 15.47

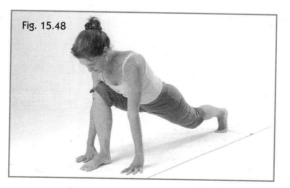
Fig. 15.48

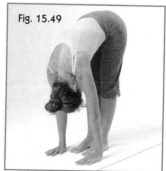
Fig. 15.49

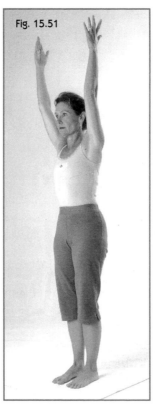

Fig. 15.51

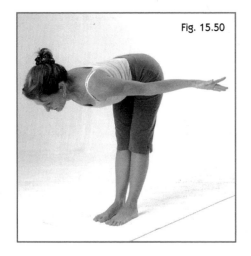

Fig. 15.50

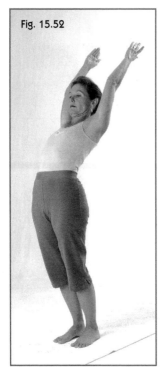

Fig. 15.52

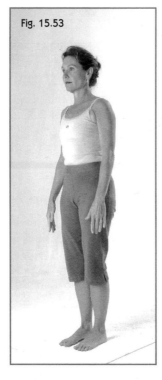

Fig. 15.53

hang in Standing Forward Bend, keep your knees slightly bent and release the weight of your torso to hang, lengthening from the tip of your tailbone through the crown of your head.

15. On an inhaling breath, press into your feet, spread your arms open to your sides, and peel your torso upward off your thighs; **(fig. 15.50)** continue lengthening the long line of your spine upward into Mountain pose, your arms extending toward the heavens **(fig. 15.51)**. Tuck your chin slightly and press your hip bones forward, lengthening the front side of your body upward from the pubic bone through the sternum and crown **(fig. 15.52)**. Pause and relax into your breath as you allow your gaze to softly focus toward the horizon and your shoulders to roll downward and back. Experience the surge of energy that streams upward from the center of the earth through the arches in your feet, upward through the core of your body and out through the crown of your head.

16. Allow your gaze to soften as you hold forward-extended Mountain pose. Hold an inhaling breath, then rotate your wrists with the palms facing down and allow your arms to float to your sides through an ocean of energy **(fig. 15.53)**. As the arms float down toward your sides, prana streams upward through the core of your body.

17. Stand in Mountain pose for as long as you desire, then begin the Salutation to the Sun again, this time stepping the left leg back into Runner's Stretch. Continue through this flow of postures for as many times as you wish, noticing how each repetition enhances the flow of prana throughout your body.

18. After several repetitions of the Sun Salutation you can bring in any other postures that you choose. When you enter the Runner's Stretch, you may want to continue into the Warrior, Side Angle Stretch, Standing Spinal Twist, Triangle, Rotated Triangle, or Intense Leg Stretch poses. From the Upward Dog position, you may want to move into Cobra, Bow, or Downward Boat. From the Mountain you can move into the balancing poses, such as Tree, Heron, Eagle, or Queen of Dancers. From Downward Dog you can come to the floor for the Pigeon, Hero, Spinal Twist, and Seated Forward Bend. Toward the end of your flow you may wish to include some inversions, such as Bridge, Half Shoulderstand, or Plow. Take this opportunity to allow your body to communicate to you what would feel balancing and energizing in this moment.

19. Before ending your practice, allow some time to enter into a posture flow in which you allow yourself to be moved spontaneously by the awakened movement of prana in your body.

20. When you are ready to complete your practice, choose one of the prana posture flows detailed below to deepen your contact with the movement of prana awakened in your practice. Allow yourself the time to fully receive the effects in every level of your being. End your practice by offering gratitude to your logical mind for creating this important time for integrating the many dimensions of your being.

Integrative Flow 4: Prana Posture Flow

How does attuning to the movement of prana invite meditative awareness?

In the course of working with this book, every time that you've followed the suggestion to close your eyes and notice what is happening inside your body you have been preparing for the Prana Posture Flow. The inquiries of Self-Awakening Yoga provide a multitude of opportunities for traveling within your interior and attuning to the sensations that are naturally awakened in your body as a result of that inquiry. Noticing sensations is a simple and direct method for developing the power of concentrating your logical mind to witness prana at work in your body.

Each time you have followed the urges of your body into the phase of an inquiry in which you let go of the conscious control over a new movement pattern, you have entered into a Prana Posture Flow. The more you respond to the promptings of prana within your organism, the more you develop the capacity for observing the intelligence of this primal energy as it unlocks vast creative potentials that are awakening within your whole being. When you let everything go to follow the intelligence of your organism as it invents a new way to do a movement, a way that you have never done it before, you are surrendering to inborn instinctual guidance, as opposed to willfully controlling your movements. Each time you have asked yourself the question, "What wants to happen; what wants to let go through my organism?" you have been building a bridge between the rational intelligence of your mind and the primal wisdom of prana at work in your being. This happens by simply becoming fascinated in the mysterious creativity that surfaces as you pause to get interested in the authentic presence of this power residing within yourself.

Learning to use your capacities for movement by entering the inquiries is like learning to play the scales on a musical instrument. Integrating the movements and postures of Self-Awakening Yoga into posture flows, or vinyasas, is similar to reading and playing the music of other composers. When new and unexpected movements emerge that open the doorway to surprising or unpremeditated experiences, you have entered the domain of prana showing you the way into your own music. In a Prana Posture Flow, your experience will probably alternate between following movements you already know and are familiar with and following the urges of prana into spontaneously generated new movements. As you develop greater skill, flexibility, and ease during the more familiar movement patterns, you will probably begin to experience greater satisfaction emerging from following the unchoreographed and sometimes astonishing positions that happen through you. By following this practice, you will come to know the origin of all yoga postures and realize that you have a direct connection to the intelligent source of wisdom that stimulates the unfoldment and the evolution of all organisms.

The methods for entering a Prana Posture Flow vary from person to person and may even vary from day to day for the same person. The suggestions included in the explorations below may be used individually or combined at different times within your flow. You will notice that they each begin with a willful way to enter into experiences that carry you over the threshold for surrendering into movement guided by the intelligence of prana. The primary condition that fosters your ability to enter this experience is your intention to let go into ever-deepening levels of trust in the wisdom of your organism to guide your way into self-awakening.

Prana Opening 1: Attuning to the Sound and Rhythm of Breath

1. Come into a position that allows you to relax into the sensation of breathing deeply. Suggest to your logical mind that it is safe, desirable, and pleasurable to move across a time boundary into the time of following the stream of your breath.

2. Without expecting any particular effects to arise, begin to notice how your breathing happens throughout your body. Listen for the sound and cadence of rhythms as your breath touches interior surfaces that float up into awareness. As you continue to submerge into gradations of sensation, notice how it is possible for the breath to reach into places where you have never breathed before.

3. Imagine or sense how the dense, physical structures of your body become fluid, giving way to the swelling current of prana that streams through you. As your body melts into the river of breath, allow your body to move without thinking. As you allow your breath to move you, observe how you can let go into the unknown by releasing control over the impulses that arise. How would it feel to be carried beyond the familiarity of here and now into vast expanses that have no limits?

4. Suspend the reflex to analyze or to rationalize the unfolding movements that arise by continuously returning to and attuning to the rhythm and pulse of your breath.

5. When you are ready, gradually return to stillness. In this place of deep, relaxed awareness, notice how you feel when you are at home in the center of your being, receiving from the wisdom of your organism.

Prana Opening 2: Attuning to the Pulses of Your Organism

1. Lie down on the ground, taking the time you need to make any adjustments that allow you to settle into your body. As you become aware of your mind, notice the speed and momentum of your thoughts and thinking. What is the speed or pulse of your thoughts and thinking? Do you notice any particular thoughts arising in this moment? Allow whatever thoughts are present to simply be.

2. Invite your logical mind to remain present to help you to witness the dimensions of your experience that open as you attune to the presence of prana moving in your body. Notice how you begin to cross over a time boundary to enter the time in which the body actually lives. The body lives in a time that is much slower than mental time. Where does your awareness travel as your body relaxes and your mind slows down?

3. Now travel into the deep core of your belly. What is your internal mood in this moment? What are the colors, textures, and shapes of any feelings that are present? Do you notice any particular feelings or emotions that are present? Suggest to your logical mind that it is safe, desirable, and pleasurable to expand awareness to include all of your thoughts, feelings, and emotions arising in every level of your being.

4. Using the power of your awareness, sense or imagine the pulsing in your belly. Imagine that you are connected to the warmth of the sun through an umbilical cord into your navel.

5. As you breathe in, inhale warm, glowing sun into the core of your belly. Sense the pulse in your belly growing stronger and warmer. As the heat in your belly expands, imagine warm, glowing energy streaming through the entire interior space of your body. Be aware of the glowing sensation becoming so concentrated that liquid warmth starts to stream through the pores of your skin, radiating through the body wall to envelop all of the space around you.

6. Now allow your body to begin to move in response to the pulsing energy of prana, streaming though every cell of your physical body. Sense how prana is moving you, with ever-increasing potency, from the center of your being.

7. Notice how prana-generated movement is connecting you to the surrounding universe. Let go into the pulse of being. Allow the movement to continue for as long as you are feeling engaged.

8. When you are ready, gradually return to stillness. In this place of deep, relaxed awareness, notice how you feel when you are at home in the center of your being, receiving from the wisdom of your organism.

Prana Opening 3: Holding and Releasing into Counterbalancing Movement of Prana

1. Begin by moving into a flow of stretches, movements, and postures that feel good to you in this moment. Slow down to a pace that allows you to synchronize your breath with your movement.

2. When you come to a posture that you want to hold for an extended period of time, deepen your breath and consciously relax into the areas of your body that are being affected. Where are you feeling the stretch? What parts of your body are being compressed as you hold the posture? Does any trembling or vibration arise?

3. Deepen your resolve to stay in the posture, allowing the sensations to intensify. With the increasing potency of prana accumulating in this posture, notice the conversations that arise in your mind. What is your mind saying about allowing this much sensation to intensify in your body? As you hold the posture, do you notice insights arising that will reassure your mind that it is safe and desirable to hold this posture longer than usual? Does your mind really know what might happen if you pass through the limitations you may have experienced in the past?

4. At the precise moment you are guided to release from holding, allow the wisdom of your body to move you into a counterbalancing posture or flow of movement. As you let go of control over your movement, witness how prana carries you into the experiences that open deeper dimensions of your physical and emotional being. If feelings or sounds or insights arise while you let go into prana, allow them to be expressed through the spontaneous tears, laughter, or whole-body mudras that may arise through the continuous movement.

5. When you are ready, gradually return to stillness. In this place of deep, relaxed awareness, notice how you feel when you are at home in the center of your being, receiving from the wisdom of your organism.

Prana Opening 4: Speeding Up to Heighten Prana Consciousness

1. Begin by moving into a flow of stretches, movements, and postures that feel good to you in this moment. Slow down to a pace that allows you to synchronize your breath with your movement. Enter into a sequence of movements that involves your whole body and that you can repeat for several repetitions, such as Salutation of the Child or Sun Salutation.

2. When your breath opens to allow deeper movement, begin to speed up the pace of your flow, increasing the number of repetitions and adding to the overall length of time you are repeating the sequence. Gradually increase the speed of your movement until you feel the movements taking over; notice that you do not have to think about what is coming next.

3. Allow your body to be moved by the rhythm and momentum of the flow. Notice the place in your awareness that is witnessing the flow. Do you sense how the movement comes to feel effortless, even though you are using increasing levels of physical energy? As such velocity drives your body, can you sense another source of energy beginning to take over or the feeling of perpetual-motion rocking beginning to arise? Is there a place of stillness in the center of your movement? Observe how it feels to release the control over your movement to prana.

4. Gradually begin to slow down and allow prana to guide your body into whatever actions or postures arise. What wants to happen through your body at this time? Traveling through the sensations, feelings, and insights that are stimulated by heightened prana movement, experience how your body conveys the workings of prana through sound and whole-body motion.

5. When you are ready, gradually return to stillness. In this place of deep, relaxed awareness, notice how you feel when you are at home in the center of your being, receiving from the wisdom of your organism.

Prana Opening 5: Slowing Down to Heighten Prana Consciousness

1. Begin by moving into a flow of stretches, movements, and postures that feel good to you in this moment. Slow down to a pace that allows you to synchronize your breath with your movement. Enter into a sequence of movements that involves your whole body that you can repeat for several repetitions, such as Salutation of the Child or Sun Salutation.

2. When your breath opens to allow deeper movement, begin to slow the pace of your flow, repeating the same sequence for a longer period of time than usual. Gradually reduce the speed of your movement until you feel the movements are happening in slow motion.

3. Exaggerate the deliberate, unhurried momentum of your movement until you enter a pace that is so slow that it seems as though you are watching a slow-motion video of yourself. Notice the place in your awareness that is witnessing the flow. Do you sense how the movement comes to feel effortless, even though you are increasing concentration on the heightened flow of physical energy? As such slowness drives your body, can you sense another source of energy beginning to take over, or the feeling of perpetual-motion rocking beginning to arise? Is there a place of stillness in the center of your movement? Observe how it feels to release control over your movement to prana.

4. As movement becomes slower and slower, allow prana to guide your body into whatever actions or postures arise. What wants to happen through your body at this time? Traveling through the sensations, feelings, and insights that are stimulated by heightened prana activation, experience how your body expresses the workings of prana through sound and through whole-body motion.

5. When you are ready, gradually return to stillness. In this place of deep, relaxed awareness, notice how you feel when you are at home in the center of your being, receiving from the wisdom of your organism.

Integration: Surrendering to Your Body's Prana Prayer

1. Contemplate the experiences you have had in which the benevolent presence of prana has guided you into expanded awareness of yourself. With reverent regard for your journey of awakening and in a prayerful attitude for receiving the power of prana at work in your life, create an intention to be present in this moment to allow prana to communicate its wisdom directly through your body.

2. Begin in stillness by doing nothing at all. Suggest to your logical mind that, for however long you need to remain still, you will suspend the reflex to use your will to make something happen. The impulse to move from prana does not come from any familiar or known part of you.

3. Notice the bodily sensations that arise in the vacuum as you wait for prana to move you. How does any particular sensation that you are noticing intensify when you allow it to manifest precisely as it is? How does a sensation transform when you suspend the reflex to shift or move in a habitual way to relieve the discomfort? Is there a place in your being that expands to include all of your bodily sensations?

4. Notice whatever mental conversations arise as you are waiting for prana to move you. Who are you when you are not willfully engaged in any purposeful activity? As your awareness discerns deeper and deeper layers of perception about who you are in this moment, is there a place in your being that accepts and includes all of your thoughts about who you are?

5. When you forget not to move and instead notice that movement is happening, allow it to continue. Experience how prana takes over your movement when you are not thinking. As though you are in communion with your highest source of inner wisdom, allow your movement to become a prayer in motion. Humbly surrender into a deeper yearning that arises for exploring the ultimate creative force at work your body's movement. What wants to open through you at this time? Allow your body's Prana Prayer to continue as long as you are engaged in the moving meditation

6. When stillness returns, receive the effects of your meditation. Notice where you have gone within yourself. Are there insights, inspirations, or messages that are revealed to you in this moment that may inform the choices you have available in your current life context? Do you notice any alterations in your mood or any feelings that call your attention?

7. Before you begin your return, offer gratitude to your logical mind for participating in this event of consciousness by allowing the focus of concentration to flow to the intelligence of prana that is awakening every dimension of your being.

8. Begin your return by vigorously rubbing your palms together until the friction creates radiant, glowing heat. Draw your palms to your face, reaching through the layers of muscle and flesh to allow the heat to melt all expressions from your face. Notice the way your face looks and feels when all the masks and roles of all previous identities have been dissolved.

9. Circle your tongue around your mouth, stimulating a fresh flow of saliva to lubricate the interior surfaces of your teeth, lips, and gums. Notice the taste in your mouth. Is it familiar or is it difficult to describe? What is the fragrance you smell in this moment? Is it recognizable? surprising? exotic?

10. When you are ready, allow the windows of your eyes to open to receive the world. Invite the colors and forms into your inner world. Has your vision altered in any way? Is your sense of self altered in any way? What do you want to consciously carry in your heart about your body's Prana Prayer?

Before Moving On . . .

The inquiries of this chapter have provided a variety of methods that build upon a combination of explorations in the inquiries of all preceding chapters. From experimenting with these suggestions, you may have already begun to design your own ongoing practice. A question to ask yourself that can support your intention for continuing your yoga practice is this: "What helps me attune to the workings of prana in my body?" Considering your needs and interests, what time of day suits the rhythms of your energy? What is the appropriate time frame that appeals to you for a yoga practice, and how often during the week is reasonable for supporting your active engagement?

In order to sustain a personal practice that is suitable to your needs and interests, it is crucial that you return to your personal experience to review the effects of these explorations, periodically checking in to assess what is making the most difference for nurturing your continued inquiry. What are some creative ways to interact with yourself that allow for a balance between commitment to your practice and the flexibility to change with the shifts you begin to experience? Remind yourself continuously that there is no "right" way to practice your yoga. What will make your practice a constant source of energetic regeneration is that you are passionate about the connection your practice provides to engaging with your internal wisdom.

Epilogue: As You Prepare to Journey On . . .

The privelege of a lifetime is being who you are.

JOSEPH CAMPBELL

YOU MAY RECALL THAT AT THE BEGINNING OF THIS BOOK you were invited into a personal inquiry that promised to yield a friendlier relationship between your mind and body by learning to listen to the language of sensation through which your body is speaking. Like sharing a cozy seat in front of a hearth with your most trusted friend, the journey to expanded consciousness is nothing less than establishing a trusting relationship with yourself that respects the wisdom of your organism with equal value to your mental and emotional intelligence. As you learn to learn through your body's wisdom, you are able to take into account the unpredictability and often surprising realities of each unfolding moment. With your body as your best friend you will always dwell at the source of your creativity.

Another name for creativity is self-love. With self-love flowing from your home within, creative solutions will always be revealed in the way that you are willing to be transformed in the moment.

When it comes to choosing and committing to a personal practice for the purpose of continuing to develop the communication between body and mind, your practice itself will need to change as your consciousness expands to include greater levels of insight into your vast capacities. At the times when your practice becomes routine, you can be assured that, having nurtured your deepest intentions along the way, you will be propelled toward inventing new ways of inquiring into your experience of self.

Each and every time you return to the wisdom of your inner counsel will be a genuine homecoming.

Nurturing your relationship to self through expanding awareness is a means for taking refuge from the dynamic and changing circumstances of life, refuge in infinite self-love. On this journey there is no failure, even when the landscape turns desolate and strange. The knowledge that this is your unique and personal journey provides its own comforting peace.

Ultimately, it is our innate intuition of *samadhi*, the unity and interconnectedness with all things, that guides us away from mistakenly identifying the fluxuating realities of the moment as being absolute. Self-Awakening Yoga presents a method for moving beneath the surface appearances of reality to witness the underlying unity. This quest is something that we must discover within ourselves. Until we make this quest our life's purpose, we will always be living against the flow of the universe.

What about samadhi? If you've ever noticed how your body instinctively stretches when you first wake up, before getting out of bed, you've had an experience of natural samadhi. There are many blissful experiences and moments of great equanimity that occur throughout life. These are not just glimpses of samadhi; they are actual experiences of that state. It is precisely because we have already experienced samadhi that we have the intuition that it exists as a possibility. From this perspective, we actually begin our yoga practice because we already have experienced samadhi. Cycling back through the other limbs, or dimensions, of the yoga practices give us an expanded access to the unity of our inner being. Samadhi is not a privileged state for a gifted few. It is a birthright for human beings. The gift of your yoga practice is that it will yield greater points of reference for establishing balance and harmony in the midst of your life.

With Self-Awakening Yoga, you have access to the benefits and results of consciousness from the very beginning of your journey. As you continue your journey into self, fresh infusions of creativity will arise each and every moment that move beyond techniques. Techniques are not a substitute for consciousness. With an ever-deepening consciousness—an awareness of your capacity to become aware—you will have unlimited access to prana as a trustworthy guide and companion in life. May you dwell in the center of your being in the counsel of your best friend—your own inner knowing.

Resources

Desai, Yogi Amrit. *Kripalu Yoga: Meditation in Motion.* Summit Station, Penn.: Kripalu Publications, 1981.

Desikachar, T.K.V. *The Heart of Yoga: Developing a Personal Practice..* Rochester, Vt.: Inner Traditions International, 1995.

Feldenkrais, Moshe. *Awareness through Movement.* New York, N.Y.: Harper and Row, 1972.

Hanna, Thomas. *Somatics.* Boston, Mass.: Addison-Wesley Publishing Co., Inc., 1988.

Hartsuiker, Dolf. *Sadhus: Holy Men of India.* Rochester, Vt.: Inner Traditions, 1993.

Khalili, Nader. *Ceramic Houses: How to Build Your Own.* San Francisco, Calif.: Harper and Row, 1986.

Knaster, Mirka. *Discovering the Body's Wisdom.* New York, N.Y.: Bantam Books, 1996.

Kramer, David, and Alstad, Diana. *The Guru Papers: Masks of Authoritarian Power.* Berkeley, Calif.: North Atlantic Books, 1993.

Lowenfeld, Viktor. *Creative and Mental Growth.* New York: McGraw, Hill, 1983.

Muni, Swami Rajarshi. *Awakening Life Force: The Philosophy and Psychology of "Spontaneous Yoga."* St. Paul, Minn.: Llewellyn Publications, 1994.

Taimni, I.K. *The Science of Yoga.* Wheaton, Ill.: The Theosophical Publishing House, 1961.

Yoga As Is: An Oasis of Experiences for Self-Awakening by Don Stapleton. Based on the principles of Self-Awakening Yoga, this twelve-session audiotape series of thirty-minute guided inquiries supports your yoga practice and enhances awareness of movement patterns throughout your body. Order through Nosara Yoga Institute.

Nosara Yoga Institute, located on the Pacific coast of Costa Rica, is dedicated to professional training and advanced career development for teachers and practitioners in the fields of yoga and bodywork. Internationally acclaimed cofounders and codirectors Don and Amba Stapleton are known for their ability to create educational environments that support inquiry, experiential learning, and teacher creativity. The 200-hour and 500-hour Yoga Alliance-approved teacher training programs are offered year-round in the institute's pristine tropical surroundings that draw from the power of nature to support a prana-filled experience of self-awakening. For detailed descriptions and program calendar, contact:

website: www.nosarayoga.com • email: info@nosarayoga.com
U.S. toll free: 1-806-439-4704